Semisolid Dosage

Semisolid Dosage

Editors

Rolf Daniels
Dominique Lunter

MDPI • Basel • Beijing • Wuhan • Barcelona • Belgrade • Manchester • Tokyo • Cluj • Tianjin

Editors
Rolf Daniels
University of Tübingen
Germany

Dominique Lunter
University of Tübingen
Germany

Editorial Office
MDPI
St. Alban-Anlage 66
4052 Basel, Switzerland

This is a reprint of articles from the Special Issue published online in the open access journal *Pharmaceutics* (ISSN 1999-4923) (available at: https://www.mdpi.com/journal/pharmaceutics/special_issues/semi_solid).

For citation purposes, cite each article independently as indicated on the article page online and as indicated below:

LastName, A.A.; LastName, B.B.; LastName, C.C. Article Title. *Journal Name* **Year**, *Article Number*, Page Range.

ISBN 978-3-03936-948-5 (Hbk)
ISBN 978-3-03936-949-2 (PDF)

Contents

About the Editors . . . vii

Dominique Jasmin Lunter and Rolf Daniels
Semisolid Dosage
Reprinted from: *Pharmaceutics* **2020**, *12*, 315, doi:10.3390/pharmaceutics12040315 . . . 1

Yali Liu and Dominique Jasmin Lunter
Systematic Investigation of the Effect of Non-Ionic Emulsifiers on Skin by Confocal Raman Spectroscopy—A Comprehensive Lipid Analysis
Reprinted from: *Pharmaceutics* **2020**, *12*, 223, doi:10.3390/pharmaceutics12030223 . . . 5

Antonella Casiraghi, Chiara Grazia Gennari, Umberto Maria Musazzi, Marco Aldo Ortenzi, Susanna Bordignon and Paola Minghetti
Mucoadhesive Budesonide Formulation for the Treatment of Eosinophilic Esophagitis
Reprinted from: *Pharmaceutics* **2020**, *12*, 211, doi:10.3390/pharmaceutics12030211 . . . 21

Kashif Ahmad Ghaffar and Rolf Daniels
Oleogels with Birch Bark Dry Extract: Extract Saving Formulations through Gelation Enhancing Additives
Reprinted from: *Pharmaceutics* **2020**, *12*, 184, doi:10.3390/pharmaceutics12020184 . . . 33

Diana Berenguer, Maria Magdalena Alcover, Marcella Sessa, Lyda Halbaut, Carme Guillén, Antoni Boix-Montañés, Roser Fisa, Ana Cristina Calpena-Campmany, Cristina Riera and Lilian Sosa
Topical Amphotericin B Semisolid Dosage Form for Cutaneous Leishmaniasis: Physicochemical Characterization, Ex Vivo Skin Permeation and Biological Activity
Reprinted from: *Pharmaceutics* **2020**, *12*, 149, doi:10.3390/pharmaceutics12020149 . . . 43

Seeprarani Rath and Isadore Kanfer
A Validated IVRT Method to Assess Topical Creams Containing Metronidazole Using a Novel Approach
Reprinted from: *Pharmaceutics* **2020**, *12*, 119, doi:10.3390/pharmaceutics12020119 . . . 59

Selenia Ternullo, Laura Victoria Schulte Werning, Ann Mari Holsæter and Nataša Škalko-Basnet
Curcumin-In-Deformable Liposomes-In-Chitosan- Hydrogel as a Novel Wound Dressing
Reprinted from: *Pharmaceutics* **2020**, *12*, 8, doi:10.3390/pharmaceutics12010008 . . . 73

Yanling Zhang, Chin-Ping Kung, Bruno C. Sil, Majella E. Lane, Jonathan Hadgraft, Michael Heinrich and Balint Sinko
Topical Delivery of Niacinamide: Influence of Binary and Ternary Solvent Systems
Reprinted from: *Pharmaceutics* **2019**, *11*, 668, doi:10.3390/pharmaceutics11120668 . . . 87

Chin-Ping Kung, Bruno C. Sil, Jonathan Hadgraft, Majella E. Lane, Bhumik Patel and Renée McCulloch
Preparation, Characterization and Dermal Delivery of Methadone
Reprinted from: *Pharmaceutics* **2019**, *11*, 509, doi:10.3390/pharmaceutics11100509 . . . 101

Juho Lee, Shwe Phyu Hlaing, Jiafu Cao, Nurhasni Hasan, Hye-Jin Ahn, Ki-Won Song and Jin-Wook Yoo
In Situ Hydrogel-Forming/Nitric Oxide-Releasing Wound Dressing for Enhanced Antibacterial Activity and Healing in Mice with Infected Wounds
Reprinted from: *Pharmaceutics* **2019**, *11*, 496, doi:10.3390/pharmaceutics11100496 . . . . **115**

Fiorenza Rancan, Hildburg Volkmann, Michael Giulbudagian, Fabian Schumacher, Jessica Isolde Stanko, Burkhard Kleuser, Ulrike Blume-Peytavi, Marcelo Calderón and Annika Vogt
Dermal Delivery of the High-Molecular-Weight Drug Tacrolimus by Means of Polyglycerol-Based Nanogels
Reprinted from: *Pharmaceutics* **2019**, *11*, 394, doi:10.3390/pharmaceutics11080394 . . . . **133**

Markus Schmidberger, Ines Nikolic, Ivana Pantelic and Dominique Lunter
Optimization of Rheological Behaviour and Skin Penetration of Thermogelling Emulsions with Enhanced Substantivity for Potential Application in Treatment of Chronic Skin Diseases
Reprinted from: *Pharmaceutics* **2019**, *11*, 361, doi:10.3390/pharmaceutics11080361 . . . . **147**

Stella Zsikó, Kendra Cutcher, Anita Kovács, Mária Budai-Szűcs, Attila Gácsi, Gabriella Baki, Erzsébet Csányi and Szilvia Berkó
Nanostructured Lipid Carrier Gel for the Dermal Application of Lidocaine: Comparison of Skin Penetration Testing Methods
Reprinted from: *Pharmaceutics* **2019**, *11*, 310, doi:10.3390/pharmaceutics11070310 . . . . **161**

About the Editors

Rolf Daniels is Professor and Head of the Department of Pharmaceutical Technology at the University of Tübingen, Germany. He studied Pharmacy at the University of Regensburg (Germany) and received a Ph.D. in Pharmaceutical Technology from the same University. Then, he worked in the pharmaceutical development department of Pfizer (Illertissen) and was a postdoctoral fellow at the University of Regensburg before he completed his "Habilitation" thesis. He was appointed as Full Professor at the University of Braunschweig (1995–2005) before he moved to his current position.

Dominique Lunter was appointed Full Professsor of Pharmaceutical Technology in 2020. She studied Pharmacy at the University of Tuebingen and received a Ph. D. in Pharmaceutical Technology from the same university. In 2019, she held the position of Guest Professor at PMU Salzburg, Austria. In the same year she completed her "Habilitation" thesis at the University of Tuebingen, Germany.

pharmaceutics

MDPI

Editorial

Semisolid Dosage

Dominique Jasmin Lunter * and Rolf Daniels *

Department of Pharmaceutical Technology, Eberhard Karls University, Auf der Morgenstelle 8, 72076 Tuebingen, Germany

* Correspondence: dominique.lunter@uni-tuebingen.de (D.J.L.); rolf.daniels@uni-tuebingen.de (R.D.); Tel.: +49-7071-2974558 (D.J.L.); +49-7071-2978790 (R.D.)

Received: 19 March 2020; Accepted: 26 March 2020; Published: 1 April 2020

Already in ancient times, semisolid preparations for cutaneous application, popularly known as ointments, played an important role in human society. An advanced scientific investigation of "ointments" as dosage forms was set off in the late fifties of the previous century. It was only from then on that the intensive physico-chemical characterization of ointments as well as the inclusion of dermatological aspects led to a comprehensive understanding of the various interactions between the vehicle, the active ingredient, and the skin.

In the meantime, many researchers have been involved in optimizing semisolid formulations with respect to continuously changing therapeutic and patient needs. Aspects that have been dealt with are the optimization of dermato-biopharmaceutical properties and many different issues related to patient's compliance, such as skin tolerance, applicability, and cosmetic appeal. Moreover, processing technology has been improved and analytical techniques developed and refined in order to enable improved characterization of the formulation itself as well as its interaction with the skin.

This Special Issue serves to highlight and capture the contemporary progress and current research on semisolid formulations such as dermal drug delivery systems. We gathered articles on different aspects of semisolid formulations highlighting the research currently undertaken to improve and better understand these complex drug delivery systems, in particular with respect to formulation, processing, and characterization issues.

This Special Issue comprises 12 articles featuring the various aspects of semisolids, which mainly comprise but are not limited to cutaneous application.

Three papers in this Special Issue deal with formulations intended to treat wounds. In particular, the paper by Ghaffar et al. describes a concept to enhance the gelling ability of an oleogel consisting of sunflower oil and a birch bark extract where the triterpene extract functions as the active substance as well as the gelling agent [1]. In order to save the extract, the authors studied several additives, which can act as linkers between the extract particles and thereby enhance the formation of a particulate network. The most pronounced effect was observed in diols with terminal hydroxyl groups, e.g., 1,6-Hexanediol. In contrast, 1,2-diols impaired gel formation by blocking superficial OH groups on the extract particles.

The contribution of Ternullo et al. describes "Curcumin-In-Deformable Liposomes-In-Chitosan-Hydrogel as a Novel Wound Dressing" that utilizes the wound-healing potential of both curcumin and chitosan [2]. Most promising results were achieved with positively charged deformable liposomes. They proved to stabilize the formulation's bioadhesiveness and allowed sustained permeation of curcumin through ex-vivo fullthickness-human skin. The developed advanced dermal delivery system therefore seems to be a promising candidate as a wound dressing.

As third article on wound healing, Lee et al. present results of "In-Situ Hydrogel-Forming/Nitric Oxide-Releasing Wound Dressing for Enhanced Antibacterial Activity and Healing in Mice with Infected Wounds" [3]. The formulation is a dry powder consisting of alginate, pectin, PEG, and S-nitrosoglutathione, which shows good storage stability. When applied to wounds, it absorbs wound fluid and transforms it into an adhesive hydrogel that enables a controlled NO release property for the effective treatment of infected wounds.

The paper of Liu et al. is entitled "Systematic Investigation of the Effect of Non-Ionic Emulsifiers on Skin by Confocal Raman Spectroscopy—A Comprehensive Lipid Analysis" [4]. The article deals with the effect of topically applied emulsifiers on the qualitative and quantitative composition of the stratum corneum lipids. Using confocal Raman spectroscopy (CRS), the authors could demonstrate that polyethylene glycol (PEG) sorbitan esters revealed no alteration of intercellular lipid properties, while PEG-20-ethers appeared to have the most significant effects on reducing lipid content and interrupting lipid organization. Thus, CRS was shown to be a valuable tool to characterize the molecular effects of nonionic emulsifiers on skin lipids and further deepen the understanding of enhancing substance penetration with reduced skin barrier properties and increased lipid fluidity.

Formulation development for treatment of various skin diseases is the topic of the following three papers.

Schmidberger et al. present a study dealing with the "Optimization of Rheological Behaviour and Skin Penetration of Thermogelling Emulsions with Enhanced Substantivity for Potential Application in Treatment of Chronic Skin Diseases" [5]. The aim of this study was to find an innovative formulation with increased substantivity allowing for a controlled cutaneous drug release, reduced application frequency, and diminished contamination of patients' environment with the active ingredients. This was achieved by adding high amounts of methyl cellulose to a cream, which changes the formulation into a predominantly elastic body at skin surface temperature.

Berenguer and coworkers present results on a "Topical Amphotericin B (AmB) Semisolid Dosage Form for Cutaneous Leishmaniasis: Physicochemical Characterization, Ex-Vivo Skin Permeation and Biological Activity" [6]. The study describes an AmB gel that proved to be stable for 60 days at 4 °C and showed characteristics that made it favorable for cutaneous application. As desired, ex-vivo permeation experiments revealed that neither application to damaged nor to nondamaged skin produced detectable concentration of AmB in the receptor fluid. Furthermore, no cytotoxic effects were observed in the macrophage or in the keratinocyte cell lines. This makes the AmB gel a promising candidate for further evaluation of its activity and efficacy in the treatment of cutaneous leishmaniasis.

Finally, the article of Rancan and coworkers deals with "Dermal Delivery of the High-Molecular-Weight Drug Tacrolimus by Means of Polyglycerol-Based Nanogels" [7]. The authors show that tacrolimus formulated as ointment or nanogel suspension penetrates skin with different efficiency in dependence on SC thickness and integrity. Irritation effects of tacrolimus ointment and nanogel formulations, reflected by the released inflammatory cytokines IL-6 and IL-8, were more pronounced in barrier-disrupted and immuno-activated skin. The results support the key role of the SC as barrier for drug and nanocarrier penetration and underline the critical balance of penetration enhancement and potential increase of side effects. All in all, the results suggest that nanogel suspensions are valuable dermal delivery systems for high molecular weight, poorly water-soluble drugs like tacrolimus.

Four of the remaining articles deal with the investigation of skin penetration and permeation.

Zsikó et al. provide a "Comparison of Skin Penetration Testing Methods based on a Nanostructured Lipid Carrier (NLC) Gel for the Dermal Application of Lidocaine" [8]. As expected, drug release profiles of the Lidocaine-NLC gel obtained with the different techniques were not fully equivalent. The various tested synthetic membranes were shown to be useful tools to examine the permeation/release of an active from a dermal formulation. The presented results can be used to guide formulators in selecting appropriate vehicles. However, no general recommendation can be made and it is still a challenging task for researchers to select the most suitable membrane to be used with Franz cells for topical product testing.

Rath et al. present in their article "A Validated In-Vitro Release Test (IVRT) Method to Assess Topical Creams Containing Metronidazole Using a Novel Approach" [9]. The reported IVRT method was carefully developed and comprehensively validated to assess the release of metronidazole from cream products, taking into account the various parameters that may affect the API release rate. The presented data indicate that the developed IVRT method can be applied to accurately and precisely assess "sameness" and differences between various metronidazole cream products as a valuable procedure in formulation development.

Zhang et al. summarize in their article results on the "Influence of Binary and Ternary Solvent Systems on the Topical Delivery of Niacinamide" [10]. Binary systems consisting of propylene glycol (PG) and some fatty acids showed enhanced skin penetration. However, the correlation for the permeation data of binary and ternary systems in Skin (Parallel Artificial Membrane Permeability Assay) PAMPA and in porcine skin was limited. It could be clearly improved by excluding the PG-Oleic Acid and PG-Linoleic Acid systems, indicating that there is still a lack of knowledge concerning specific interactions between the Skin PAMPA model and penetration-enhancing excipients.

"Preparation, Characterization and Dermal Delivery of Methadone" is the title of the article by Kung et al. [11]. They tested a range of solvents using ex-vivo permeation and mass balance method in porcine skin. Their data identified octyl salicylate, d-limonene, Transcutol®, and ethyl oleate as the most promising penetration enhancer for methadone base. Furthermore, maximum skin flux was estimated. Although the study confirms skin permeation of methadone base, the outcome was suboptimal as the majority of the active remained on the skin surface after 24 h under finite dose conditions.

Last but not least, the article that does not deal with dermal application describes a "Mucoadhesive Budesonide Formulation for the Treatment of Eosinophilic Esophagitis (EE)" [12]. The authors present results from a study that revealed a standardized budesonide oral formulation intended to improve the resistance time of the drug on the esophageal mucosa for EE treatment. The development focused on the formulation's physicochemical stability and the main critical quality attributes of the formulation, e.g., rheological properties, syringeability, mucoadhesiveness, and in-vitro penetration of budesonide in porcine esophageal tissue. The optimized formula demonstrated that the used gums enable a prolonged residence time in the esophagus.

The purpose of this Special Issue was to provide an overview of recent advances in the field of semisolid formulations. Following the results of the interesting articles collected for this Special Issue, we can conclude that although semisolids already played an important role in human society in ancient times there is still innovative research in this field adding new pieces to the jigsaw puzzle.

Conflicts of Interest: The authors declare no conflict of interest.

References

1. Ghaffar, K.A.; Daniels, R. Oleogels with Birch Bark Dry Extract: Extract Saving Formulations through Gelation Enhancing Additives. *Pharmaceutics* **2020**, *12*, 184. [CrossRef] [PubMed]
2. Ternullo, S.; Werning, L.V.S.; Holsæter, A.M.; Škalko-Basnet, N. Curcumin-In-Deformable Liposomes-In-Chitosan Hydrogel as a Novel Wound Dressing. *Pharmaceutics* **2020**, *12*, 8. [CrossRef] [PubMed]
3. Lee, J.; Hlaing, S.P.; Cao, J.; Hasan, N.; Ahn, H.-J.; Song, K.-W.; Yoo, J.-W. In Situ Hydrogel-Forming/Nitric Oxide-Releasing Wound Dressing for Enhanced Antibacterial Activity and Healing in Mice with Infected Wounds. *Pharmaceutics* **2019**, *11*, 496. [CrossRef] [PubMed]
4. Liu, Y.; Lunter, D.J. Systematic Investigation of the Effect of Non-Ionic Emulsifiers on Skin by Confocal Raman Spectroscopy—A Comprehensive Lipid Analysis. *Pharmaceutics* **2020**, *12*, 223. [CrossRef] [PubMed]
5. Schmidberger, M.; Nikolic, I.; Pantelic, I.; Lunter, D. Optimization of Rheological Behaviour and Skin Penetration of Thermogelling Emulsions with Enhanced Substantivity for Potential Application in Treatment of Chronic Skin Diseases. *Pharmaceutics* **2019**, *11*, 361. [CrossRef] [PubMed]
6. Berenguer, D.; Alcover, M.M.; Sessa, M.; Halbaut, L.; Guillén, C.; Boix-Montañés, A.; Fisa, R.; Calpena-Campmany, A.C.; Riera, C.; Sosa, L. Topical Amphotericin B Semisolid Dosage Form for Cutaneous Leishmaniasis: Physicochemical Characterization, Ex Vivo Skin Permeation and Biological Activity. *Pharmaceutics* **2020**, *12*, 149. [CrossRef] [PubMed]

7. Rancan, F.; Volkmann, H.; Giulbudagian, M.; Schumacher, F.; Stanko, J.I.; Kleuser, B.; Blume-Peytavi, U.; Calderón, M.; Vogt, A. Dermal Delivery of the High-Molecular-Weight Drug Tacrolimus by Means of Polyglycerol-Based Nanogels. *Pharmaceutics* **2019**, *11*, 394. [CrossRef] [PubMed]
8. Zsikó, S.; Cutcher, K.; Kovács, A.; Budai-Szűcs, M.; Gácsi, A.; Baki, G.; Csányi, E.; Berkó, S. Nanostructured Lipid Carrier Gel for the Dermal Application of Lidocaine: Comparison of Skin Penetration Testing Methods. *Pharmaceutics* **2019**, *11*, 310. [CrossRef] [PubMed]
9. Rath, S.; Kanfer, I. A Validated IVRT Method to Assess Topical Creams Containing Metronidazole Using a Novel Approach. *Pharmaceutics* **2020**, *12*, 119. [CrossRef] [PubMed]
10. Zhang, Y.; Kung, C.-P.; Sil, B.C.; Lane, M.E.; Hadgraft, J.; Heinrich, M.; Sinko, B. Topical Delivery of Niacinamide: Influence of Binary and Ternary Solvent Systems. *Pharmaceutics* **2019**, *11*, 668. [CrossRef] [PubMed]
11. Kung, C.-P.; Sil, B.C.; Hadgraft, J.; Lane, M.E.; Patel, B.; McCulloch, R. Preparation, Characterization and Dermal Delivery of Methadone. *Pharmaceutics* **2019**, *11*, 509. [CrossRef] [PubMed]
12. Casiraghi, A.; Gennari, C.G.; Musazzi, U.M.; Ortenzi, M.A.; Bordignon, S.; Minghetti, P. Mucoadhesive Budesonide Formulation for the Treatment of Eosinophilic Esophagitis. *Pharmaceutics* **2020**, *12*, 211. [CrossRef] [PubMed]

pharmaceutics

MDPI

Article

Systematic Investigation of the Effect of Non-Ionic Emulsifiers on Skin by Confocal Raman Spectroscopy—A Comprehensive Lipid Analysis

Yali Liu and Dominique Jasmin Lunter *

Department of Pharmaceutical Technology, Eberhard Karls University, Auf der Morgenstelle 8, 72076 Tuebingen, Germany; cpuyali@gmail.com

* Correspondence: dominique.lunter@uni-tuebingen.de; Tel.: +49-7071-297-4558; Fax: +49-7071-295-531

Received: 20 January 2020; Accepted: 29 February 2020; Published: 2 March 2020

Abstract: Non-ionic emulsifiers are commonly found in existing pharmaceutical and cosmetic formulations and have been widely employed to enhance the penetration and permeation of active ingredients into the skin. With the potential of disrupting skin barrier function and increasing fluidity of stratum corneum (SC) lipids, we herein examined the effects of two kinds of non-ionic emulsifiers on intercellular lipids of skin, using confocal Raman spectroscopy (CRS) with lipid signals on skin CRS spectrum. Non-ionic emulsifiers of polyethylene glycol alkyl ethers and sorbitan fatty acid esters were studied to obtain a deep understanding of the mechanism between non-ionic emulsifiers and SC lipids. Emulsifier solutions and dispersions were prepared and applied onto excised porcine skin. Water and sodium laureth sulfate solution (SLS) served as controls. SC lipid signals were analysed by CRS regarding lipid content, conformation and lateral packing order. Polyethylene glycol (PEG) sorbitan esters revealed no alteration of intercellular lipid properties while PEG-20 ethers appeared to have the most significant effects on reducing lipid content and interrupting lipid organization. In general, the polyoxyethylene chain and alkyl chain of PEG derivative emulsifiers might indicate their ability of interaction with SC components. HLB values remained critical for complete explanation of emulsifier effects on skin lipids. With this study, it is possible to characterize the molecular effects of non-ionic emulsifiers on skin lipids and further deepen the understanding of enhancing substance penetration with reduced skin barrier properties and increased lipid fluidity.

Keywords: non-ionic emulsifiers; intercellular lipids; confocal Raman spectroscopy (CRS); polyethylene glycol alkyl ethers; polyethylene glycol sorbitan fatty acid esters

---

1. Introduction

Skin represents the largest organ of the human organism and forms the outermost barrier film that protects the human body from external environment impacts and exogenous irritations and corrosions. Stratum corneum (SC) is the uppermost layer of the skin, composed of a highly ordered, multilamellar lipid matrix with embedded flattened, keratin-filled corneocytes [1,2]. The particular intercellular lipids in SC consist of ceramides, free fatty acids and cholesterol in an approximately equimolar ratio [3,4]. It has been well accepted that intercellular lipids in SC play an important role in maintaining skin barrier function and keeping the skin in a proper hydration state [5]. The removal and organizational alteration of intercellular lipids would disrupt the barrier function from multiple aspects and deteriorate into some chronic skin diseases [6,7]. With the importance of assuring the solid structures and ordered properties of skin lipids, it is essential to monitor the molecular lipid interactions with exposed substances and maintain the protective barrier state for further optimization of dermatological treatments.

In everyday life, the skin is exposed to different environments and mostly exposed to various sanitary and cosmetic products and cleansers. Among the main components of them, non-ionic emulsifiers have been widely used and become the potential class to be exposed on the skin and may simultaneously interact with molecular skin components [8,9]. Although non-ionic emulsifiers are usually considered to be relatively safe and better tolerated in comparison to cationic and anionic emulsifiers, they have been proved having the potential to interact with biological membranes, especially skin, with their increasing applications [10–12]. In particular, recent studies from our group found that polyethylene glycol (PEG)-20 glycerol monostearate displayed negative effects on skin lipid extraction and structural disruption while polysorbate 80 reflected no such effects [13,14]. For this reason, the selection and usage of non-ionic emulsifiers in pharmaceutical and cosmetic formulations are currently of high interest. In order to gain mechanistic insights into their skin effects, PEG alkyl ethers and sorbitan fatty acid esters (e.g., polysorbate or Tween) were taken into consideration which are both non-ionic PEG derivatives. They are composed of a hydrophilic polyoxyethylene head group and a lipophilic alkyl chain. Keeping constant either of these two parts, the other part of size and chain length etc. would be potential parameters to monitor the governing rules [15]. Furthermore, these two groups of emulsifiers are widely applied in cosmetic and dermal products due to their solubility and viscosity properties with low toxicity according to the existing safety assessments identified in previous studies [16,17]. We therefore chose to further investigate these two groups of emulsifiers in a systematic approach and evaluate their possibilities for prospective development of skin products with relatively mild effects on skin lipids [18].

Up to now, considerable number of studies have made efforts on obtaining more information about the quantitative and structural properties of skin lipids [19–21]. The means of small- and wide-angle X-ray scattering, neutron scattering, and liquid chromatography coupled with mass spectrometry have been intensively applied. However, those methodologies have potential risks of sample contamination, being time-consuming and sample destruction [22,23]. In this area confocal Raman spectroscopy (CRS) has emerged as a promising non-invasive tool in skin research and caught increasing attention for skin characterizations such as skin penetration and permeation of topically applied materials [24,25]. CRS is also an efficient and label-free method and has been increasingly used to study the macroscopic alterations of skin properties with humidity changes, age difference and hair removal comparisons [26–28]. Detailed information about biochemical molecules can be obtained from CRS, including the chemical structure, phase and molecular interactions. Recent findings from our group have demonstrated that CRS could be used as an alternative method to analyze lipid extraction and conformation in SC [13,14]. Based on this proof and listed advantages, CRS was used in this study as a useful and convenient approach for lipid analysis.

For studying the physiological parameters of SC lipids, many researchers have focused on finding spectral signals in CRS for skin research [29,30]. Those spectral signals in this study are the identified Raman bands associated with molecular vibrations of lipids inside the skin. They are originated from the methylene ($-CH_2-$) and methyl ($-CH_3$) groups in lipid molecular structures. Using them a comprehensive study measuring lipid content, conformational order, lateral packing order and SC thickness could be conducted at the same time. However, the skin CRS spectrum is extremely complex and the lipid-derived Raman bands usually overlap with bands originating from molecular vibrations of proteins [19,31]. In order to track the individual lipid-related spectral signals, a Gaussian-function based mathematical procedure could be applied on account of a previous report from Choe et al. [32].

As we know, many hypotheses regarding the interactions between emulsifiers and skin are still not well grounded [33], making it essential to perform a systematic investigation of non-ionic emulsifiers. Therefore, the aim of this study is to use different lipid-related spectral signals to analyse the interactions between non-ionic emulsifiers and intercellular lipids. PEG alkyl ethers and sorbitan fatty acid esters were selected. To the best of our knowledge, this is the first systematic report considering PEG derivatives with different number of oxyethylene groups and different hydrophobic alkyl chain lengths using CRS to better understand their mechanism of influence on skin components.

Results should be helpful to find a rule for further selections of non-ionic emulsifiers which is beneficial to the development of skin products.

2. Materials and Methods

2.1. Materials

PEG alkyl ethers including PEG-2 oleyl ether (O2), PEG-10 oleyl ether (O10), PEG-20 oleyl ether (O20), PEG-2 stearyl ether (S2), PEG-10 stearyl ether (S10), PEG-20 stearyl ether (S20), PEG-2 cetyl ether (C2), PEG-10 cetyl ether (C10), PEG-20 cetyl ether (C20) were purchased from Croda GmbH, (Nettetal, Germany). PEG sorbitan fatty acid esters containing PEG-20 sorbitan monopalmitate (Polysorbate 40, PS40), PEG-20 sorbitan monostearate (Polysorbate 60, PS60), PEG-20 sorbitan monooleate (Polysorbate 80, PS80) were obtained from Caesar & Loretz GmbH (Hilden, Germany). Sodium lauryl sulfate (SLS) was obtained from Cognis GmbH & Co. KG (Düsseldorf, Germany). Trypsin type II- S (lyophilized powder) and trypsin inhibitor (lyophilized powder) were obtained from Sigma-Aldrich Chemie GmbH (Steinheim, Germany). Parafilm® was from Bemis Company Inc., (Oshkosh, WI, USA). Sodium chloride, disodium hydrogen phosphate, potassium dihydrogen phosphate, and potassium chloride were of European Pharmacopoeia grade. All aqueous solutions were prepared with ultra-pure water (Elga Maxima, High Wycombe, UK). Porcine ear skins (German land race; age: 15 to 30 weeks; weight: 40 to 65 kg) were provided by Department of Experimental Medicine at the University of Tuebingen. The Department of Pharmaceutical Technology at the University of Tuebingen has been registered for the use of animal products [13].

2.2. Preparation of Dermatomed Porcine Ear Skin

Porcine ear skin was selected as substitute for human skin in this study due to their histologically and morphologically similarity with human skin [34,35]. Porcine ears used in this study were achieved from the Department of Experimental Medicine of the University Hospital Tuebingen. The live animals used were kept at the Department of Experimental Medicine and sacrificed in the course of their experiments, which are approved by the ethics committee of the University Hospital Tuebingen. Those ears were received directly after the death of the animals. Prior to study start, the Department of Pharmaceutical Technology has registered for the use of animal products at the District Office of Tuebingen (registration number: DE 08 416 1052 21). Fresh porcine ears were cleaned with isotonic saline. Full-thickness skin was removed from cartilage and gently cleaned from blood with cotton swabs and isotonic saline. The obtained postauricular skin sheets were then dried with soft tissue, wrapped with aluminium foil and stored in freezer at −30 °C. On the day of experiment, skin sheet was thawed to room temperature, cut into strips of approximately 3 cm width and stretched onto a Styrofoam plate (wrapped with aluminium foil) with pins to minimize the effect of furrows. Skin hairs were trimmed to approximately 0.5 mm with electric hair clippers (QC5115/15, Philips, Netherlands). Subsequently, the skin was dermatomed to a thickness of 0.8 mm (Dermatom GA 630, Aesculap AG & Co. KG, Tuttlingen, Germany) and punched out for circles to a diameter of 25 mm.

2.3. Incubation of Porcine Ear Skin in Franz Diffusion Cells

Franz diffusion cells have been commonly used as a specific analytical setup for ex vivo determination of skin absorption. Here, degassed, prewarmed (32 °C) phosphate buffered saline (PBS) was used as receptor fluid and filled in the Franz diffusion cells of 12 mL. The stirring speed of the receptor fluid was 500 rpm. The dermatomed skin circles were mounted onto the cells with donor compartment on above. The equipped Franz diffusion cells were put into water bath with temperature of 32 °C. After a short equilibrium of 30 min, 1 mL of each emulsifier solution/dispersion was applied to each skin sample (all non-ionic emulsifiers used in this study are listed in Table 1 with detailed information). Then, a piece of parafilm was capped onto each donor compartment to prevent evaporation. After 4 h incubation, skin samples were removed from cells and each skin surface was gently washed and cleaned with isotonic saline and cotton swabs for 30 times in order to remove the remaining samples and avoid erroneous measuring result. Finally, the actual application area (15 mm in diameter) was punched out and patted dry with cotton swabs. This part of the method has been detailly described by our group [13].

Table 1. Characteristics of non-ionic emulsifiers including polyethylene glycol (PEG) alkyl ethers and PEG sorbitan esters used in this study.

Non-Ionic Emulsifiers	Alkyl Chain	Alkyl Chain LENGTH and Saturation	Number of Oxyethylene Group	Abbreviations	HLB Value
PEG-2 oleyl ether	Oleyl alcohol	C18, C9–C10 unsaturated	2	O2	5.0
PEG-10 oleyl ether	Oleyl alcohol	C18, C9–C10 unsaturated	10	O10	12.4
PEG-20 oleyl ether	Oleyl alcohol	C18, C9–C10 unsaturated	20	O20	15.3
PEG-2 stearyl ether	Stearyl alcohol	C18	2	S2	4.9
PEG-10 stearyl ether	Stearyl alcohol	C18	10	S10	12.4
PEG-20 stearyl ether	Stearyl alcohol	C18	20	S20	15.3
PEG-2 cetyl ether	Cetyl alcohol	C16	2	C2	5.3
PEG-10 cetyl ether	Cetyl alcohol	C16	10	C10	12.9
PEG-20 cetyl ether	Cetyl alcohol	C16	20	C20	15.7
PEG-20 sorbitan monopalmitate	Palmitic acid	C16	20	PS40	15.6
PEG-20 sorbitan monostearate	Stearic acid	C18	20	PS60	14.9
PEG-20 sorbitan monooleate	Oleic acid	C18, C9–C10 unsaturated	20	PS80	15

2.4. Isolation of Stratum Corneum

The stratum corneum was isolated following the trypsin digestion process as described by Kligman et al. and Zhang [14,36]. This isolation procedure has been proved to have no influence on the lamellar lipid organization [37]. The obtained skin circles (with diameter of 15 mm) from last step were placed dermal side down on filter paper soaked with a 0.2% trypsin and PBS solution. After the incubation of skin sample for overnight at room temperature, digested SC was peeled off gently and immersed into 0.05% trypsin inhibitor solution for 1 min. Afterwards, the isolated SC was washed with fresh purified water for min. five times to remove the underlayer tissues. The final obtained SC sheet was then placed onto glass slide and stored in desiccator to dry for min. three days.

2.5. Confocal Raman Spectroscopy (CRS)

In order to investigate the effects of different non-ionic emulsifiers on SC, CRS served as the primary instrument to detect their differences. After drying, the SC sheets were taken out of the desiccator and fitted onto the scan table of alpha 500 R confocal Raman microscope (WITec GmbH, Ulm, Germany). This CRS device was equipped with a 532-nm excitation laser, UHTS 300 spectrometer and DV401-BV CCD camera. To avoid the damage of skin sample due to higher laser intensity, the laser power used was 10 mW, which could be adjusted using the optimal power meter (PM100D, Thorlabs GmbH, Dachau, Germany). A 100× objective with numerical aperture of 0.9 (EC Epiplan-neofluor, Carl Zeiss, Jena, Germany) was used to focus the light on skin surface. The backscattered light from the skin was then dispersed by an optical grating (600 g/mm) to achieve the spectral range from 400–3800 cm^{-1}. Collected scattered light was analysed on a charge-coupled device (DV401-BV CCD detector) which had been cooled down to −60 °C in advance. The CRS measurements were performed based on a method developed by Zhang et al. [13,14].

2.6. Determination of Skin Surface and Thickness

In order to achieve spectral signals of lipids from skin surface and measure SC thickness at the same time, the spectra were detected with the focus point moving from −50 μm beneath the skin to

50 μm above the skin. The spectra were recorded with the step size of 1 μm. The skin surface was determined using the intensity difference of keratin signal (ν (CH_3), 2920–2960 cm^{-1}). The area under the curve (AUC) of the keratin peak was calculated and plotted against depth. While the intensity of the keratin signal reaches the half maximum, the laser spot would be located at the boundary between glass slide and skin bottom or the boundary between skin surface and air [13,38]. So that the spectrum extracted from the boundary between skin surface and air was regarded as skin surface and used for lipid signal analysis. Moreover, with the description above, the full width of half maximum (FWHM) could serve as the thickness of skin sample.

2.7. Lipid Signals in Fingerprint Region

2.7.1. C–C Skeleton Vibration Mode

The first three small peaks in Figure 1 highlighted in red are assigned to the vibration of C–C skeleton. They are sensitive to the trans–gauche conformational order of long chain hydrocarbons which exist mostly in intercellular lipids [39,40]. The peaks located at 1060 cm^{-1} and 1130 cm^{-1} arise from all-trans conformation which stand for a more ordered state of lipids. The peak at 1080 cm^{-1} corresponds to the gauche conformation which represents a more disordered state of lipids [41,42]. In this case, PCA analysis and polynomial background subtraction are needed to remove the noise and obtain a more precise result. On the other hand, the band at 1130 cm^{-1} contains part of the contribution of keratin at 1125 cm^{-1}. As a result, an adequate integration area is selected to eliminate the influence of keratin peak. Then, the conformational order could be calculated with the ratio of AUC of those three peaks: conformational order = AUC_{1080} / (AUC_{1060} + AUC_{1130}) as originally described by Snyder, et al. [43]. Thus, a higher value of conformational order represents an indication to the gauche conformation and disordered state of lipids.

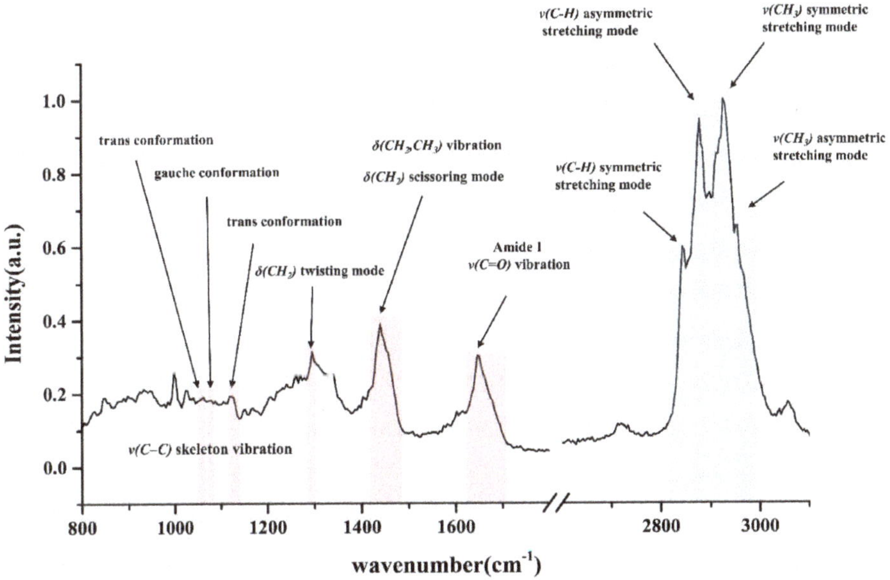

Figure 1. Major band assignments of CRS spectrum obtained from skin sample. The red/blue areas represent the specific peak referring to different molecular vibrations. The break on the axis of wavenumber separates the fingerprint region (left side) and high wavenumber region (right side). The peaks assigned to trans and gauche conformations are both originated from C–C skeleton vibration.

2.7.2. CH_2 Twisting and Scissoring Mode

The peak located at about 1300 cm^{-1} in Figure 1 is assigned to the CH_2 twisting mode. The shift of this peak could also indicate the order or disorder of lipid conformations because of the sensitivity of this peak to hydrocarbon chains [44]. The broadening and shift to a higher wavenumber of this peak indicates a tendency of intercellular lipids turning into a more disordered and gauche conformation state.

Apart from the detection of conformational order on Raman spectra, vibrational characteristics are also convenient to determine the lateral packing state (orthorhombic order, hexagonal order, and liquid-like chain packing) influenced by the intramolecular interactions [44]. The CH_2 scissoring band at 1430–1470 cm^{-1} reflects the nature of lateral packing between ceramide molecules. The shift of this peak to a higher wavenumber in the Raman spectrum stands for a more hexagonal or even liquid like packing state.

2.7.3. CH_2 and CH_3 Stretching and C=O Vibration Mode

The last two bands marked in fingerprint region of Figure 1 are assigned to δ (CH_2, CH_3)– mode at 1425–1490 cm^{-1} and ν (C=O)– mode at 1630–1710 cm^{-1} respectively. The band at 1630–1710 cm^{-1} arises from the Amide I mode which showed the least variation within one donor or among different donors. Thus, this band has been often used in the normalization of other Raman peaks derived from SC [30,42]. The band at 1425–1490 cm^{-1} originates from both keratins and lipids. In this study, this band was regarded as "lipids-peak" for calculation of lipid content.

Based on the equation of Normalized lipids = $AUC_{1425-1490}/AUC_{1630-1710}$, the lipid-keratin peak was normalized by the amide I peak. The final calculated result would indicate the content variation of lipids. Therefore, the lipid content in fingerprint region in this study was calculated as equation above.

2.8. *Lipid Signals in High Wavenumber Region*

In order to achieve further information about lipid content and lateral packing order state for a more precise and forceful result, the lipid-keratin peak (2800–3030 cm^{-1}) in the HWN region was taken into consideration. This band is also derived from the CH_2 and CH_3 vibrations.

2.8.1. Gaussian Deconvolution Process

As depicted in Figure 1, it is obvious that the peaks originated from lipids and keratins overlapped and formed a peak with higher intensity and broad width. In order to track the information of each peak individually, a mathematical process based on Gaussian functions was employed. As described by Choe, the Gaussian function type exhibited the least fitting error and demonstrated to be the best fitting function for Raman spectra of the skin [32].

In this study, the obtained spectrum of SC was deconvoluted into four Gaussian peaks automatically with the application of curve fitting toolbox on Matlab software (version R2019a, MathWorks GmbH, Natick, MA, USA). The summation of four Gaussian functions was used as the fitting formula. In order to achieve reproducible result and reduce the fitting error, the Gaussian peak maximum positions and FWHMs were allowed to vary in defined intervals only. Afterwards, a non-linear iteration process was applied. It can be seen from Figure 2 that each fitted peak was labelled in different colour. The goodness of fitting results could also be generated automatically with all R^2 above than 0.98.

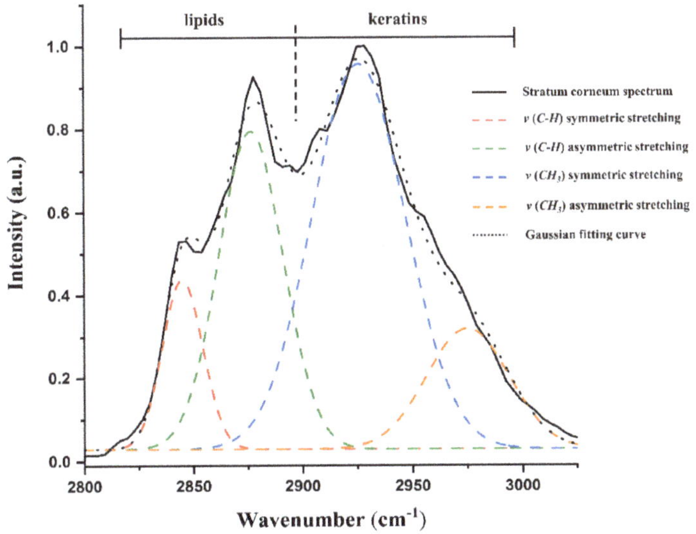

Figure 2. Deconvolution of lipid-keratin peak from skin spectrum by using four Gaussian peaks in high wavenumber region. The assignments were labelled with different colours.

2.8.2. ν (C–H) Symmetric and Asymmetric Stretching

As illustrated in Figure 2, peaks located at 2850 cm^{-1} and 2880 cm^{-1} stand for the ν (C–H) symmetric and ν (C–H) asymmetric stretching mode respectively which are both derived from the vibration of lipids. These two peaks are sensitive to the packing order of alkyl chains of lipids. Based on some research, the ratio of the intensities of these two peaks could be used as a sign of crystalline phase of intercellular lipids [39,45]. In this study, peak areas after deconvolution were applied for the calculation of lateral packings $Ratio_{lat} = AUC_{2880}/AUC_{2850}$ according to ref. [46]. This procedure has effectively eliminated the influence of multi-peak overlap phenomenon. Hereby, the higher $Ratio_{lat}$ represents a prevalence towards highly crystalline and orthorhombic phase. The lower $Ratio_{lat}$ reveals a tendency towards disordered and liquid-like phase.

2.8.3. ν (CH_3) Symmetric and Asymmetric Stretching

As is shown in Figure 2, the blue and orange peaks at 2930 cm^{-1} and 2980 cm^{-1} arise from the contribution of keratins and originated from the ν (CH_3) symmetric and ν (CH_3) asymmetric stretching separately. Previous studies often use the area of these two keratin related peaks to normalize lipid related peaks in order to determine the lipid content [47,48]. As described in this study, the AUC extracted directly in high wavenumber would contain the contribution of adjacent peaks. The deconvolution process would exclude the influence of peak superposition. As a result, the Gaussian areas after deconvolution were employed for calculation of lipid content: Normalized lipid = $(AUC_{2880} + AUC_{2850})/(AUC_{2930} + AUC_{2980})$.

2.9. Data Analysis

2.9.1. Raman Spectra Pre-Processing

The initial processing step of Raman spectra usually included the spectral cosmic ray removal, smoothing as well as background subtraction which were all performed by the WITec Project Software (WITec GmbH). Referring to the smoothing process, Savitzky-Golay (SG) filter was applied with third polynomial order and nine smoothing point. For the type of background subtraction, an automatic polynomial function was fitted to the spectrum and subtracted. Furthermore, the AUC extracted in this study is the integrated area under a specified peak of the spectrum and could be calculated using trapezoidal method on WITec Project Software or MatLab software.

2.9.2. Principle Component Analysis

Multivariate data analysis was also performed on the WITec Project Software. For the study, Principle component analysis (PCA) was employed to further analysis the grouped spectra and reduce minor variations. PCA is the underlying method for many multivariate methods and could effectively obtain a reduced data set from multiple dimensions. Among the grouped Raman spectra, the first three principle components (PCs) are selected for reconstruction since they have contained most of essential information. In this study, PCA was applied for lipid conformation analysis.

2.9.3. Statistical Analysis

Spectra data were obtained from repeated measurements ($n \geq 18$). The graphs were shown with mean values ± standard deviations (mean ± SD). Statistical differences were determined using one-way or two-way analysis of variance (ANOVA) followed by Student-Newman-Keuls (SNK) which were employed by GraphPad Prism 7.0 (GraphPad Software Inc., La Jolla, CA, USA). Diagrams and statistical differences were ultimately generated. Significant differences were marked with different number of asterisks: * $p < 0.05$, ** $p < 0.01$, *** $p < 0.001$.

3. Results

3.1. Lipid Content Analysis with Normalized Lipid Signal

Lipid content in SC was analysed in the fingerprint and HWN regions by using lipid signals normalized by keratin signals. With the aim of detecting their impacts on lipids, different non-ionic emulsifiers were used to treat the SC, respectively. The alterations of lipid content are shown in Figure 3a,b. As can be seen, the red bars indicate the relative lipid content in fingerprint region while the blue bars represent the content in HWN region. It is evident that most of the PEG ethers cause a reduction of lipid content (Figure 3a) while all the polysorbate emulsifiers show no effects on SC lipid content (Figure 3b). Specifically speaking, the group of PEG ethers treated SC shows different extent of lipid reduction. Among them, only O2 and S2 treated SCs indicate no effects on SC lipid content. Focusing on the rest of the emulsifiers, all the PEG-20 alkyl ethers display to dramatically reduce lipid content. Regarding the PEG-10 alkyl ethers, O10 shows a relatively smaller difference compared to S10 and C10 which both indicate a greater reduction of skin lipid content. Interestingly, only C2 in PEG-2 alkyl ethers shows a slight impact on reducing lipid content. In contrast, polysorbate emulsifiers reflect completely no extraction of lipids. It turns out a part of this outcome is correlated with a previous result in our group that showed 5% of polysorbate 60 had no effects on lipids [13]. In general, the result of lipid content analysis in fingerprint region is complementary to that in HWN region and exhibited the same tendency of emulsifier effects.

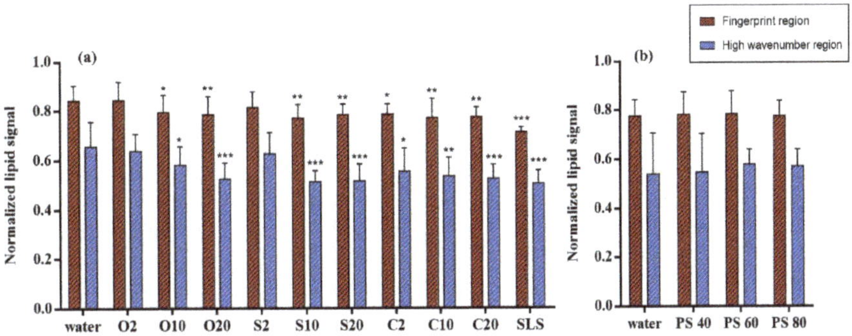

Figure 3. Normalized lipid signals in fingerprint and HWN region for lipid composition analysis of (**a**) PEG alkyl ethers treated SC and (**b**) PEG sorbitan esters treated SC. Mean ± SD, $n = 18$. * $p < 0.05$; ** $p < 0.01$; *** $p < 0.001$.

3.2. CH_2 *Twisting and Scissoring Mode Analysis*

CH_2 twisting mode in fingerprint region was selected in this study. It is also feasible to analyse the lipid conformational order. The band derived from CH_2 twisting mode is located at about 1300 cm^{-1}. The band shift is sensible to the conformation of hydrocarbon chains of lipids, so that it could be used as another conformational signal. Figure 4 shows the comparison of twisting mode between emulsifier treated and water treated skin samples. The peak location is in between 1285–1303 cm^{-1}. It can be clearly seen that SLS has the most significant effect on SC lipid as the band shifts from about 1293 cm^{-1} to about 1299 cm^{-1}. Among PEG ethers, relatively higher effects on lipids are caused by the PEG ether emulsifiers with the average number of oxyethylene groups of 20 as well as O10 and S10. Interestingly, C10 only shows small effects on lipid conformation. Nevertheless, in lipid content and C–C skeleton conformation analysis presented above, C10 has been determined to strikingly extract lipids and change conformational order. Apart from this slight discordance, the result is still a confirmation of emulsifier effects on lipid signals. Further, no significant effects are noted in polysorbate emulsifier treated SCs.

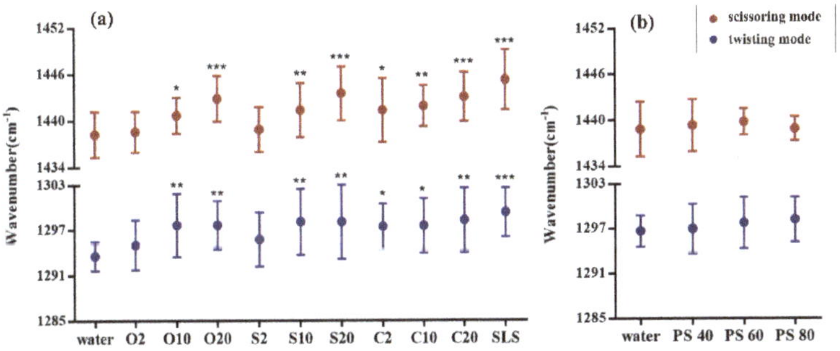

Figure 4. Lipid signals of CH_2 twisting and scissoring mode for analyzing (**a**) PEG alkyl ethers treated SC and (**b**) PEG sorbitan esters treated SC. Mean ± SD, $n = 18$. * $p < 0.05$; ** $p < 0.01$; *** $p < 0.001$.

Except for the detailed information of hydrocarbon chains of lipids, CRS is also available to determine the lateral packing of lipids with CH_2 scissoring mode in fingerprint region. Using the peak at 1434–1452 cm^{-1}, Figure 4 shows the differences of scissoring mode when comparing emulsifier treated and water treated skin samples. It can be observed that some bands strikingly shift to higher wavenumbers after treatment with emulsifiers such as PEG-20 alkyl ethers and SLS. It means that the lateral packing tends to be transformed from orthorhombic phase to hexagonal or liquid-like phase. C10 and S10 shows to moderately lower the lateral packing density. However, the influence of O10 on SC is slightly lower than what we expected but similar to the impact of C10 on SC. In line with results from C–C skeleton vibration mode analysis, the results from scissoring mode analysis show no significant difference for polysorbate emulsifiers treated SCs.

3.3. C–C Skeleton Conformation Analysis

C–C skeleton vibrations in fingerprint region contain the all-*trans* signal (1060 cm^{-1} and 1130 cm^{-1}) and *gauche* signal (1080 cm^{-1}) of SC lipids. With the application of non-ionic emulsifiers, lipid conformation in SC was influenced to different degree. As displayed in Figure 5a, most of the PEG ethers show significant effects on lipid conformation when compared with water treated SC. Especially S10 and S20 as well as C10 and C20 present huge effects on SC lipid conformation, indicating the intercellular lipids have more gauche conformation (more disorder state). Surprisingly, O10 and O20 only show small influence on altering lipid conformation which is even less than the impact of C2. Whereas O2 and S2 show no effects on turning lipids into a more *gauche* conformation. Focusing on the investigation of the polysorbate group, it can be seen from Figure 5b that no significant difference has been found in polysorbate emulsifiers-treated SCs. It turns out that, with the application of polysorbate emulsifiers, lipid conformation remains in a more *trans* and ordered state.

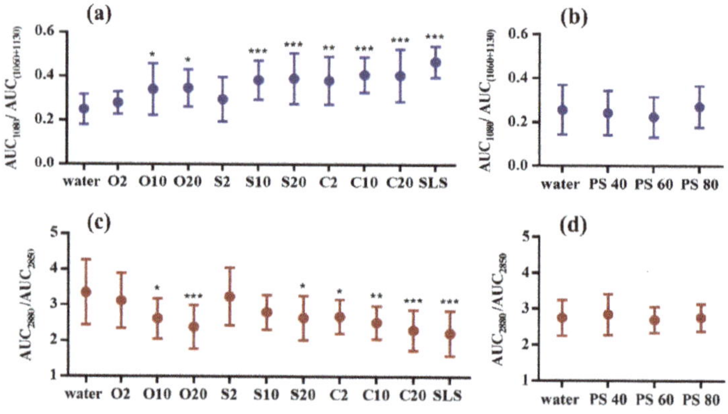

Figure 5. C–C skeleton vibration mode for lipid conformation analysis of (**a**) PEG alkyl ethers treated SC and (**b**) PEG sorbitan esters treated SC; lateral packing order analysis by AUC ratio of band 2850 cm^{-1} and 2880 cm^{-1}: (**c**) PEG alkyl ethers treated SC and (**d**) PEG sorbitan esters treated SC. Mean ± SD, $n = 18$. * $p < 0.05$; ** $p < 0.01$; *** $p < 0.001$.

3.4. Lateral Packing Analysis in HWN Region

Commonly, the broad shaped lipid-keratin peak originated from C–H vibration in HWN region is used to calculate lipid content and lipid lateral packing. The ratio of AUCs of 2880/2850 cm^{-1} has been defined to evaluate the lateral packing density of intercellular lipids. In this spectral region, peaks reflecting vibrations of SC lipids overlap with peaks derived from keratin. After the deconvolution process of lipids-keratin signals, the calculation of lateral packing in HWN is more precise owing to the exclusion of keratin peak influences.

As the results shown in Figure 5c, O20 and C20 have the highest effects on decreasing the lateral packing density which are nearly the same as the effect of SLS. C10 tends to transform the lipid structure to hexagonal phase (more disordered structure). In addition, O10, S20 as well as C2 treated SC only indicate relatively lower effects. Whereas S10 treated SC unexpectedly presents no statistical difference which is unlike the lateral packing result shown in the scissoring mode analysis. The results depicted in Figure 5d reconfirmed that polysorbate emulsifiers appeared to exert no significant effects on SC lipids and maintained the orthorhombic structure of intercellular lipids.

3.5. Skin Thickness Measurement

The thickness of skin samples was measured after the treatment with different emulsifiers. It has to be noted that SC thickness was measured on dried SC sheets and will thus give lower values as in (hydrated) full thickness skins. With the comparison to references, the results are shown in Figure 6. It is apparent from Figure 6a that the water treated SC was measured to be the thickest with the average thickness of 4.50 ± 0.64 μm. In contrast, SLS treated SC exhibited the thinnest skin samples (2.55 ± 0.54 μm), followed by the C20 and C10 treated SC with thickness of 2.84 ± 0.69 μm and 3.27 ± 1.20 μm respectively. O10 and O20 treated SC showed a tendency towards a reduced thickness as well. Unexpectedly, no indication was found of reduction of SC thickness after treatment with S10. In another experiment depicted in Figure 6b, the water treated SC was measured to have the thickness of 4.04 ± 1.16 μm, while the polysorbate emulsifiers treated SCs showed no significant difference when compared with water treated SC.

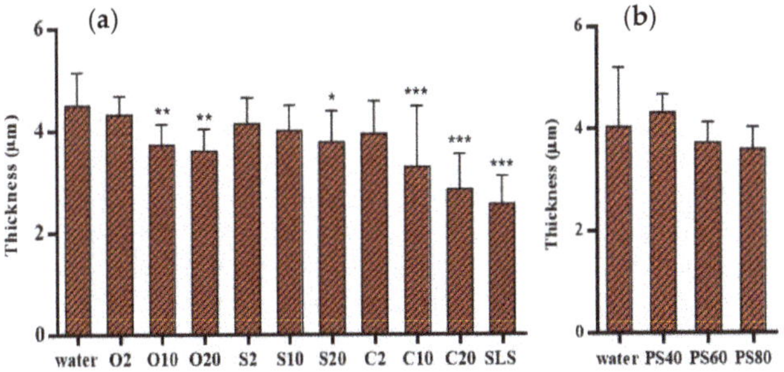

Figure 6. Thickness of SC after treatment with (**a**) PEG alkyl ethers treated SC and (**b**) PEG sorbitan esters treated SC. Mean ± SD, $n = 18$. * $p < 0.05$; ** $p < 0.01$; *** $p < 0.001$.

4. Discussion

Throughout this study, different spectral signals were utilized to analyse the effects of non-ionic emulsifiers on SC lipids. The result of lipid content analysis was achieved with the combination of lipid spectral signals from fingerprint region and HWN region. We could clearly see that PEG ethers were more capable to extract the lipids from SC than polysorbate emulsifiers. Meanwhile, both results of lipid content analysis were in good correlation with each other. It proved that after curve fitting process, the lipid-keratin peak ratio could serve as a sensitive lipid signal to calculate the lipid content. As an alternative, the lipid-keratin peak ratio in fingerprint region may be used and gives similar results.

The conformational analysis was evaluated in this study with the band shift of the twisting mode and calculated by the ratio of three small peaks related to *gauche/trans* conformation which originated from the C–C skeleton vibration bands. In view of the same tendency of detected emulsifier effects, both of the lipid spectral signals are capable to analyse lipid conformation accurately. However, comparing a series of complicated data processing steps in C–C skeleton vibration features, the prominent peak shift related to CH_2 twisting mode at about 1300 cm^{-1} would be a better choice and less time-consuming.

There was a slightly difference in lipid analysis of lateral packing density. The ratio calculated by 2880/2850 cm^{-1} revealed that S10 had no significant effect. Whereas the results of scissoring mode indicated significant difference ($p < 0.01$). Although the deconvolution process has eliminated the influence of the keratin signal in the HWN region, the differences between results from S10 treated SC and water treated SC are not large enough to reach statistical significance. With the consideration of minor errors may result from the curve fitting process, the signal of scissoring mode might provide a more sensitive and efficient detection in our further study.

As the preliminary study of our group presented, the thinning of SC was assumptively caused by the extraction of lipids, subsequently leading to a loosened cohesion of SC and thereby fascinating keratinocytes removal [13]. In the skin thickness analysis of present work, most results complied with expectations and previous findings although the results of S10 and C2 reflected inconsistent with former lipid signals which may be triggered by the influence of different donors. The thinner the SC thickness originally, the less accurate the measuring result. Besides, the isolation of SC may also induce measurement errors.

Since this systematic study has proved that non-ionic emulsifiers have the potential to interact with SC lipids, we may find some rules or mechanisms to explain the ability of them to extract lipid components and decrease lipid order of SC. First, their capability to affect SC lipids might be governed by their structural properties as they contain both polar head region of hydrophilic chain and nonpolar tail region of hydrophobic chain. The characteristics of non-ionic emulsifiers used in this study has been listed in Table 1. As the influence of PEG ethers on SC shown, we may suggest that the higher the average number of oxyethylene groups, the stronger the interaction between PEG ethers and SC lipids. Meanwhile, the alkyl chain was highlighted in the potency of emulsifier interaction with SC lipid as well. With the results shown in this study, C2 appeared to be the only emulsifier to reduce lipid content and increase lipid disorder compared to other PEG-2 ethers. As they own the same number of oxyethylene groups, we may speculate that PEG derivatives with less carbon numbers of alkyl chain present higher ability to disturb SC lipid properties. Furthermore, keeping constant the number of carbon atoms in hydrophobic chain, similar effects of PEG oleyl ethers (unsaturated alkyl chain, C18) and PEG stearyl ethers (saturated alkyl chain, C18) on SC lipids were observed. We might then assume that with the same length of alkyl chain, the double bound only show little impact on SC lipids.

In the present study of polysorbate emulsifiers, they have been confirmed to have no influence on SC lipids, although they have longer polyoxyethylene chain ($n = 20$) and different length of alkyl chain. In this case, the molecular weight and structures could also serve as underlying factors for explaining the effects of polysorbate emulsifiers. The molecular structures of PEG ethers and esters used in this study are given in Table 2. It is apparent that polysorbate emulsifiers have larger molecular structure sizes which are expected to make it difficult for them to penetrate the skin and interact with SC lipids. Furthermore, although a recent finding from another group revealed a slight toxicity of polysorbate emulsifiers towards skin cells, it is not contradictory to our results that presented more friendly effects of them on skin lipids [49]. Our investigation suggests that polysorbates do not penetrate the skin and thus do not reach the deeper levels of the skin where living cells are located. Thus, it can be concluded that they may be regarded as safe excipients as long as they are not taken up into viable cell layers. Meanwhile, the emulsifier incorporated in various formulations may also display different influence on skin properties [13,49].

Last, according to the HLB values listed in Table 1, we first expect that the HLB values of non-ionic emulsifiers correlate to their effects on SC lipids. We could suggest from the result of PEG ethers that the higher the HLB value, the more intensive effects of emulsifiers on SC lipids. However, C2 with HLB value of 5.3 sometimes revealed relatively similar influence with O10 and S10 (HLB value 12.4). More strikingly is that all polysorbate emulsifiers present no effects on SC lipids with HLB values all around 15. Therefore, we may conclude that HLB value alone is not a reliable predictor of interactions between non-ionic emulsifiers and SC lipids. On the other hand, the molecular weight and structures may be the main factor of polysorbate emulsifiers to interact with skin lipids. Concerning these debatable factors, further research needs to be done for deeper understandings of possible mechanisms to describe how non-ionic emulsifiers penetrate the skin and interact with skin components.

Table 2. Chemical structures of PEG alkyl ethers and PEG sorbitan fatty acid esters.

PEG Alkyl Ethers	Chemical Structures	PEG Sorbitan Fatty Acid Esters	Chemical Structures
PEG-n oleyl ether	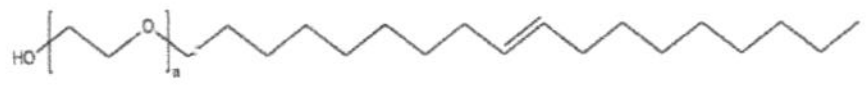	PEG-20 sorbitan monopalmitate (Polysorbate 40)	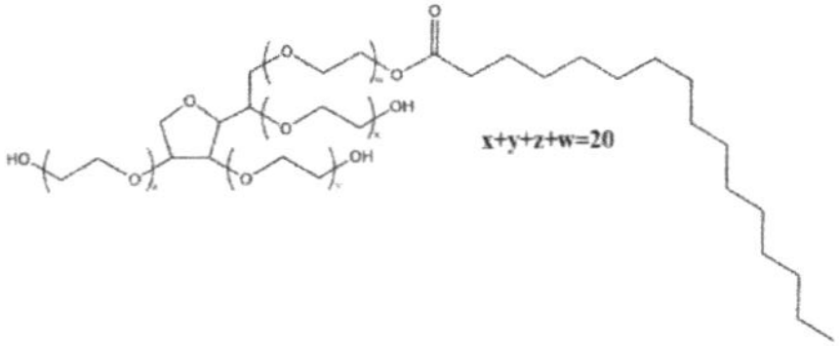
PEG-n stearyl ether	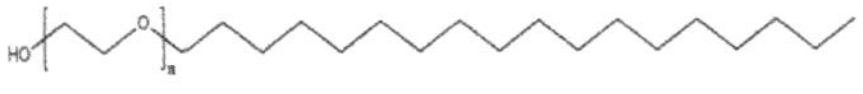	PEG-20 sorbitan monostearate (Polysorbate 60)	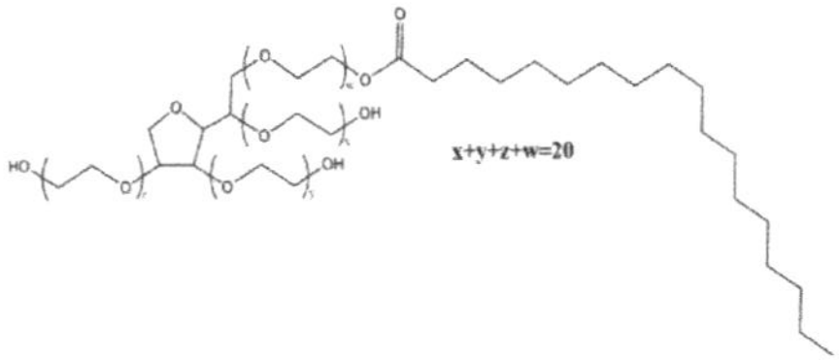
PEG-n cetyl ether	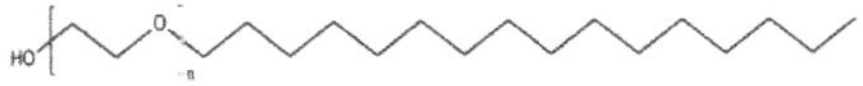	PEG-20 sorbitan monooleate (Polysorbate 80)	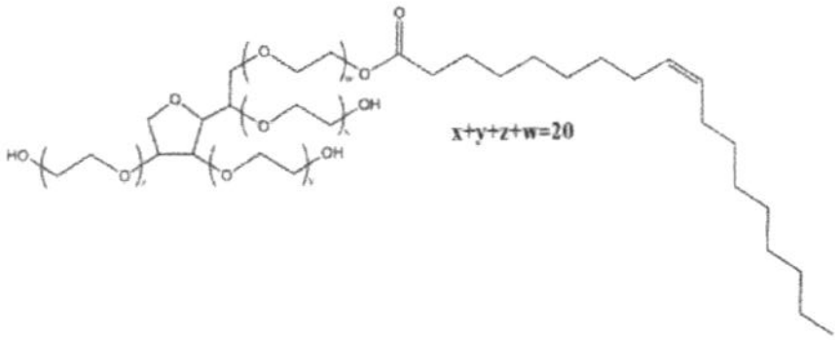

5. Conclusions

This study systematically examined the effects of non-ionic emulsifiers, including PEG alkyl ethers and PEG sorbitan fatty acid esters, on SC lipids. CRS was employed in this study as a non-invasive, efficient and versatile instrument. Different spectral signals of CRS in both fingerprint and HWN regions were applied to assess the alteration of lipid content, conformation, lateral packing order and SC thickness which caused by the interaction of non-ionic emulsifiers with SC. To sum up, it has been demonstrated that the results of conformation and lateral packing order analysis were basically correlated with the results of content analysis, indicating that the extraction of lipids from SC may disturb the lipid structures in SC, and to some extent weaken the skin structural integrity. Furthermore, our results so far implied that non-ionic emulsifiers of polysorbates as well as PEG ethers with a smaller number of oxyethylene groups would be better choices to incorporate into topical formulations due to their lower effects regarding extraction of lipids, interruption of lipid organizations and further damage of skin barrier functions.

Overall, based on these findings, the assessment of different lipid signals played a meaningful role to filtrate more effective spectral features for deeper differentiations. This research on non-ionic emulsifiers could also serve as a basis and be helpful to screen suitable emulsifiers for further formulation development.

Author Contributions: Conceptualization, Y.L. and D.J.L.; Data curation, Y.L.; Funding acquisition, Y.L. and D.J.L.; Investigation, Y.L.; Methodology, Y.L. and D.J.L.; Project administration, D.J.L.; Supervision D.J.L.; Writing—original draft, Y.L.; Writing—review & editing, D.J.L. All authors have read and agreed to the published version of the manuscript.

Funding: This project was supported by the European Social Fund and by the Ministry of Science, Research and the Arts Baden-Wuerttemberg and the China Scholarship Council. The University library of Tuebingen is thanked for covering part of the publication fee.

Acknowledgments: PD Martin Schenk is acknowledged for the donation of pig ears.

Conflicts of Interest: The authors declare no conflict of interest.

References

1. Bouwstra, J.A.; Gooris, G.S. The Lipid Organisation in Human Stratum Corneum and Model Systems. *Open Dermatol. J.* **2014**, *4*, 10–13. [CrossRef]
2. Bouwstra, J.A. The skin barrier in healthy and diseased state. *Biochim. Biophys. Acta-Biomembr.* **2006**, *1758*, 2080–2095. [CrossRef] [PubMed]
3. Weerheim, A.; Ponec, M. Determination of stratum corneum lipid profile by tape stripping in combination with high-performance thin-layer chromatography. *Arch. Dermatol. Res.* **2001**, *293*, 191–199. [CrossRef] [PubMed]
4. Caussin, J.; Gooris, G.S.; Janssens, M.; Bouwstra, J.A. Lipid organization in human and porcine stratum corneum differs widely, while lipid mixtures with porcine ceramides model human stratum corneum lipid organization very closely. *Biochim. Biophys. Acta-Biomembr.* **2008**, *1778*, 1472–1482. [CrossRef]
5. Warner, R.R.; Boissy, Y.L.; Lilly, N.A.; Spears, M.J.; McKillop, K.; Marshall, J.L.; Stone, K.J. Water disrupts stratum corneum lipid lamellae: Damage is similar to surfactants. *J. Investig. Dermatol.* **1999**, *113*, 960–966.
6. Van Smeden, J.; Janssens, M.; Boiten, W.A.; Van Drongelen, V.; Furio, L.; Vreeken, R.J.; Hovnanian, A.; Bouwstra, J.A. Intercellular Skin Barrier Lipid Composition and Organization in Netherton Syndrome Patients. *J. Investig. Dermatol.* **2014**, *134*, 1238–1245. [CrossRef]
7. Broere, F.; Gooris, G.; Schlotter, Y.M.; Rutten, V.P.M.G.; Bouwstra, J.A. Altered lipid properties of the stratum corneum in Canine Atopic Dermatitis. *Bba-Biomembr.* **2018**, *1860*, 526–533.
8. Kumar, G.P.; Rajeshwarrao, P. Nonionic surfactant vesicular systems for effective drug delivery—An overview. *Acta Pharm. Sin. B* **2011**, *1*, 208–219. [CrossRef]
9. Ghanbarzadeh, S.; Khorrami, A.; Arami, S. Nonionic surfactant-based vesicular system for transdermal drug delivery. *Drug Deliv.* **2015**, *22*, 1071–1077. [CrossRef]

10. Park, E.S.; Chang, S.Y.; Hahn, M.; Chi, S.C. Enhancing effect of polyoxyethylene alkyl ethers on the skin permeation of ibuprofen. *Int. J. Pharm.* **2000**, *209*, 109–119. [CrossRef]
11. Bárány, E.; Lindberg, M.; Lodén, M. Unexpected skin barrier influence from nonionic emulsifiers. *Int. J. Pharm.* **2000**, *195*, 189–195. [CrossRef]
12. Silva, S.M.C.; Hu, L.; Sousa, J.J.S.; Pais, A.A.C.C.; Michniak-Kohn, B.B. A combination of nonionic surfactants and iontophoresis to enhance the transdermal drug delivery of ondansetron HCl and diltiazem HCl. *Eur. J. Pharm. Biopharm.* **2012**, *80*, 663–673. [CrossRef] [PubMed]
13. Zhang, Z.; Lunter, D.J. Confocal Raman microspectroscopy as an alternative method to investigate the extraction of lipids from stratum corneum by emulsifiers and formulations. *Eur. J. Pharm. Biopharm.* **2018**, *127*, 61–71. [CrossRef] [PubMed]
14. Zhang, Z.; Lunter, D.J. Confocal Raman microspectroscopy as an alternative to differential scanning calorimetry to detect the impact of emulsifiers and formulations on stratum corneum lipid conformation. *Eur. J. Pharm. Sci.* **2018**, *121*, 1–8. [CrossRef] [PubMed]
15. Walters, K.A.; Walker, M.; Olejnik, O. Non-ionic Surfactant Effects on Hairless Mouse Skin Permeability Characteristics. *J. Pharm. Pharmacol.* **1988**, *40*, 525–529. [CrossRef]
16. Fiume, M.M.; Heldreth, B.; Bergfeld, W.F.; Belsito, D.V.; Hill, R.A.; Klaassen, C.D.; Liebler, D.; Marks, J.G.; Shank, R.C.; Slaga, T.J.; et al. Safety Assessment of Alkyl PEG Ethers as Used in Cosmetics. *Int. J. Toxicol.* **2012**, *31*, 169S–244S. [CrossRef]
17. Fruijtier-Pölloth, C. Safety assessment on polyethylene glycols (PEGs) and their derivatives as used in cosmetic products. *Toxicology* **2005**, *214*, 1–38. [CrossRef]
18. Chiappisi, L. Polyoxyethylene alkyl ether carboxylic acids: An overview of a neglected class of surfactants with multiresponsive properties. *Adv. Colloid Interface Sci.* **2017**, *250*, 79–94. [CrossRef]
19. Czamara, K.; Majzner, K.; Pacia, M.Z.; Kochan, K.; Kaczor, A.; Baranska, M. Raman spectroscopy of lipids: A review. *J. Raman Spectrosc.* **2015**, *46*, 4–20. [CrossRef]
20. Ali, S.M.; Bonnier, F.; Ptasinski, K.; Lambkin, H.; Flynn, K.; Lyng, F.M.; Byrne, H.J. Raman spectroscopic mapping for the analysis of solar radiation induced skin damage. *Analyst* **2013**, *138*, 3946–3956. [CrossRef]
21. Stamatas, G.N.; de Sterke, J.; Hauser, M.; von Stetten, O.; van der Pol, A. Lipid uptake and skin occlusion following topical application of oils on adult and infant skin. *J. Dermatol. Sci.* **2008**, *50*, 135–142. [CrossRef] [PubMed]
22. Van Smeden, J.; Janssens, M.; Kaye, E.C.J.; Caspers, P.J.; Lavrijsen, A.P.; Vreeken, R.J.; Bouwstra, J.A. The importance of free fatty acid chain length for the skin barrier function in atopic eczema patients. *Exp. Dermatol.* **2014**, *23*, 45–52. [CrossRef]
23. Ibrahim, S.A.; Li, S.K. Chemical enhancer solubility in human stratum corneum lipids and enhancer mechanism of action on stratum corneum lipid domain. *Int. J. Pharm.* **2010**, *383*, 89–98. [CrossRef] [PubMed]
24. Lunter, D.; Daniels, R. Confocal Raman microscopic investigation of the effectiveness of penetration enhancers for procaine delivery to the skin. *J. Biomed. Opt.* **2014**, *19*, 126015. [CrossRef] [PubMed]
25. Lunter, D.; Daniels, R. Measuring skin penetration by confocal Raman microscopy (CRM): Correlation to results from conventional experiments. In Proceedings of the Medical Imaging 2016: Biomedical Applications in Molecular, Structural, and Functional Imaging, San Diego, CA, USA, 1–3 March 2016; Volume 9788, p. 978829.
26. Choe, C.S.; Schleusener, J.; Lademann, J.; Darvin, M.E. Age related depth profiles of human Stratum Corneum barrier-related molecular parameters by confocal Raman microscopy in vivo. *Mech. Ageing Dev.* **2018**, *172*, 6–12. [CrossRef] [PubMed]
27. Pany, A.; Klang, V.; Peinhopf, C.; Zecevic, A.; Ruthofer, J.; Valenta, C. Hair removal and bioavailability of chemicals: Effect of physicochemical properties of drugs and surfactants on skin permeation ex vivo. *Int. J. Pharm.* **2019**, *567*, 118477. [CrossRef]
28. Vyumvuhore, R.; Tfayli, A.; Duplan, H.; Delalleau, A.; Manfait, M.; Baiilet-Guffroy, A. Effects of atmospheric relative humidity on Stratum Corneum structure at the molecular level: Ex vivo Raman spectroscopy analysis. *Analyst* **2013**, *138*, 4103–4111. [CrossRef]
29. Vyumvuhore, R.; Tfayli, A.; Duplan, H.; Delalleau, A.; Manfait, M.; Baillet-Guffroy, A. Raman spectroscopy: A tool for biomechanical characterization of Stratum Corneum. *J. Raman Spectrosc.* **2013**, *44*, 1077–1083. [CrossRef]

30. Tfayli, A.; Guillard, E.; Manfait, M.; Baillet-Guffroy, A. Raman spectroscopy: Feasibility of in vivo survey of stratum corneum lipids, effect of natural aging. *Eur. J. Dermatol.* **2012**, *22*, 36–41. [CrossRef]
31. Rygula, A.; Majzner, K.; Marzec, K.M.; Kaczor, A.; Pilarczyk, M.; Baranska, M. Raman spectroscopy of proteins: A review. *J. Raman Spectrosc.* **2013**, *44*, 1061–1076. [CrossRef]
32. Choe, C.S.; Lademann, J.; Darvin, M.E. Gaussian-function-based deconvolution method to determine the penetration ability of petrolatum oil into in vivo human skin using confocal Raman microscopy. *Laser Phys.* **2014**, *24*, 105601. [CrossRef]
33. Savić, S.; Weber, C.; Savić, M.M.; Müller-Goymann, C. Natural surfactant-based topical vehicles for two model drugs: Influence of different lipophilic excipients on in vitro/in vivo skin performance. *Int. J. Pharm.* **2009**, *381*, 220–230. [CrossRef] [PubMed]
34. Jacobi, U.; Kaiser, M.; Toll, R.; Mangelsdorf, S.; Audring, H.; Otberg, N.; Sterry, W.; Lademann, J. Porcine ear skin: An in vitro model for human skin. *Ski. Res. Technol.* **2007**, *13*, 19–24. [CrossRef] [PubMed]
35. Tfaili, S.; Gobinet, C.; Josse, G.; Angiboust, J.F.; Manfait, M.; Piot, O. Confocal Raman microspectroscopy for skin characterization: A comparative study between human skin and pig skin. *Analyst* **2012**, *137*, 3673–3682. [CrossRef] [PubMed]
36. Kligman, A.M. Preparation of Isolated Sheets of Human Stratum Corneum. *Arch. Dermatol.* **2011**, *88*, 702. [CrossRef] [PubMed]
37. Van Smeden, J.; Janssens, M.; Gooris, G.S.; Bouwstra, J.A. The important role of stratum corneum lipids for the cutaneous barrier function. *Biochim. Biophys. Acta-Mol. Cell Biol. Lipids* **2014**, *1841*, 295–313. [CrossRef]
38. Bridges, T.E.; Houlne, M.P.; Harris, J.M. Spatially Resolved Analysis of Small Particles by Confocal Raman Microscopy: Depth Profiling and Optical Trapping. *Anal. Chem.* **2004**, *76*, 576–584. [CrossRef]
39. Hathout, R.M.; Mansour, S.; Mortada, N.D.; Geneidi, A.S.; Guy, R.H. Uptake of microemulsion components into the stratum corneum and their molecular effects on skin barrier function. *Mol. Pharm.* **2010**, *7*, 1266–1273. [CrossRef]
40. Hoppel, M.; Baurecht, D.; Holper, E.; Mahrhauser, D.; Valenta, C. Validation of the combined ATR-FTIR/tape stripping technique for monitoring the distribution of surfactants in the stratum corneum. *Int. J. Pharm.* **2014**, *472*, 88–93. [CrossRef]
41. Choe, C.; Lademann, J.; Darvin, M.E. A depth-dependent profile of the lipid conformation and lateral packing order of the stratum corneum in vivo measured using Raman microscopy. *Analyst* **2016**, *141*, 1981–1987. [CrossRef]
42. Williams, A.C.; Edwards, H.G.M.; Barry, B.W. Raman spectra of human keratotic biopolymers: Skin, callus, hair and nail. *J. Raman Spectrosc.* **1994**, *25*, 95–98. [CrossRef]
43. Snyder, R.G.; Hsu, S.L.; Krimm, S. Vibrational spectra in the CH stretching region and the structure of the polymethylene chain. *Spectrochim. Acta Part A Mol. Spectrosc.* **1978**, *34*, 395–406. [CrossRef]
44. Tfayli, A.; Guillard, E.; Manfait, M.; Baillet-Guffroy, A. Thermal dependence of Raman descriptors of ceramides. Part I: Effect of double bonds in hydrocarbon chains. *Anal. Bioanal. Chem.* **2010**, *397*, 1281–1296. [CrossRef] [PubMed]
45. Schwarz, J.C.; Klang, V.; Hoppel, M.; Mahrhauser, D.; Valenta, C. Natural microemulsions: Formulation design and skin interaction. *Eur. J. Pharm. Biopharm.* **2012**, *81*, 557–562. [CrossRef]
46. Wallach, D.F.H.; Verma, S.P.; Jeffrey, F. Application of laser Raman and infrared spectroscopy to the analysis of membrane structure. *Biochim. Biophys. Acta-Rev. Biomembr.* **1978**, *559*, 153–208. [CrossRef]
47. Choe, C.; Lademann, J.; Darvin, M.E. Analysis of Human and Porcine Skin in vivo/ex vivo for Penetration of Selected Oils by Confocal Raman Microscopy. *Ski. Pharmacol. Physiol.* **2015**, *28*, 318–330. [CrossRef]
48. Choe, C.; Lademann, J.; Darvin, M.E. Confocal Raman microscopy for investigating the penetration of various oils into the human skin in vivo. *J. Dermatol. Sci.* **2015**, *79*, 176–178. [CrossRef]
49. Vater, C.; Adamovic, A.; Ruttensteiner, L.; Steiner, K.; Tajpara, P.; Klang, V.; Elbe-Bürger, A.; Wirth, M.; Valenta, C. Cytotoxicity of lecithin-based nanoemulsions on human skin cells and ex vivo skin permeation: Comparison to conventional surfactant types. *Int. J. Pharm.* **2019**, *566*, 383–390. [CrossRef]

pharmaceutics

MDPI

Article

Mucoadhesive Budesonide Formulation for the Treatment of Eosinophilic Esophagitis

Antonella Casiraghi [1,*], Chiara Grazia Gennari [1], Umberto Maria Musazzi [1], Marco Aldo Ortenzi [2,3], Susanna Bordignon [4] and Paola Minghetti [1]

1 Department of Pharmaceutical Sciences, Università degli Studi di Milano, Via G. Colombo 71-20133 Milan, Italy; chiara.gennari@unimi.it (C.G.G.); umberto.musazzi@unimi.it (U.M.M.); paola.minghetti@unimi.it (P.M.)

2 CRC Materiali Polimerici (LaMPo), Department of Chemistry, Università degli Studi di Milano, Via Golgi 19-20133 Milan, Italy; marco.ortenzi@unimi.it

3 Department of Chemistry, Università degli Studi di Milano, Via Golgi 19-20133 Milan, Italy

4 Student of Specialization School in Pharmacy, Department of Pharmaceutical Sciences, Università degli Studi di Milano, Via G. Colombo 71-20133 Milan, Italy; susanna.bordignon@gmail.com

* Correspondence: antonella.casiraghi@unimi.it

Received: 20 December 2019; Accepted: 23 February 2020; Published: 1 March 2020

Abstract: Eosinophilic esophagitis (EE) is a chronic immune/antigen-mediated esophageal inflammatory disease for which off-label topical corticosteroids (e.g., budesonide) are widely used in clinic. In general, thickening excipients are mixed with industrial products to improve the residence time of the drug on the esophageal mucosa. The compounding procedures are empirical and the composition is not supported by real physicochemical and technological characterization. The current study aimed to propose a standardized budesonide oral formulation intended to improve the resistance time of the drug on the esophageal mucosa for EE treatment. Different placebo and drug-loaded (0.025% *w/w*) formulations were prepared by changing the percentage of xanthan gum alone or in ratio 1:1 with guar gum. Both excipients were added in the composition for their mucoadhesive properties. The formulative space was rationalized based on the drug physicochemical stability and the main critical quality attributes of the formulation, e.g., rheological properties, syringeability, mucoadhesiveness and in vitro penetration of budesonide in porcine esophageal tissue. The obtained results demonstrated that gums allowed a prolonged residence time. However, the concentration of the mucoadhesive polymer has to be rationalized appropriately to permit the syringeability of the formulation and, therefore, easy dosing by the patient/caregiver.

Keywords: eosinophilic esophagitis; budesonide; xanthan gum; guar gum; mucoadhesion; esophagus permeability; rheological characterization; pediatric medicine; compounded preparation

1. Introduction

Eosinophilic esophagitis (EE) is a chronic immune/antigen-mediated esophageal inflammatory disease associated with esophageal dysfunction resulting from severe eosinophil-predominant inflammation [1,2]. EE treatment is mainly based on dietary and pharmacological interventions. The diet of patients having EE is a highly restricted regimen based on the elimination of specific allergen components for a limited number of weeks. Removal of harmful food allergens results in clinical remission of EE. After the elimination period, foods can be reintroduced in the diet sequentially in order to identify food triggers of esophageal eosinophilia and to establish a less restrictive, long-term, therapeutic diet for the effective disease management [3]. Elemental formulas and other types of elimination diets are safe and efficacious approaches for EE treatment [4], but the severe restrictions markedly reduce patient compliance [5]. The main drawbacks are the scant palatability of the highly restricted diet regimen, the marked weight loss and the high costs for the patient [6]. Therefore, pharmacological treatments are often necessary. First line therapy is based on oral proton pump inhibitors (PPIs) [7], which are effective, safe and not so expensive for the patients. If the patient does not respond to PPIs, corticosteroids are useful alternative therapeutics, since they can inhibit maturation and activation of eosinophils through suppression of the release of their stimulating cytokines. Inhaled budesonide (BU) and fluticasone are the most investigated drugs of this class [8–10]. However, the benefit-risk balance of such medicinal products may be affected by significant secondary side effects due to systemic drug absorption after pulmonary administration. It may also be affected by a low patient adherence, due to the complexity of the administration devices (e.g., metered-dose inhaler). Therefore, the interest in developing topically applied therapeutics is increasing [11,12]. In this context, off-label topical corticosteroids are frequently used in clinic: patients are trained to swallow asthma medicinal products designed initially to be inhaled or viscous oral formulations extemporaneously compounded in pharmacies. Recently, European regulatory authorities have authorized an orodispersible tablet loaded with BU indicated for the treatment of EE in adults older than 18 years of age. This medicinal product is not suitable for pediatric patients since they require adjustments in strength and dosage form in comparison to adults [13–15].

When an authorized medicinal product is not available on the market, the compounding of extemporaneous preparations by the community and hospital pharmacists is crucial to meet the special needs of patients [16,17]. The compounding activities should be based on the provisions of the Good Compounding Practice and other available technical guidelines to assure the required quality of the magistral preparation [18].

In the case of the BU for EE, a certain number of studies in the literature suggested the clinical efficacy of viscous preparations. Frequently, they have been prepared by mixing a commercial sterile suspension of BU to be nebulized, which is indicated in the treatment of bronchial asthma and in infants and children with croup, with a thickening agent (e.g., sucralose) [19–21]. Alternatively, cellulose derivatives [22] or gums [23,24] have also been added. Hefner et al. [25] compared the technological performances of different types of thickening agents like sucralose, xanthan gum or honey, demonstrating that the gum permitted a better residence time of the active pharmaceutical ingredients (API) on the esophageal mucosa. However, such pieces of evidence have been obtained using a medicinal product as an API source instead of the API. Although such an approach seems practical to meet patient's needs, the use of a medicinal product can determine the presence of unnecessary excipients in the final preparation and can cause problems of physical compatibility to arise with all the adopted substances. Moreover, the exact quantitative composition of the medicinal product is generally unknown. In this light, it is preferable that compounding starts from the raw materials (pure active principle and excipients). Alternatively, a proprietary excipient mixture can be used as a formulation base (e.g., Mucolox™) [26].

The development of standardized formulations can be a valid strategy to support pharmacists in their activities, reducing heterogenicity and uncertainty in compounding procedures, improving the quality of the final preparation, at the same time. Indeed, the availability of well set up and validated operating procedures is instrumental in assuring the quality of the magistral preparation.

The aim of this work is to propose a standardized BU oral formulation to improve the residence time of the drug on the esophageal mucosa. Starting from a formulation already in use in hospital pharmacies, based on xanthan gum, six pharmacists were enrolled in the compounding process to verify its reproducibility. On the bases of these results, the formulation and the compounding procedures were optimized. Considering the evidence, reported in the literature, on the combined use with galactomannans, guar gum was selected to compare its performances, when in ratio 1:1, as opposed to xanthan gum alone. The formulative space was rationalized based on the drug's physicochemical stability and the main critical quality attributes of the formulation, such as rheological properties, mucoadhesiveness and in vitro penetration of BU in porcine esophageal tissue.

2. Materials and Methods

2.1. Materials

Micronized Budesonide (BU) was obtained from Farmabios, Gropello Cairoli, PV, Italy. Guar Gum (GG, viscosity min 5000 mPas) was kindly gifted by Lamberti spa, Albizzate, VA, Italy. All other materials were obtained from the named supplier: Xanthan Gum (XG, viscosity more than 1200 mPas), (ethylenedinitrilo)tetraacetic acid disodium salt dihydrate (EDTA), sodium benzoate, sodium saccharin (Farmalabor, Canosa di Puglia, BAT, Italy), glycerin, sodium dihydrogen phosphate, orthophosphoric acid, ethanol chemical grade (VWR International, Milan, Italy).

Acetonitrile was HPLC-gradient grade. Purified water was obtained from the purification system Milli-Q, according to Ph. Eur. 10.0 ed.

2.2. Preparation of Oral Formulations

The exact amount of glycerin (23.6 mL) was weighed on an analytical balance and poured into a beaker. Sodium saccharin, EDTA and sodium benzoate were crushed to a fine powder with mortar and pestle, then, the exact amount of each was weighted and the powders were transferred into the same beaker. Then, XG or the mixture of gums (XG:GG) 1/1 *w/w* was added. All substances were mixed to form a homogeneous mixture, then, the exact weighted amount of BU (1 mg/4 mL) was added and carefully mixed. Purified water was weighed and added, then stirred until a uniform system was obtained. Different percentages of gums were used: F1P was prepared using XG 2% *w/w*, F2P with XG:GG 2% *w/w*, F3P with XG 1.5% *w/w* and F4P with XG:GG 1.5% *w/w*. Placebo formulations were prepared for rheological and technological evaluation. BU was added only to obtain final loaded formulations F1, F2 and F4. The composition of the formulations is reported in Table 1.

Table 1. Composition (expressed in grams) of the formulations for 240 mL (four doses each of 60 mL).

Excipients	F1P	F1	F2P	F2	F3P	F4P	F4
Budesonide (BU)	-	0.06	-	0.06	-	-	0.06
Xanthan gum (XG)	4.80	4.80	2.40	2.40	3.60	1.80	1.80
Guar gum (GG)	-	-	2.40	2.40	-	1.80	1.80
Sodium saccharin	0.24	0.24	0.24	0.24	0.24	0.24	0.24
Glycerin	29.74	29.74	29.74	29.74	29.74	29.74	29.74
EDTA	0.24	0.24	0.24	0.24	0.24	0.24	0.24
Sodium benzoate	0.45	0.45	0.45	0.45	0.45	0.45	0.45
Water up to (mL)	240	240	240	240	240	240	240

2.3. Measurements of pH Values of the Formulations

The pH was measured at time $T = 0$, using a pHmeter CyberScan 1100 (Eutech Instruments/Thermo Fisher Scientific, Waltham, MA, USA).

2.4. Drug Content

About two grams of each formulation were exactly weighed and transferred into a 10 mL amber glass volumetric flask, bringing up to volume with ethanol. Then, the flask was placed in an ultrasound bath for 20 min. The sample was then centrifuged for 5 min at 3500 rpm. A portion of the supernatant was diluted to 2:5 with the mobile phase composed of phosphate buffer pH 3.2:acetonitrile:ethanol (68:30:2 *v/v/v*) and analyzed [23]. The remaining supernatant was completely and accurately removed and 10 mL of fresh ethanol were added to repeat the same extraction procedure. For each preparation, extraction was performed twice.

2.5. Stability Study

Samples of F1 were stored in an incubator (INCU-Line, VWR International, Milan, Italy) at 40 °C. The drug content was measured at time T = 0, T = 10, 20, 60 days. Evaluation of BU content was also performed after T = 30 days at room temperature exposed to light.

2.6. Determination of Rheological Properties

The steady and dynamic shear rheological properties of the formulations were carried out using a controlled stress/strain rheometer Anton Paar MCR 302 (Anton Paar GmbH, Graz, Austria) equipped with a plate-plate geometry (25 mm diameter and 500 μm gap). The temperature was controlled by a Peltier system on the bottom plate. Each sample was transferred to the rheometer plate and was then equilibrated at 25 °C for 5 min before steady and dynamic shear rheological measurements were taken.

2.6.1. Steady Shear Measurements

Flow behavior was evaluated at controlled strain mode to obtain flow rheological data (shear stress and shear rate) over a shear rate range of 0.1–100 s^{-1} at 25 °C. The shear stress-shear rate data were fitted to the well-known power law and Casson models [27] to describe the flow properties of the samples.

2.6.2. Dynamic Shear Measurements

Dynamic rheological data were obtained from frequency sweeps over the range of 0.628–62.8 rad s^{-1} at 2% strain using a small-amplitude oscillatory rheological measurement. The applied 2% strain was confirmed within the linear viscoelastic region by strain sweep measurement. Frequency sweep tests were also performed at 25 °C. The RheoCompass software (Anton Paar GmbH, Graz, Austria) was used to obtain the experimental data and to calculate the storage (or elastic) modulus (G′), loss (or viscous) modulus (G″) and loss factor (tan δ = G″/G′).

2.7. Quantitative Determination of Syringeability

The measurement of the injection force was performed in compression mode by using a software-controlled texture analyzer (Instron 5965, ITW Test and Measurement Italia S.r.l., Trezzano sul Naviglio, Italy). A 10 mL syringe (SOFT-JECT®, VWR International, Milan, Italy) filled with 9 mL formulation was positioned in the dynamometer holder, downward needle. The plunger end of the syringe was placed in contact with a 50 N loading cell. Testing was carried out at the crosshead speed of 0.5 mm/s. The loading force required to displace the plunger was measured as a function of plunger displacement. The following parameters were also determined from the force-displacement plot:

- Plunger-stopper break loose force (or "initial glide force," PBF): the force required to initiate the movement of the plunger;
- Maximum force (MF): the highest force measured before the plunger finishes its course at the front end of the syringe;
- Dynamic glide force (DGF): the force required to sustain the movement of the plunger to expel the content of the syringe.

A schematic representation of the syringeability test setting and a general force-displacement plot are illustrated in Figure 1. The registered force values were normalized by dividing them for the cross-sectional area of the cylindrical plunger. The experiments were performed in triplicate.

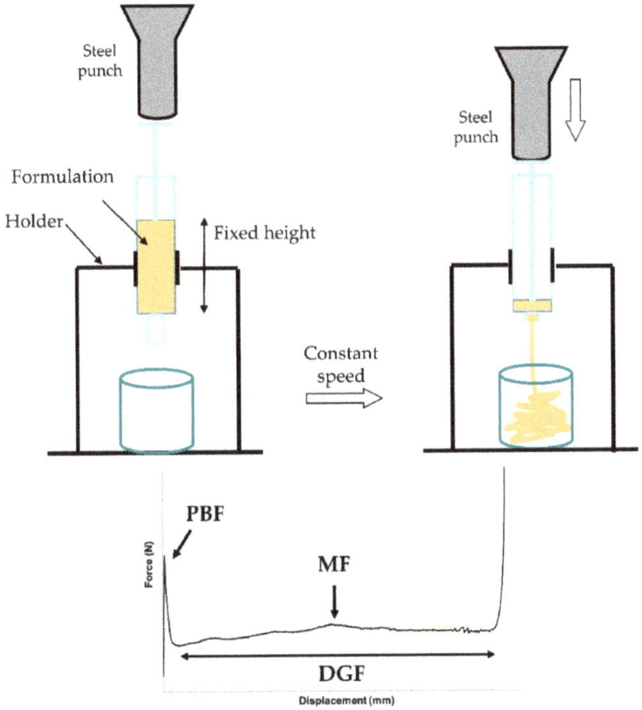

Figure 1. Syringeability test setting and a general force versus displacement curve (PBF: plunger-stopper break loose force; MF: Maximum force; DGF: Dynamic glide force).

2.8. Mucoadhesive Properties and In Vitro Esophagus Penetration

The in vitro mucosal penetration study was performed adapting the flow-through test described by Cilurzo et al. [28] by using fresh porcine esophageal tissue obtained by a local slaughterhouse. The mucosa epithelium was separated by mucosal specimens using a scalpel.

In-house equipment of three components was built up (Figure 2): (a) in series mucosa supports set at an angle of 45°, (b) peristaltic pump and (c) collector of fractions. The apparatus was designed to investigate at the same time the elution of the preparation from the mucosal surface and the drug penetration into the tissue.

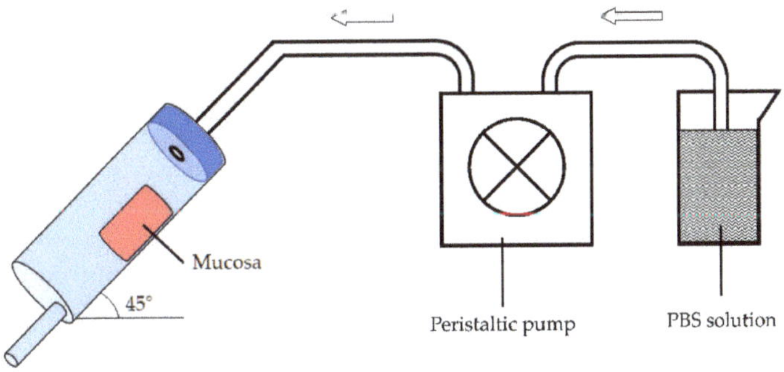

Figure 2. Apparatus used to evaluate mucoadhesive properties and mucosal penetration in vitro.

A dose of the selected formulation was deposited onto a 3 × 2 cm mucosal surface corresponding to a total amount of about 500 mg. Then, the porcine esophageal membrane was placed on the sample support and pH 6.8 phosphate buffer solution (PBS) was dropped at a rate of 1 mL/min to simulate the physiological environment and the saliva swallowing. The test was performed at room temperature.

The residence time was qualitatively estimated by checking the time required for each formulation to be thoroughly washed away from the surface of the mucosa exposed to the washing medium. In all cases, after 30 min from the beginning of the experiment, the apparatus was dismantled, and the applied test sample was peeled away using an adhesive tape strip [28]. The mucosa samples were then washed from both sides with 5 mL of purified water and homogenized. The amount of the penetrated drug was extracted with 2 mL methanol and assayed by HPLC.

2.9. *Drug Content Analysis*

The analysis was carried out by HPLC-DAD (Agilent 1100, Agilent, Santa Clara, CA, USA) using an RP-C18 column (LC 150 × 4.6 mm, 5 µm) with pre-column (Phenomenex, Torrance, CA, USA). The mobile phase was composed of phosphate buffer pH 3.2:acetonitrile:ethanol [29]. The elution was carried out in gradient (Table 2). The flow rate was 1.7 mL/min, the wavelength was set at 240 nm and the injection volume at 10 µl. The retention times of the 22R and 22S epimers were 8.8 min and 9.1 min, respectively. A calibration curve was prepared twice solubilizing in ethanol 10 mg of BU in a 100 mL volumetric flask. Dilution to obtain 0.1, 0.2, 0.5, 1 and 2 µg/mL concentration were performed (22R: R^2 = 0.99930; 22S: R^2 = 0.99999).

Table 2. The gradient of the mobile phase.

Time (min)	Phosphate Buffer pH 3.2 (% *v/v*)	Acetonitrile (% *v/v*)	Ethanol (% *v/v*)
0–10	68→50	30→48	2
10–11	50	48	2
11–16	50→68	48→30	2

2.10. *Statistical Analysis*

Tests for significant differences between means were performed by the one-way ANOVA followed by Turkey-Kramer post-analyses. Differences were considered significant at the $p < 0.05$ level.

3. Results and Discussion

As the number of patients suffering from EE is increasing, among both adults and young population, the need to have a standardized topical dosage form has grown. Moreover, the widespread habit of mixing the industrial inhalation product with sweeteners (among them is largely used an artificial sweetener based on sucralose in maltodextrin/glucose) should not be the first choice. Instead, the use of a viscous preparation as a vehicle is well established in improving the efficacy of topical corticosteroid administration. The proprietary blend Mucolox™ gave good results [26], but it is composed of a very complex blend. For these reasons, other simpler compositions, already in use in hospital pharmacies, deserve to be investigated. Quite diffused is the use of viscous formulation containing XG as a thickening and rheological agent (F1P and F1, Table 1).

XG is a polysaccharide, largely applied in the food industry. It is highly stable in a wide range of pH and ionic strength, and, dispersed in water at moderate temperatures, it increases its viscosity even at low concentration [30,31]. Temperature preparation can modify the ordered or disordered state of xanthan chains, as this state is controlled by temperature.

According to the already in use hospital preparation (F1, Table 1), six pharmacists were enrolled and each of them compounded a batch. At the end of the preparation process, performed at room temperature, BU was completely dispersed, and the gel-like liquid appeared homogeneous. Dispersion is due to the low BU solubility in water [32]; good improvement of solubilization could be obtained using mixtures with ethanol, but this approach must be discarded in the pediatric population for limitations in the use of this excipient [33]. The use of glycerin, usually foreseen in mixture with rheological agents, can contribute in improving BU solubility, but this is not enough to obtain its complete solubilization. The measured pH and drug content are reported in Table 3. pH values were close to 5 and no significant changes in pH were observed during the storage period. To exactly measure the drug content, the extraction procedure reported in the literature [23] was performed twice, as a too high amount of BU remained not extracted after a single exposure to solvent. Variability among operators was low (CV% = 2.7) and immediately after preparation, the mean content was within the range of acceptability, fixed in ±10% *w/w*, according to the Italian Pharmacopoeia (Table 3). The chemical stability study showed that the preparation has good stability, as evidenced by the accelerated stability study (storage for over 60 days in an incubator at 40 °C; Table 3) and confirmed the need to avoid the exposure to light for long period when the preparation is handled by caregivers or patients. Indeed, preparations left at room temperature for over 30 days at the light showed a reduction of more than 50% in strength (Table 3). The addition of sodium benzoate allows to avoid microbiological contamination [23].

Table 3. Chemical characterization of the in-use preparation in the hospital pharmacy (F1: XG 2%). pH values and drug content at preparation time (T = 0) and at the end of the storage period in an incubator in dark condition (T = 60 days). Drug content determined after 30 days at room temperature (r.t.) exposed at the light.

Batch	**pH**		**Micronized Budesonide Content (mg/mL, *n* = 6)**		
	T = 0	**60 days**	**T = 0**	**60 days, 40 °C, dark**	**30 days, r.t., light**
F1	4.629 ± 0.020	4.814 ± 0.115	0.262 ± 0.007	0.246 ± 0.018	0.103 ± 0.022

To test the technological properties of these systems, their adhesion on the site of action (i.e., esophageal tissue) or the handling during the application, F1P was modified and a mixture of XG and GG was used (F2P, Table 1). The addition of galactomannans such as locust bean gum or GG to a solution of XG at room temperature causes a synergistic increase in viscosity, both at dilute and concentrated solution [27]. GG is a galactomannan that forms colloidal solutions with elevated viscosity even at very low concentrations. It is anionic in nature and it remains stable and gives consistent viscosity over a wide pH range [34]. The viscosity of XG:GG mixtures depends on operational properties such as the dissolution temperature of gums, polymer concentration and relationship between XG and galactomannan. Indeed, with the polymer concentration and the ratio between the gums being fixed, in case of extemporaneous preparation, attention must be paid to the temperature at which each polysaccharide has been solved [35].

Rheological characterization was performed on the placebo samples based on XG (F1P and F3P) and XG:GG (F2P and F4P), mixed at room temperature. They have different behaviors: formulations containing the mixture of the gums have higher shear stress in comparison to those containing only XG, as already reported in the literature [35], but the shear sensitivity is different. As shown in Figure 3, XG samples have a linear stress-strain dependence, whereas XG:GG samples have a pseudoplastic behavior, with the stress vs. strain lowering at higher shear rates. When reaching the highest shear rates, XG:GG 1.5% (F4P) starts having lower stress than XG 2% (F1P). Given the slope of the curves (i.e., pseudoplastic vs. linear dependence), the behavior is expected to be confirmed at shear rates higher than 100 s^{-1}, which is the highest that can be reached with the experimental setup used. In addition, samples loaded with the active principle were investigated and it was concluded that the behavior was not influenced by the presence of BU (F1 and F4, Table 4). The pseudo-plastic behavior of XG:GG samples indicates that physicochemical properties of such formulations are similar to the ones of linear polymers, i.e., the effect of ionic interactions or other weak bonds (such as hydrogen or van der Waals bonds) creating branching and reversible crosslinking between the macromolecular chains of the gums and other ingredients of the formulations is negligible. This behavior is in agreement with the one previously observed by Jo et al. on gum mixtures [27]. The same authors evidenced a pseudoplastic behavior also for the single gums in water solution. In our work, the presence of glycerin, adding a lot of –OH groups in the formulation, seems to increase the formation of entanglements and weak bonds in the formulation of XG alone, within the shear range tested. Table 4 also shows the difference in viscosity of the samples at the highest shear rates, confirming that the XG:GG sample viscosity has a far less marked increase than that of XG samples in the 50–100 s^{-1} range. This trend is due to the pseudoplastic behavior of XG:GG samples.

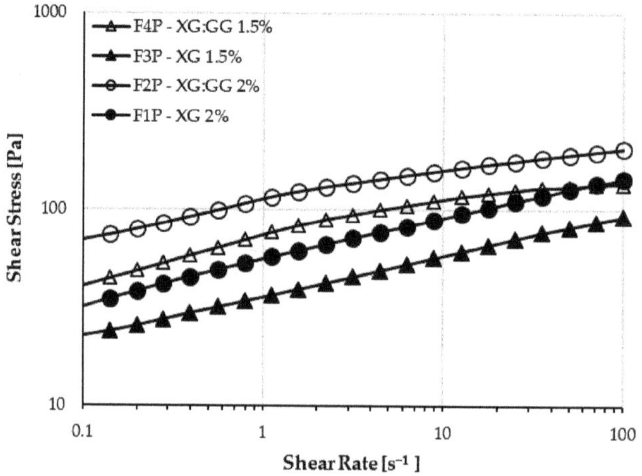

Figure 3. Plots of shear stresses versus shear rates of XG and XG:GG mixtures.

Table 4. Viscosity values and injection force measurements of each formulation.

Form.	Viscosity (Pa*s)			Δη 100 vs. 50 s^{-1} (%)	Loss factor °	Injection force		
	50.1 (s^{-1})	70.8 (s^{-1})	100 (s^{-1})			DGF (kPa)	MF (kPa)	PBF (kPa)
F1P	128.15	136.12	144.25	12.6	0.157 ± 0.015	90.01 ± 31.16	77.87 ± 14.50	66.25 ± 5.24
F1	127.22	135.75	144.83	13.8	0.160 ± 0.016	-*	-*	-*
F2P	190.48	197.68	204.46	7.3	0.190 ± 0.040	83.28 ± 8.68	87.08 ± 7.30	58.57 ± 14.13
F3P	81.57	87.09	92.42	13.3	0.171 ± 0.018	78.08 ± 24.23	85.00 ± 29.67	63.11 ± 19.28
F4P	130.67	134.89	135.60	3.8	0.231 ± 0.045	121.69 ± 14.75	126.39 ± 14.78	89.49 ± 27.24
F4	126.77	128.5	130.02	2.6	0.242 ± 0.047	-*	-*	-*

Note: ° average ratio and standard deviation of G″/G′ over the whole curve; * value not determined.

A different behavior among the formulations was also evidenced from the performed dynamic shear measurements. In particular, as shown in Figure 4, a markedly different trend in loss modulus is visible. In XG:GG samples, the G″ has only slight variations over the angular frequency range used, whereas in XG samples, it markedly increases as the frequency gets higher, especially at the highest frequencies.

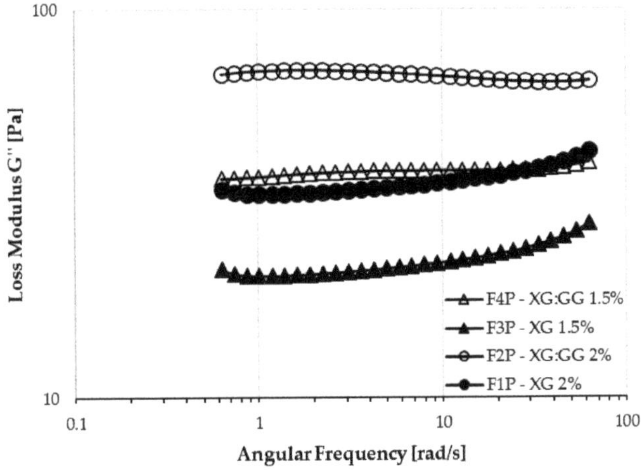

Figure 4. Plots of log ω versus log G″ of XG and XG:GG mixtures.

To identify elastic or viscous behavior, loss factor values can be calculated. When this value is smaller than the unit, a sample is more elastic than viscous, and this has been suggested as a rheological criterion for safe-swallow foods meant for dysphagia [36]. All proposed formulations had low loss factor values (Table 4). Moreover, while loss factor values for F1P, F2P and F3P were similar, F4P had a loss factor significantly higher than all the other samples ($p < 0.0001$).

The administration of this preparation in very young patients was performed by caregivers, normally the parents, by means of a big syringe containing 60 mL of the formulation. During this treatment, some difficulties due to the hard extrusion of the formulation from the syringe were described by the users. The values measured for the injection force measured for placebo formulations are reported in Table 4.

In the force vs. displacement plot of low-viscosity formulations (Figure 1), two different portions can be identified: the former is related to the force required to displace the plunger, (i.e., PBF). This event is followed by a plateau (second portion), indicating that the streamline of the formulation through the needle occurs with a constant force. In this portion, the average load required to sustain the movement of the plunger to expel the content of the syringe is calculated and reported as DGF.

PBF values were not statistically different among the tested products ($p = 0.3890$), suggesting that the force required to initiate the movement of the plunger was independent from the formulation.

The measured extrusion forces showed that F4P required a slightly higher extrusion force (in terms of DGF) with respect to the other formulations, even if the differences were not statistically significant ($p = 0.1565$). Moreover, in the shear stress plots, F4P showed also a pseudoplastic behavior that could not be detected with the syringeability test, probably because the applied force felt below the useful range of stress. In the case of this pseudoplastic formulation, taking into consideration the loss factor value, another rheological parameter, we can observe that it was higher if compared to the other formulations, suggesting that F4P has a more pronounced viscous component, even if its overall behavior was mainly elastic. However, overall results show that in any case low forces are needed to extrude the formulations from a syringe, despite the differences highlighted in the rheological studies.

The chemical and technological effects of the combination of the two gums in the revised formulations are reported in Table 5. Formulation F3 was considered of minor interest because of the lower shear stress and therefore it was not further investigated. Placebo formulations showed pH values from 4.975 (F2P) to 5.155 (F4P). As in the case of F1, the addition of BU did not change these values (Table 5). The formulations can be expected to be non-irritating to the buccal mucosa since the pH of the esophageal mucosa is reported to be 6.8 in healthy subjects [37].

Table 5. Chemical and technological characterization of the modified preparation.

Batch	pH T = 0	Permanence Time (min)	BU Penetrated the Mucosa	
			(mg/g mucosa)	(%)
F1	4.976	28 ± 4	0.790 ± 0.192	0.610 ± 0.132
F2	5.156	29 ± 2	0.783 ± 0.231	0.562 ± 0.152
F4	5.068	25 ± 5	0.901 ± 0.367	0.682 ± 0.270

As far as the mucoadhesive properties are concerned, comparing the formulations, a similar sliding time from the mucosa samples was observed for all of them. Thanks to the establishment of interactions between the mucosal layer and the bioadhesive polymer, it was possible to obtain formulations able to persist onto the mucosal surface for about 30 min.

The good mucoadhesive properties can be due to the presence of free $-COO^-$ groups of XG. As a matter of fact, it is well known that polymers that exhibit a high density of available hydrogen bonding groups ($-COO^-$ groups of XG) can interact more strongly with mucin glycoprotein [38]. Moreover, hydrogen bonds are involved in the formation of a strengthened network, thus contributing to the good bioadhesive strength of the tested formulations. The permanence time onto the mucosa samples was not influenced by the presence of the drugs into the formulations. Because of the similar residence time, the percentages of BU that penetrated the mucosa by the different formulations were not significantly different (Table 3). A very small percentage of BU loaded remained in the mucosae; therefore, to optimize the use of the corticosteroid, further evaluations could be done with formulations containing a reduced amount of the active principle with respect to that used in the present work.

As it is known, penetration of BU into the mucosa is the final combination of many events; the physicochemical characteristics of the molecule, and the mucoadhesive properties and viscosity of the formulation. The advantage of increased viscosity of the formulation is a reduced outflow from the mucosal surface, with a consequent increase in the contact time of the drug with the mucous membrane, and therefore, in its penetration into the tissue. On the other hand, an excessive viscosity could obviously create problems in the extrusion from a syringe. The results showed that the use of the two gums in combination can help to modulate the viscosity of the formulation, however, remaining within an optimal range such as to be retained onto the mucosal surface for enough time. Moreover, thanks to its pseudoplastic behavior, the extrusion of such formulations through a syringe can take place in a feasible way. Unfortunately, this aspect could not be fully investigated through the experiments carried out in this work, since the viscosity data should be collected in a higher shear range to highlight a correlation between syringeability test and viscosity measurements.

4. Conclusions

The prepared formulations showed suitable technological and rheological characteristics for the treatment of EE. As the addition of GG to XG caused an increase in viscosity, the choice of a mixture of gums allows the use of thickening agents in a reduced amount. In this case, the obtained results were not significantly different from those measured with the formulation already in use. Considering the limited percentage of BU absorbed in the in vitro penetration experiments, further evaluations should be carried out to rationalize the drug content and reduce the risk of systemic side effects.

Author Contributions: Individual contributions in this research article was as follows: conceptualization and writing—original draft preparation, A.C.; writing—original draft preparation, C.G.G. and M.A.O.; writing—review and editing, U.M.M.; formal analysis and data curation, S.B.; supervision, P.M. All authors have read and agreed to the published version of the manuscript.

Funding: This research received no external funding.

Conflicts of Interest: The authors declare no conflict of interest.

References

1. Papadopoulou, A.; Koletzko, S.; Heuschkel, R.; Dias, J.A.; Allen, K.J.; Murch, S.H.; Chong, S.; Gottrand, F.; Husby, S.; Lionetti, P.; et al. Management guidelines of eosinophilic esophagitis in childhood. *J. Pediatric Gastroenterol. Nutr.* **2014**, *58*, 107–114. [CrossRef]
2. Lucendo, A.J.; Molina-Infante, J.; Arias, Á.; von Arnim, U.; Bredenoord, A.J.; Bussmann, C.; Amil Dias, J.; Bove, M.; González-Cervera, J.; Larsson, H.; et al. Guidelines on eosinophilic esophagitis: Evidence-based statements and recommendations for diagnosis and management in children and adults. *United Eur. Gastroenterol.* **2017**, *5*, 335–358. [CrossRef]
3. Cotton, C.C.; Durban, R.; Dellon, E.S. Illuminating Elimination Diets: Controversies Regarding Dietary Treatment of Eosinophilic Esophagitis. *Digest. Dis. Sci.* **2019**, *64*, 1401–1408. [CrossRef] [PubMed]
4. Cotton, C.C.; Eluri, S.; Wolf, W.A.; Dellon, E.S. Six-food elimination diet and topical steroids are effective for eosinophilic esophagitis: A meta-regression. *Digest. Dis. Sci.* **2017**, *62*, 2408–2420. [CrossRef] [PubMed]
5. Asher Wolf, W.; Huang, K.Z.; Durban, R.; Iqbal, Z.J.; Robey, B.S.; Khalid, F.J.; Dellon, E.S. The six-food elimination diet for eosinophilic esophagitis increases grocery shopping cost and complexity. *Dysphagia* **2016**, *31*, 765–770. [CrossRef] [PubMed]
6. Peterson, K.A.; Byrne, K.R.; Vinson, L.A.; Ying, J.; Boynton, K.K.; Fang, J.C.; Gleich, G.J.; Adler, D.G.; Clayton, F. Elemental diet induces histologic response in adult eosinophilic esophagitis. *Am. J. Gastroenterol.* **2013**, *108*, 759–766. [CrossRef]
7. Molina-Infante, J.; Bredenoord, A.J.; Cheng, E.; Dellon, E.S.; Furuta, G.T.; Gupta, S.K.; Hirano, I.; Katzka, D.A.; Moawad, F.J.; Rothenberg, M.E.; et al. Proton pump inhibitor-responsive oesophageal eosinophilia: An entity challenging current diagnostic criteria for eosinophilic oesophagitis. *Gut* **2016**, *65*, 521–531. [CrossRef]
8. Aceves, S.S.; Dohil, R.; Newbury, R.O.; Bastian, J.F. Topical viscous budesonide suspension for treatment of eosinophilic esophagitis. *J. Allergy Clin. Immun.* **2005**, *116*, 705–706. [CrossRef]
9. Straumann, A.; Conus, S.; Degen, L.; Felder, S.; Kummer, M.; Engel, H.; Bussmann, C.; Beglinger, C.; Schoepfer, A.; Simon, H.-U. Budesonide is effective in adolescent and adult patients with active eosinophilic esophagitis. *Gastroenterology* **2010**, *139*, 1526–1537. [CrossRef]
10. Konikoff, M.R.; Noel, R.J.; Blanchard, C.; Kirby, C.; Jameson, S.C.; Buckmeier, B.K.; Akers, R.; Cohen, M.B.; Collins, M.H.; Assa'ad, A.H.; et al. A randomized, double blind, placebo-controlled trial of fluticasone propionate for pediatric eosinophilic esophagitis. *Gastroenterology* **2006**, *131*, 1381–1391. [CrossRef]
11. Biedermann, L.; Straumann, A. Medical and dietary treatments in eosinophilic esophagitis. *Curr. Opin. Pharmacol.* **2018**, *43*, 139–144. [CrossRef] [PubMed]
12. Dellon, E.S.; Sheikh, A.; Speck, O.; Woodward, K.; Whitlow, A.B.; Hores, J.M.; Ivanovic, M.; Chau, A.; Woosley, J.T.; Madanick, R.D.; et al. Viscous topical is more effective than nebulized steroid therapy for patients with eosinophilic esophagitis. *Gastroenterology* **2012**, *143*, 321–324.e1. [CrossRef] [PubMed]
13. Rodieux, F.; Vutskits, L.; Posfay-Barbe, K.M.; Habre, W.; Piguet, V.; Desmeules, J.A.; Samer, C.F. When the safe alternative is not that safe: Tramadol prescribing in children. *Front. Pharmacol.* **2018**, *9*, 148. [CrossRef] [PubMed]
14. Gore, R.; Chugh, P.K.; Tripathi, C.D.; Lhamo, Y.; Gautam, S. Pediatric off-label and unlicensed drug use and its implications. *Curr. Clin. Pharmacol.* **2017**, *12*, 18–25. [CrossRef] [PubMed]
15. Casiraghi, A.; Musazzi, U.M.; Franceschini, I.; Berti, I.; Paragò, V.; Cardosi, L.; Minghetti, P. Is propranolol compounding from tablet safe for pediatric use? Results from an experimental test. *Minerva Pediatr.* **2014**, *66*, 355–362.
16. Casiraghi, A.; Musazzi, U.M.; Rocco, P.; Franzè, S.; Minghetti, P. Topical treatment of infantile haemangiomas: A comparative study on the selection of a semi-solid vehicle. *Skin. Pharmacol. Physiol.* **2016**, *29*, 210–219. [CrossRef]
17. Resolution CM/Res(2016)1 on Quality and Safety Assurance Requirements for Medicinal Products Prepared in Pharmacies for the Special Needs of Patients. Available online: https://www.edqm.eu/sites/default/files/resolution_cm_res_2016_1_quality_and_safety_assurance_requirements_for_medicinal_products_prepared_in_pharmacies.pdf (accessed on 20 December 2019).
18. Minghetti, P.; Pantano, D.; Gennari, C.G.M.; Casiraghi, A. Regulatory framework of pharmaceutical compounding and actual developments of legislation in Europe. *Health Policy* **2014**, *117*, 328–333. [CrossRef]

19. Aceves, S.S.; Bastian, J.F.; Newbury, R.O.; Dohil, R. Oral viscous budesonide: A potential new therapy for eosinophilic esophagitis in children. *Am. J. Gastroenterol.* **2007**, *102*, 2271–2279. [CrossRef]
20. Dohil, R.; Newbury, R.; Fox, L.; Bastian, J.; Aceves, S. Oral viscous budesonide is effective in children with eosinophilic esophagitis in a randomized, placebo-controlled trial. *Gastroenterology* **2010**, *139*, 418–429. [CrossRef]
21. Lee, J.; Shuker, M.; Brown-Whitehorn, T.; Cianferoni, A.; Gober, L.; Muir, A.; Verma, R.; Liacouras, C.; Spergel, J.M. Oral viscous budesonide can be successfully delivered through a variety of vehicles to treat eosinophilic esophagitis in children. *J. Allergy Clin. Immunol. Pract.* **2016**, *4*, 767–768. [CrossRef]
22. Ey, C.; Hosselet, C.; Villon, B.; Marçon, F. Paediatric formulation: Budesonide 0.1 mg/mL viscous oral solution for eosinophilic esophagitis using cyclodextrins. *Pharm. Technol. Hosp. Pharm.* **2018**, *3*, 71–77. [CrossRef]
23. Bonnet, M.; Dermu, M.; Roessle, C.; Bellaiche, M.; Abarou, T.; Vasseur, V.; Benakouche, S.; Storme, T. Formulation of a 3-months stability oral viscous budesonide gel and development of an indicating stability hplc method. *Pharm. Technol. Hosp. Pharm.* **2018**, *3*, 91–99. [CrossRef]
24. Zur, E. Eosinophilic esophagitis: Treatment with oral viscous budesonide. *Int. J. Pharm. Compd.* **2012**, *16*, 288–293. [PubMed]
25. Hefner, J.N.; Howard, R.S.; Massey, R.; Valencia, M.; Stocker, D.J.; Philla, K.Q.; Goldman, M.D.; Nylund, C.M.; Min, S.B. A randomized controlled comparison of esophageal clearance times of oral budesonide preparations. *Digest. Dis. Sci.* **2016**, *61*, 1582–1590. [CrossRef] [PubMed]
26. Ip, K. Physical and chemical stability of budesonide mucoadhesive oral suspensions (MucoLox). *Int. J. Pharm. Compd.* **2017**, *21*, 322–329.
27. Jo, W.; Ha Bak, J.; Yoo, B. Rheological characterizations of concentrated binary gum mixtures with xanthan gum and galactomannans. *Int. J. Biol. Macromol.* **2018**, *114*, 263–269. [CrossRef]
28. Cilurzo, F.; Gennari, C.G.M.; Selmin, F.; Musazzi, U.M.; Rumio, C.; Minghetti, P. A novel oromucosal prolonged release mucoadhesive suspension by one step spray coagulation method. *Curr. Drug. Deliv.* **2013**, *10*, 251–260. [CrossRef]
29. Hou, S.; Hindle, M.; Byron, P.R. A stability-indicating HPLC assay method for budesonide. *J. Pharm. Biomed. Anal.* **2001**, *24*, 371–380. [CrossRef]
30. García-Ochoa, F.; Santos, V.E.; Casas, J.A.; Gómez, E. Xanthan gum: Production, recovery, and properties. *Biotechnol. Adv.* **2000**, *18*, 549–579.
31. Petri, D.F.S. Xanthan gum: A versatile biopolymer for biomedical and technological applications. *J. Appl. Polym. Sci.* **2015**, *132*, 42035. [CrossRef]
32. Ali, H.S.M.; York, P.; Blagden, N.; Soltanpour, S.H.; Acree, W.E., Jr.; Jouyban, A. Solubility of budesonide, hydrocortisone, and prednisolone in ethanol + water mixtures at 298.2 K. *J. Chem. Eng. Data* **2010**, *55*, 578–582. [CrossRef]
33. European Medicines Agency (EMA). Reflection Paper: Formulations of Choice for the Paediatric Population. Available online: https://www.ema.europa.eu/en/formulations-choice-paediatric-population (accessed on 20 December 2019).
34. George, A.; Shah, P.A.; Shrivastav, P.S. Guar gum: Versatile natural polymer for drug delivery applications. *Eur. Polym. J.* **2019**, *112*, 722–735. [CrossRef]
35. Casas, J.A.; Mohedano, A.F.; García-Ochoa, F. Viscosity of guar gum and xanthan/guar gum mixture solutions. *J. Sci. Food Agric.* **2000**, *80*, 1722–1727. [CrossRef]
36. Ishihara, S.; Nakauma, M.; Funami, T.; Odake, S.; Nishinari, K. Swallowing profiles of food polysaccharide gels in relation to bolus rheology. *Food Hydrocoll.* **2011**, *25*, 1016–1024. [CrossRef]
37. Aframian, D.J.; Davidowitz, T.; Benoliel, R. The distribution of oral mucosal pH values in healthy saliva secretors. *Oral Dis.* **2006**, *12*, 420–423. [CrossRef]
38. Andrews, G.P.; Laverty, T.P.; Jones, D.S. Mucoadhesive polymeric platforms for controlled drug delivery. *Eur. J. Pharm. Biopharm.* **2009**, *71*, 505–518. [CrossRef]

pharmaceutics

MDPI

Article

Oleogels with Birch Bark Dry Extract: Extract Saving Formulations through Gelation Enhancing Additives

Kashif Ahmad Ghaffar and Rolf Daniels *

Department of Pharmaceutical Technology, Eberhard Karls University, Auf der Morgenstelle 8, 72076 Tuebingen, Germany; kashif.ghaffar@ymail.com

* Correspondence: Rolf.Daniels@uni-tuebingen.de; Tel.: +49-7071-29-72462

Received: 10 December 2019; Accepted: 19 February 2020; Published: 21 February 2020

Abstract: Triterpenes from the outer bark of birch have many beneficial biological and pharmacological activities. In particular, its wound healing efficacy is of paramount importance. Apart from that, particles of a birch bark dry extract aggregate into a three dimensional network when they are dispersed in lipids yielding a semi-solid oleogel. However, gel formation requires high amounts of the extract, which then acts at once as the active ingredient and the gelling agent. Infrared spectra of the respective mixtures proved that hydrogen bonds play a crucial role in the formation of the gel network. Dicarboxylic acids had almost no effect on gel strength. Monoalcohols increased the firmness of the oleogel with a decreasing effect from methanol > ethanol > butanol > octanol. All tested terminal diols increased the gel strength whereas vicinal diols affected the gel strength negatively. The effect was highly dependent on their concentration. The different effects of the diols are linked to their structure and polarity. The most pronounced enhancement of gelation was found for 1,6-hexanediol, which reduced the amount of triterpene extract (TE), which is necessary for the formation of an oleogel by a factor of 10.

Keywords: birch bark extract; oleogels; hydrogen bonding; triterpene; rheology; gel strength

1. Introduction

It is well known, that triterpenoids, widespread secondary plant metabolites, have many beneficial biological and pharmacological activities [1,2]. Triterpenes from birch bark are of exceptional interest. The following triterpenes are the most common in the outer bark of the white birch: betulin, lupeol, betulinic acid, oleanolic acid, and erythrodiol (Figure 1) [3,4].

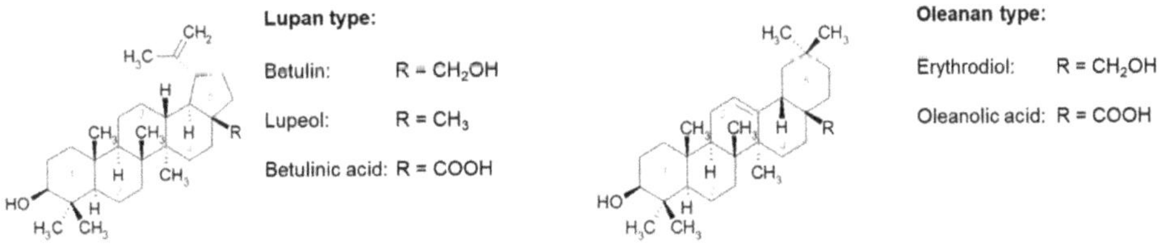

Figure 1. Chemical structure of triterpenoids with Lupan and Oleanan type skeleton.

There are different ways described in the literature to extract and isolate these triterpenes, such as extraction of triterpenoids with organic solvents like n-heptane [4,5] or ethanol [6]. Other methods used include supercritical fluid technology [3], ultrasonic-assisted extraction [7], and sublimation [8].

Triterpenes have antiviral, antibacterial, and antitumoral activities [9,10]. Moreover, a triterpene extract from the outer bark of birch was shown to enhance wound healing ex vivo as well as in vivo in humans [11–13]. In January 2016 an oleogel consisting of solely sunflower oil and birch bark extract got European marketing authorization for the treatment of partial-thickness wounds [11]. In this formulation, the triterpene extract functions as the active substance as well as an excipient. In such binary mixtures, the extract forms a three-dimensional gel network and immobilizes the liquid oil [12]. A similar aggregation of triterpenes through hydrogen bonds was also shown in organic solvents [13,14]. The aggregation of a substance and the resulting gelling effect is also described for so called organogels, where different classes of gelling agents such as glycerol ester, fatty acid, fatty alcohols, or sterols are used [15]. These are so called low-molecular-weight-gelators, and 12-hydroxystearic acid was one of the first substances investigated intensively; it was shown that both its hydroxyl and carboxyl group play a crucial role during gelation [16]. These gelators are also of exceptional interest in the food industry as an alternative to saturated triglycerides for structuring oils, in which secondary valence bonds (e.g., hydrogen bonds) play a vital role [17]. It was also shown that specific substances are able to induce the interaction of the gelling agents and thus increase the gel strength of such organogels [18,19]. In the same direction, results with triterpene extract (TE) oleogels indicated that the gel strength is affected by a complex interplay of liquid–solid interaction as well as the interaction of suspended TE particles. Up to date it is not fully understood how this kind of gelation is exactly brought about and how additives affect it. However, there are clear hints that hydrogen bonds play an essential role in this process [12]. From a formulator's point of view, the formation of a particulate gel network using the active ingredient might be problematic because it has to be added in comparably large amounts. Moreover, it is an inherent disadvantage that the concentration of the active ingredient and the gelator cannot be changed independently. Finally, the formation of a three-dimensional particulate network takes a lot of time because the rearrangement of the particles is a rather slow process.

Therefore, the aim of this study was to (1) find additives which are able to increase the gel strength and accelerate the gel formation and (2) further increase knowledge on the mechanism behind the formation of the particulate gel network. To this end, the strength of oleogels consisting of birch bark extract, sunflower oil, and several additives that might form H-bonds was studied by means of oscillation rheology. The interaction between TE particles and additives was characterized by IR spectroscopy. Furthermore, the effect of the additives on the solubility of the TE was analyzed.

2. Materials and Methods

2.1. Materials

The dry birch bark extract was a gift from Amryt AG (Niefern-Oeschelbronn, Germany). It was produced by enhanced organic solvent extraction using n-heptane [5]. The chemical and physical characterization of the extract is shown in Table 1.

Table 1. Chemical and physical characteristics of the birch bark dry extract.

Constituent	Amount (*w*/*w* %)	Specific Surface Area (m^2/g)	Particle Size (μm)
Betulin	80.0	42	5.8
Betulinic acid	3.1		
Oleanolic acid	0.5		
Lupeol	4.3		
Erythrodiol	0.8		
Undisclosed substances	11.3		

1,2-Propanediol was obtained from Caesar & Loretz GmbH (Hilden, Germany). Methanol, ethanol, butanol, octanol, ethylene glycol, 1,3-butanediol, 1,4-butanediol, 1,5-pentanediol, 1,2-hexanediol, 1,6-hexanediol, 2,5-hexanediol, 1,9-nonanediol, adipic acid, and azealic acid were purchased from Sigma Aldrich (Taufkirchen, Germany) with a purity >95%. Succinic acid was from Merck KGaA (Darmstadt, Germany) and 1,2-pentanediol was from BASF (Zurich, Switzerland).

2.2. Gel Preparation

The dry triterpene extract was sieved through a number 500 sieve before further use. Thereafter, an 8% stock oleogel was produced by homogenizing the extract for 2 min at 8500 rpm in sunflower oil by means of an Ultra Turrax (Ika Labortechnik, Staufen, Germany). The additives were added to the stock oleogel in a predetermined amount and the final formulation was again homogenized for 1 min at 8500 rpm. Oleogels were analyzed 24 h after preparation.

2.3. Rheology

Rheology of the oleogels was measured in oscillation mode using a Gemini 150 (Bohlin Instruments, Pforzheim, Germany) equipped with a 25 mm plate/plate geometry using a gap of 1 mm. After a pre-shear phase of 40 s and 5 min recovery time, an amplitude sweep was performed with a logarithmic ramp, deformation rate of 0.01–1000%, and a frequency of 1 s^{-1}. The gel strength of the oleogels was expressed as the mean of the storage modulus G′ in the linear viscoelastic range. In general, gel strength of all oleogels was measured 24 h after preparation in order to allow formation of the gel network after intense shearing during the manufacturing process.

2.4. ATR–Infrared Spectroscopy

The samples were analyzed with a Spectrum One FTIR-Spectrometer (Perkin Elmer, Rodgau, Germany). They were placed on the surface of an optical fiber and spectra were taken with a wave number ranging from 4000 cm^{-1} to 670 cm^{-1}. In total, 31 spectra were cumulated and evaluated using the software Spectrum v. 3.01 (Perkin Elmer, Rodgau, Germany).

2.5. Particle Size Measuring

The particle size distribution of the oleogels was measured through laser diffraction using a Sympatec Helos (Sympatec GmbH, Clausthal-Zellerfeld, Germany), with a lens focal length of 100 mm and measuring range of 0.9–175 µm. For these measurements oleogels were produced with light liquid paraffin and an extract concentration of 8%. After diluting the sample in a ratio of 1:10 with the oil phase, the sample was added in a cuvette where it was stirred in paraffin to get a homogeneous dispersion. Measurements were taken at an optical concentration of 25–30%.

Laser diffraction results are expressed as x_{10}, x_{50}, and x_{90} values based on a cumulative volume distribution. To ensure comparability between rheology and particle size measurements, respective oleogels for particle sizing were also stored at 25 °C.

3. Results and Discussion

3.1. Effect of Additives on Gel Strength

Previous studies dealing with oleogel formation with TE particles hypothesized that the formation of the gel network is markedly assisted by dissolved bi-functional triterpene molecules, (e.g., betulin). In order to check this, the effect of several mono- and bi-functional additives was studied systematically. Figure 2 shows the effect of the different additives on the gel strength of an oleogel consisting of sunflower oil and 8% triterpene extract.

Most tested excipients with hydroxyl functional groups were able to increase gel strength. In the series of the mono-functional alcohols, the gel strength decreased with their chain length. The addition of methanol gave the highest increase in gel strength. None of the used dicarboxylic acids (adipic acid, succinic acid, azelaic acid) affected the gel strength, which is explained by the creation of cyclic dimers of the dicarboxylic acids [20,21]. The additives prefer interacting with each other instead of the extract particles. All diols with terminal hydroxyl groups increased the gel strength. The effect was dependent on the alkyl chain length of the diols and showed maximum values with 1,6-hexanediol, leading to a 9-fold increase in viscosity when 2% of this substance were added. The gel strength decreased again when the chain length further increased. Diols with vicinal hydroxyl groups (e.g., 1,2-hexanediol), affected the gel strength negatively. Again, the effect was dependent on the chain length. Accordingly, the most prominent reduction in gel strength was seen with 1,2-hexanediol.

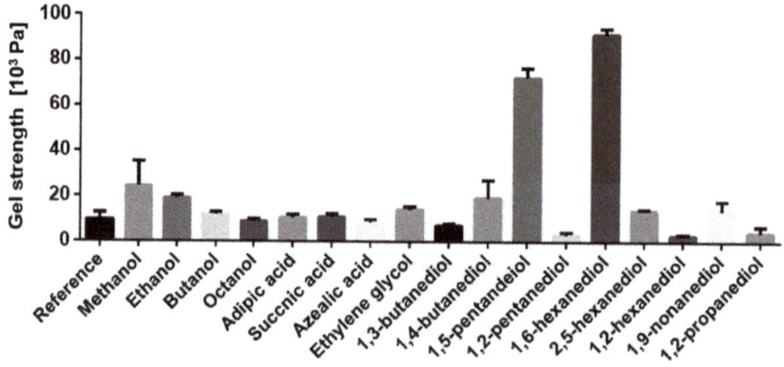

Figure 2. Gel strength of oleogels with sunflower oil, 8% triterpene extract (TE), and 2% additive; an oleogel without any additive serves as a reference; mean ± SD, $n = 3$.

3.2. *IR-Measurements*

It is well known that gel is formed through hydrogen bonds between extract particles, which is shown by IR spectroscopy [12]. Figure 3 shows IR spectra of plain TE oleogels prepared with increasing TE concentrations.

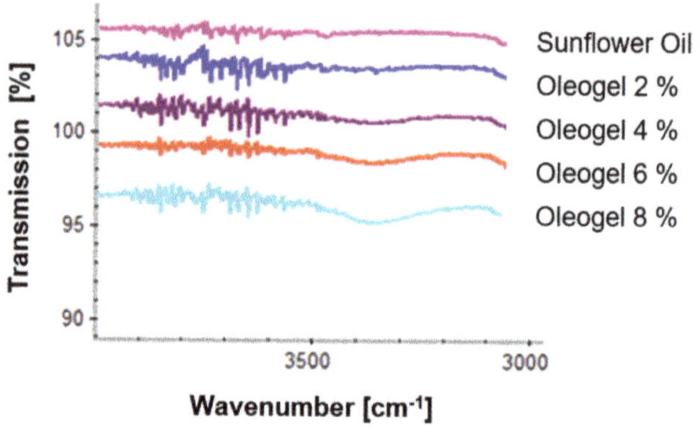

Figure 3. IR spectra of oleogels in sunflower oil with increasing TE concentration.

Free hydroxyl groups usually show an absorption band at 3700 cm^{-1}. If the hydroxyl groups are involved in hydrogen bonds the absorption band is shifted to the 3500–3200 cm^{-1} wavenumber range. In Figure 3 it is clearly seen that the absorption band at 3300 cm^{-1} increases with increasing TE concentration. This indicates an increasing number of hydrogen bonds, which is in line with an increasing gel strength [12]. Diols have been shown to markedly affect gel strength in a positive or negative manner. IR spectra were taken to further elucidate the behavior of the diols. Figure 4 shows the IR spectra of a plain 8% TE oleogel in comparison to those measured after the addition of several diols with terminal hydroxyl groups, which enhanced the gel strength.

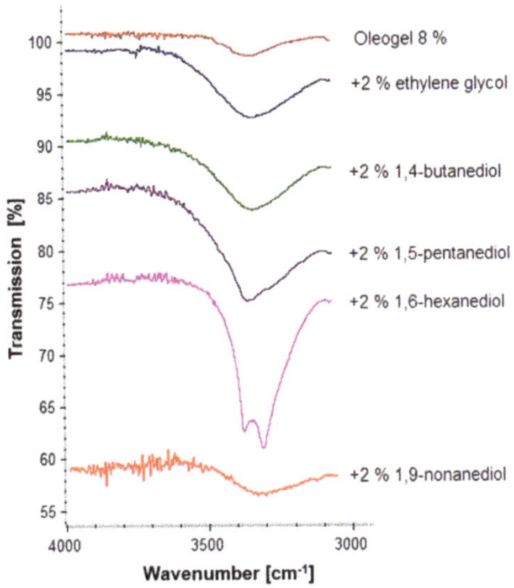

Figure 4. IR spectra of oleogels (8% TE) in sunflower oil with terminal diols (2%).

As expected, the IR spectra of the oleogels with the gel enhancing additives showed a fortified broad absorption band at 3400 cm^{-1}, indicating that these diols are able to interact intensely with the extract particles via hydrogen bonds. The characteristic absorption band increased in the series from ethylene glycol to 1,6-hexanediol, which corresponds to an increasing firmness of the oleogel. The intense interaction of 1,6-hexanediol was accompanied by a splitting of the absorption band at 3400 cm^{-1} probably due to interactions between adjacent molecules. As demonstrated by 1,9-nonanediol, a further increase in the chain length of the terminal diol resulted in a reduction of both the absorption band at 3400 cm^{-1} as well as the gel strength. Figure 5 shows IR spectra of a plain 8% TE oleogel and after the addition of pentanediols and hexanediols with either terminal or vicinal hydroxyl groups.

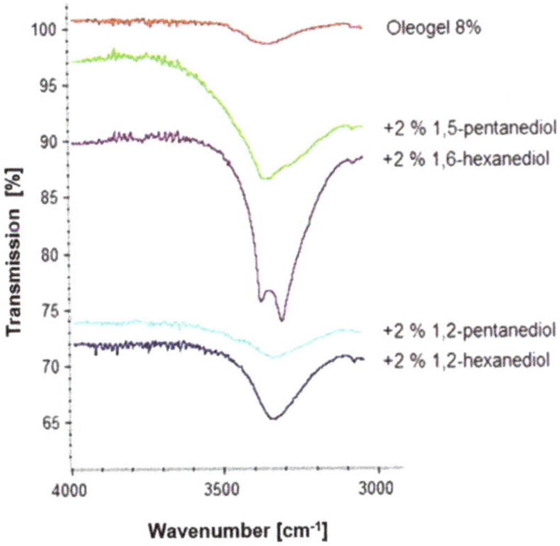

Figure 5. IR spectra of oleogels (8% TE) in sunflower oil with vicinal diols and their corresponding terminal diols (2%).

Independent from the chain length of the diols, the absorption band at 3400 cm^{-1} is significantly smaller when adding vicinal diols instead of terminal diols. However, although a marked hydrogen bonding of the vicinal diols is still detectable, they do not increase the gel strength but rather reduce the firmness of the respective oleogels. As the absorption band of oleogels with vicinal diols is still larger compared to the plain oleogel, it could be concluded that the vicinal diols interact substantially with the superficial hydroxyl groups of the TE particles, but they are not able to link the TE particles together. To the contrary, they shield the superficial hydroxyl groups of the TE particles and hence prevent them from building a three dimensional particulate gel network as exemplary visualized in Figure 6.

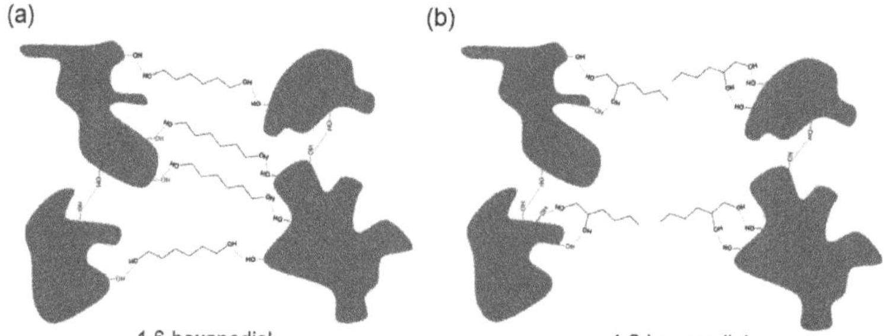

Figure 6. Schematic drawing of interaction between (**a**) 1,6-hexanediol and extract particle; (**b**) 1,2-hexanediol and extract particle (dimensions are not to scale).

Like the gel enhancing effect of the terminal diols, the gel weakening effect of the vicinal diols and the absorption band at 3400 cm^{-1} were more pronounced with increasing chain length of the diols.

3.3. *Influence of the Enhancer Concentration on the Gel Strength*

As the number of interacting superficial hydroxyl groups on the TE particles is limited it was of great interest if the effect of the additives on the gel strength depends on their concentration. To this end, oleogels were produced with terminal diols in the concentration range from 0.25–2% (corresponding to approx. 2–30 µmol m^{-2}). As shown in Figure 7, the gelation enhancing effect of terminal diols was highly dependent on their concentration, with a maximum effect mostly in the range of 0.5–1%.

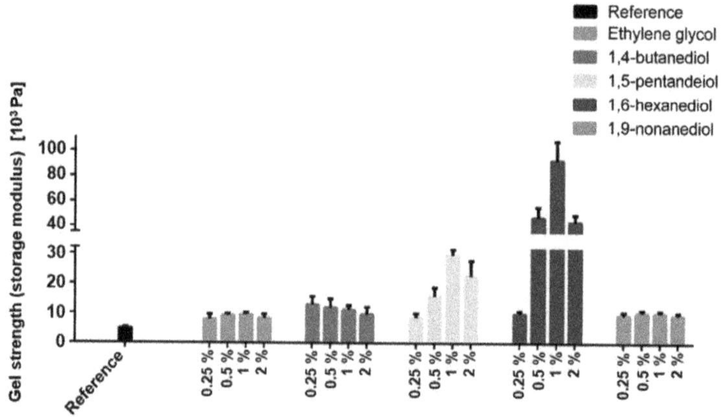

Figure 7. Gel strength of oleogels (8%) with terminal diols in a concentration range of 0.25–2%; an oleogel without any additive serves as a reference; mean ± SD, $n = 3$.

The firmness of the oleogels decreased again when the diol concentration exceeded the optimal range. However, this did not come with a decreasing absorption band at 3400 cm^{-1} (data not shown). Therefore, it is hypothesized that the surplus of diol forms hydrogen bonds with other diol molecules instead of the TE particles, leading to a less rigid three-dimensional network.

3.4. Particles Size of Oleogels

Fumed silica particles are comparable to gel oils by forming a three dimensional network [22]. The gelling mechanism is very similar compared to the triterpene oleogels. In oleogels using silica particles, the particles grow during storage because of further aggregation of the particles. This leads to a higher gel strength. We expected a similar particle growth with the TE oleogels. Moreover, 1,2-hexanediol was expected to have a negative effect, and 1,6-hexanediol to have a positive effect, on the growth of particle aggregates in line with the observed effect on gel strength. Figure 8 shows the particle size distribution and the gel strength of a plain oleogel during its one month storage at 25 °C.

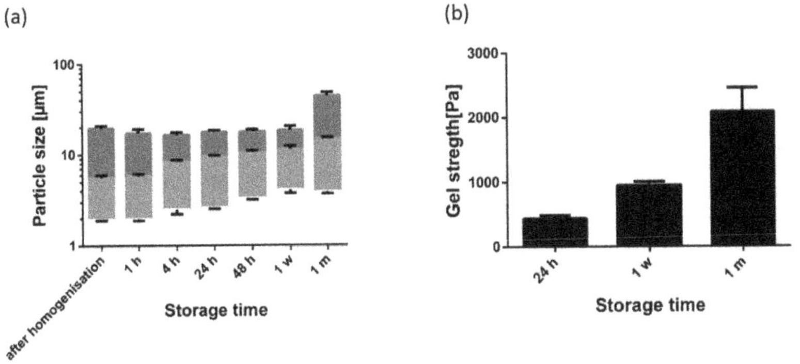

Figure 8. (**a**) Particle size distribution (x_{10}, x_{50}, and x_{90} values) and (**b**) gel strength of an oleogel (8% TE in paraffin) during one month of storage; mean ± SD, $n = 3$.

As can be seen, laser diffraction revealed minimal particle size directly after homogenization. Due to aggregation, the measured particle size (x_{10} and x_{50} value) subsequently increased steadily during storage. This aggregation of the particle is in line with measurements of the gel strength of the oleogel which also rises during storage. During storage, the x_{90} values remained almost unaffected within the first week of storage and showed a significant increase after 1 month. This indicates that the interaction forces increased during storage to such an extent that the small shear forces during sample preparation were not sufficient to further disaggregate the larger aggregates completely.

This behavior changed substantially in the presence of 1,2-hexanediol and 1,6-hexanediol (Figure 9). While 1,2-hexanediol inhibited particle aggregation during one month of storage, the measured particle size in the presence of 1,6-hexanediol was significantly larger directly after homogenization. Four hours after preparation, the particle size distribution was already comparable to the plain oleogel after one month of storage. The firmness of the oleogel with 1,6-hexanediol was too high to allow a particle size measurement after 4 h. Obviously, 1,6-hexandiol extensively promotes the interaction of TE particles.

Again, the gel strength of the oleogels were in line with the results of the particle size measurements (Figure 10).

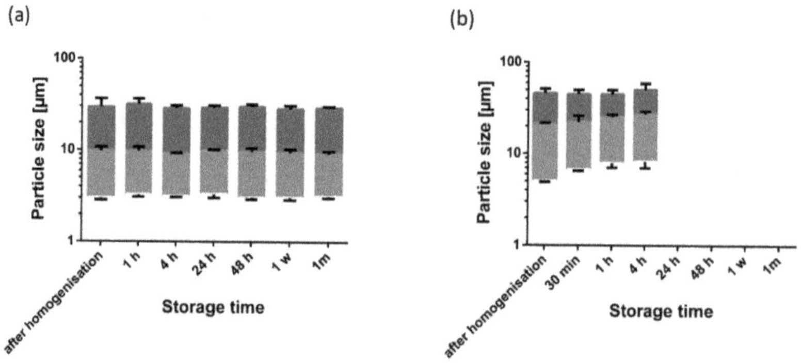

Figure 9. Particle size distribution of oleogels (8% TE in paraffin) during one month of storage with (**a**) 2% 1,2-hexanediol and (**b**) 2% 1,6-hexanediol; mean ± SD, $n = 3$.

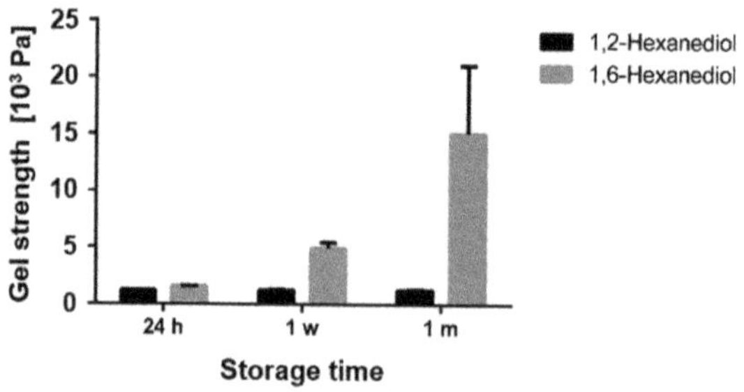

Figure 10. Gel strength of oleogels (8% TE in paraffin) during one month of storage with 2% 1,2-hexanediol and 1,6-hexanediol; mean ± SD, $n = 3$.

During one month of storage, the gel strength in the presence of 1,2-hexanediol remained almost constant at a low level due to insufficient interaction of the TE particles. In contrast, oleogels with 1,6-hexanediol showed a marked increase in the gel strength during one month of storage. At first sight, this behavior is comparable to plain oleogels, however, the absolute values of the gel strength are much higher in the presence of 1,6-hexanediol.

The mechanism behind these huge differences between 1,2-hexanediol and 1,6-hexanediol is already illustrated schematically in Figure 7. 1,6-Hexanediol with its terminal OH groups has the ability to act very effectively as a linker between the TE particles. Due to its much smaller size compared to the TE particles, 1,6-hexanediol is able to link the particles faster and more flexibly and thus more efficiently lead to a pronounced activation of the gel network. 1,2-Hexanediol with its vicinal OH groups has an amphiphile and adsorbs to the superficial functional groups of the TE particles. Consequently, the hydrocarbon chain is oriented to the continuous phase and prevents the formation of hydrogen bonds. This is comparable to the negative impact on the aggregation of silica particles dispersed in DMSO when the number of sites for hydrogen bonding of silanol groups was reduced by surface modification [22].

3.5. Extract Saving Effect of Additives

In the oleogels, TE represents the active component as well as the gel forming excipient. This brings about that higher amounts of TE are required than probably necessary for the intended therapeutic effect. In this context, supplementing the oleogel with 1,6-hexanediol as the most effective gelation enhancer should drastically reduce the required concentration of TE necessary for gel formation.

To this end, oleogels with different TE concentrations were produced without and with the addition of a rather low concentration (0.5%) of 1,6-hexanediol (Figure 11).

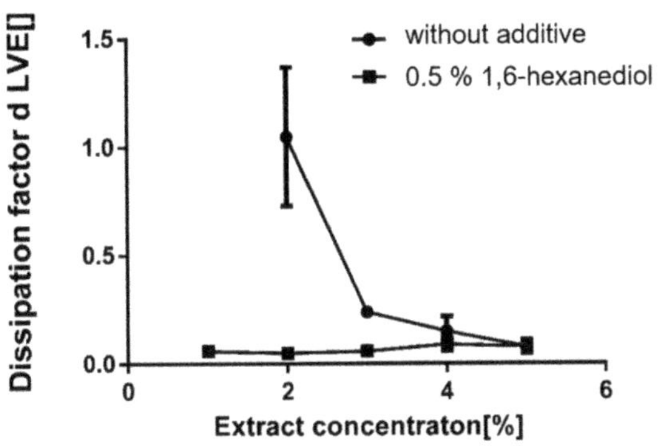

Figure 11. Dissipation factor d with different concentrations of TE with and without 1,6-hexanediol (0.5%); mean ± SD, $n = 3$.

Without additives, the critical gelation concentration of TE in sunflower oil was 3% as indicated by a dissipation factor in the linear viscoelastic region ≤1. In the presence of 0.5% 1,6-hexanediol, the critical gelation concentration dropped to <1% TE. Even at such low TE concentrations, the resulting oleogels with 1,6-hexanediol are highly elastic as indicated by a dissipation factor <0.1.

4. Conclusions

Hydrogen bonds are mainly responsible for the formation of the gel network in oleogels with birch bark dry extract. Additives, which can act as linkers between the extract particles, enhance the formation of a particulate network. The most pronounced effect was observed in diols with terminal hydroxyl groups. 1,6-Hexanediol gave the best results and allowed the formation of an oleogel with a drastically reduced concentration of TE. This effect depends on the concentration of the gelation enhancer. A concentration in the range of 0.5% to 1% was found to be optimal. In contrast, 1,2-diols impaired gel formation by blocking superficial OH groups on the extract particles and preventing them from building a three dimensional particulate network.

Author Contributions: Conceptualization, K.A.G. and R.D.; data curation, K.A.G.; investigation, K.A.G.; methodology, K.A.G. and R.D.; project administration, R.D.; supervision, R.D.; writing—original draft, K.A.G.; writing—review and editing, R.D. All authors have read and agreed to the published version of the manuscript.

Funding: This research received no external funding.

Acknowledgments: The authors would like to thank Amryt AG for the kind donation of the triterpene extract.

Conflicts of Interest: The authors declare no conflict of interest.

References

1. Dzubak, P.; Hajduch, M.; Vydra, D.; Hustova, A.; Kvasnica, M.; Biedermann, D.; Markova, L.; Urban, M.; Sarek, J. Pharmacological Activities of Natural Triterpenoids and Their Therapeutic Implications. *Nat. Prod. Rep.* **2006**, *23*, 394–411. [CrossRef] [PubMed]
2. Alqahtani, A.; Hamid, K.; Kam, A.; Wong, K.; Abdelhak, Z.; Razmovski-Naumovski, V.; Chan, K.; Li, K.; Groundwater, P.; Li, G. The Pentacyclic Triterpenoids in Herbal Medicines and Their Pharmacological Activities in Diabetes and Diabetic Complications. *Curr. Med. Chem.* **2012**, *20*, 908–931.
3. Armbruster, M.; Mönckedieck, M.; Scherließ, R.; Daniels, R.; Wahl, M. Birch Bark Dry Extract by Supercritical Fluid Technology: Extract Characterisation and Use for Stabilisation of Semisolid Systems. *Appl. Sci.* **2017**, *7*, 292. [CrossRef]

4. Laszczyk, M.; Jäger, S.; Simon-Haarhaus, B.; Scheffler, A.; Schempp, C. Physical, Chemical and Pharmacological Characterization of a New Oleogel-Forming Triterpene Extract from the Outer Bark of Birch (Betulae Cortex). *Planta Med.* **2007**, *72*, 1389–1395. [CrossRef] [PubMed]
5. Scheffler, A. Triterpene-Containing Oleogel-Forming Agent, Triterpene-Containing Oleogel and Method for Producing a Triterpene-Containing Oleogel. U.S. Patent 8,536,380, 17 September 2013.
6. Kuznetsova, S.A.; Skvortsova, G.P.; Maliar, I.N.; Skurydina, E.S.; Veselova, O.F. Extraction of betulin from birch bark and study of its physico-chemical and pharmacological properties. *Russ. J. Bioorganic Chem.* **2014**, *40*, 742–747. [CrossRef]
7. Xia, Y.-G.; Yang, B.-Y.; Liang, J.; Wang, D.; Yang, Q.; Kuang, H. Optimization of simultaneous ultrasonic-assisted extraction of water-soluble and fat-soluble characteristic constituents from Forsythiae Fructus Using response surface methodology and high-performance liquid chromatography. *Pharmacogn. Mag.* **2014**, *10*, 292–303. [CrossRef] [PubMed]
8. Guidoin, M.-F.; Yang, J.; Pichette, A.; Roy, C. Betulin isolation from birch bark by vacuum and atmospheric sublimation. A thermogravimetric study. *Thermochim. Acta* **2003**, *398*, 153–166. [CrossRef]
9. Suksamrarn, S.; Panseeta, P.; Kunchanawatta, S.; Distaporn, T.; Ruktasing, S.; Suksamrarn, A. Ceanothane- and Lupane-Type Triterpenes with Antiplasmodial and Antimycobacterial Activities from Ziziphus cambodiana. *Chem. Pharm. Bull.* **2006**, *54*, 535–537. [CrossRef] [PubMed]
10. Mishra, T.; Arya, R.; Meena, S.; Joshi, P.; Pal, M.; Meena, B.; Upreti, D.; Rana, T.; Datta, D. Isolation, Characterization and Anticancer Potential of Cytotoxic Triterpenes from Betula utilis Bark. *PLoS ONE* **2006**, *11*, e0159430. [CrossRef] [PubMed]
11. EMA: Marketing Authorisation Episalvan. Available online: https://www.ema.europa.eu/en/medicines/human/EPAR/episalvan (accessed on 20 February 2020).
12. Grysko, M.; Daniels, R. Evaluation of the mechanism of gelation of an oleogel based on a triterpene extract from the outer bark of birch. *Die Pharm.* **2013**, *68*, 572–577.
13. Bag, B.; Dash, D. Hierarchical Self-Assembly of a Renewable Nanosized Pentacyclic Dihydroxy-triterpenoid Betulin Yielding Flower-Like Architectures. *ACS Langmuir* **2015**, *31*, 13664–13672. [CrossRef] [PubMed]
14. Bag, B.; Dash, D. First self-assembly study of betulinic acid, a renewable nano-sized, 6-6-6-6-5 pentacyclic monohydroxy triterpenic acid. *Nanoscale* **2011**, *3*, 4564–4566. [CrossRef] [PubMed]
15. Pernetti, M.; Malssen, K.; Flöter, E.; Bot, A. Structuring edible oils by alternatives to crystalline fat. *Curr. Opin. Colloid Interface Sci.* **2007**, *12*, 221–231. [CrossRef]
16. Daniel, J.; Rajasekharan, R. Organogelation of Plant Oils and Hydrocarbons by Long-Chain Saturated FA, Fatty Alcohols, Wax Esters, and Dicarboxylic Acids. *J. Am. Oil Chem. Soc.* **2003**, *80*, 417–421. [CrossRef]
17. Patel, A. *Edible Oil Structuring: Concepts, Methods and Applications*; The Royal Society of Chemistry: London, UK, 2018.
18. Shchipunov, Y.; Shumilina, E. Lecithin bridging by hydrogen bonds in the organogel. *Mater. Sci. Eng. C* **1995**, *3*, 43–50. [CrossRef]
19. Buerkle, L.; Rowan, S. Supramolecular gels formed from multi-component low molecular weight species. *Chem. Soc. Rev.* **2012**, *41*, 6089–6102. [CrossRef] [PubMed]
20. Vahid, A.; Elliott, J. Transferable Intermolecular Potentials for Carboxylic Acids and Their Phase Behavior. *Thermodynamics* **2010**, *56*, 485–505. [CrossRef]
21. Tsivintzelis, I.; Kontogeorgis, G.; Panayiotou, C. On the Dimerization of Carboxylic Acids: An Equation of State Approach. *J. Phys. Chem. B* **2017**, *121*, 2153–2163. [CrossRef] [PubMed]
22. Nordström, J.; Matic, A.; Sun, J.; Forsyth, M.; MacFarlane, D. Aggregation, ageing and transport properties of surface modified fumed silica dispersions. *Soft Matter* **2010**, *6*, 2293–2299. [CrossRef]

pharmaceutics

MDPI

Article

Topical Amphotericin B Semisolid Dosage Form for Cutaneous Leishmaniasis: Physicochemical Characterization, Ex Vivo Skin Permeation and Biological Activity

Diana Berenguer [1], Maria Magdalena Alcover [1], Marcella Sessa [2], Lyda Halbaut [2], Carme Guillén [1], Antoni Boix-Montañés [2], Roser Fisa [1], Ana Cristina Calpena-Campmany [2], Cristina Riera [1] and Lilian Sosa [2,*]

1 Department of Biology, Health and Environment, Laboratory of Parasitology, Faculty of Pharmacy and Food Sciences, University of Barcelona, 08028 Barcelona, Spain; berenguer.diana@gmail.com (D.B.); mmagdalenaalcoveramengual@ub.edu (M.M.A.); carmeguillen@ub.edu (C.G.); rfisa@ub.edu (R.F.); mcriera@ub.edu (C.R.)

2 Department of Pharmaceutical Technology and Physicochemistry, Faculty of Pharmacy and Food Sciences, University of Barcelona, 08028 Barcelona, Spain; marcellass93@gmail.com (M.S.); halbaut@ub.edu (L.H.); antoniboix@ub.edu (A.B.-M.); anacalpena@ub.edu (A.C.C.-C.)

* Correspondence: liliansosa2012@gmail.com; Tel.: +34-4024560

Received: 30 December 2019; Accepted: 10 February 2020; Published: 12 February 2020

Abstract: Amphotericin B (AmB) is a potent antifungal successfully used intravenously to treat visceral leishmaniasis but depending on the *Leishmania* infecting species, it is not always recommended against cutaneous leishmaniasis (CL). To address the need for alternative topical treatments of CL, the aim of this study was to elaborate and characterize an AmB gel. The physicochemical properties, stability, rheology and in vivo tolerance were assayed. Release and permeation studies were performed on nylon membranes and human skin, respectively. Toxicity was evaluated in macrophage and keratinocyte cell lines, and the activity against promastigotes and intracellular amastigotes of *Leishmania infantum* was studied. The AmB gel remained stable for a period of two months, with optimal properties for topical use and no apparent toxic effect on the cell lines. High amounts of AmB were found in damaged and non-damaged skin (1230.10 ± 331.52 and 2484.57 ± 439.12 μg/g/cm^2, respectively) and they were above the IC_{50} of AmB for amastigotes. Although there were no differences in the in vitro anti-leishmanial activity between the AmB solution and gel, the formulation resulted in a higher amount of AmB being retained in the skin, and is therefore a candidate for further studies of in vivo efficacy.

Keywords: Amphotericin B; Sepigel 305®; *Leishmania infantum*; cutaneous leishmaniasis; topical treatment

1. Introduction

Leishmaniasis are a group of diseases caused by species of *Leishmania* protozoan parasites and transmitted by the bite of *Phlebotomine* sand flies. Nearly 12 million people are infected in 98 countries worldwide [1]. There are three main forms of the disease and the manifestations depend on the infecting species, the immunological system of the patient and the area of inoculation [2,3]. Cutaneous leishmaniasis (CL), the most common form, can appear as single or multiple skin lesions, starting as a papule and potentially evolving into an ulcer; mucocutaneous leishmaniasis involves the destruction of mucous membranes; and visceral leishmaniasis (VL) is a fatal form affecting internal organs [4]. In the Mediterranean area, *Leishmania infantum* is the main causal agent of VL and CL [5], and particularly in Spain, *L. infantum* is the responsible for the endemic CL cases [6,7].

Although there is no universal consensus on the treatment of CL [8], pentavalent antimonials still remain the first-line therapy, frequently used in combination with pentoxifylline or paromomycin to maximize treatment efficacy despite the toxic side effects and the development of resistances [9]. Pentavalent antimonials (meglumine antimoniate and sodium stibogluconate) are administered intravenously or by painful intralesional injections which are frequently discontinued by patients, which promotes resistances [10].

Amphotericin B (AmB) is a polyene macrolide antibiotic that opens ion channels and aqueous pores in the *Leishmania* membrane by binding to ergosterol, making the bilayer thinner and increasing the permeability and loss of intracellular compounds, thereby triggering lysis and parasite death [11]. AmB intravenous injections are used as a second-line treatment for CL, but they cause severe toxicity, particularly nephrotoxocity in the case of conventional AmB. Liposomal AmB (Ambisome®) has been demonstrated to be more effective and less toxic, but its high cost makes its use difficult in developing countries [12,13].

In the last five years, research directed to improve delivery systems for the treatment of leishmaniasis has focused considerable attention on AmB as an active component [14], mainly using a parenteral administration approach. PLGA polymeric nanoparticles have been studied for intralesional and intravenous administration of AmB [4,15], as well as diverse emulsions and micelle formulations for intravenous use [16,17]. Considerable research is also being directed into the development of oral or topical formulations, as they imply greater patient compliance and fewer side effects. Chitosan has been investigated as a nanocarrier for oral administration [18], as well as an ingredient in an emulsion of nanoparticles [19]. Dermal delivery has been achieved with microneedles that generate micropores in the epidermis for the administration of an AmB solution [20]. For the topical treatment of CL, a combination of cyclodextrin plus AmB has been studied in a gel formulation [21], and ultradeformable liposomes have also been postulated [22].

Pharmaceutical gels are semisolid dosage forms consisting of a solvent thickened by the addition of colloidal substances. Colloids are polymers with gelling capacity and constitute a dispersed phase, and the liquid solvent is the continuous phase. The most common solvents used in gel formulation are water or hydroalcoholic solutions that form hydrogels.

Hydrogels form cross-linked polymer chain networks able to capture large quantities of water in the spaces between chains and are widely used as vehicles in topical drug delivery [23]. They provide a refreshing sensation on the skin, are not sticky and have an optimal appearance. Sepigel 305®, which is composed of the fatty oil isoparaffin, the gelation-promoting polymer polyacrylamide and the non-ionic emulsifier laureth-7, forms hydrogels that permit the addition of hydrophilic and lipophilic substances.

The objective of this work was to develop a topical formulation incorporating AmB for CL therapy. AmB is a very hydrophobic molecule and is poorly soluble in water and most organic solvents. Using the capacity of Sepigel 305® to include hydrophobic substances, we developed an AmB hydrogel-based formulation with optimal organoleptic characteristics. The stability was assessed by examining the physicochemical properties of the gel for two months. Permeation and retention studies were performed ex vivo in human skin, tolerance was checked in healthy volunteers, and toxicity and leishmanicidal activity were examined in vitro in promastigotes and intracellular amastigotes of *Leishmania infantum*.

2. Materials and Methods

2.1. Reagents

Amphotericin B and Sepigel 305® were purchased from Acofarma (Barcelona, Spain). Dimethyl sulfoxide (DMSO) and NaOH were obtained from Sigma-Aldrich (Darmstadt, Germany). TranscutolP® was provided by Gattefossé (Barcelona, Spain). The distilled water used to perform the assays was acquired from a Mili-Q® Plus System (Millipore Co., Burlington, MA, USA).

2.2. Parasite Strains and Cultures

For the parasitology experiments, the *Leishmania infantum* strain (MHOM/ES/2016/CATB101) was isolated from a patient with CL in Spain, and promastigotes were maintained at 26 °C in supplemented Schneider complete medium at pH 7.0 with 20% heat-inactivated fetal calf serum, 25 μg/mL gentamicin solution (Sigma, St. Louis, MO, USA), and 1% penicillin (100 U/mL)–streptomycin (100 mg/mL) solution (Sigma, St. Louis, MO, USA).

2.3. Gel Preparation

Briefly, the gel-based 1% Sepigel 305® formulation was prepared with constant mechanical stirring (solution A). Subsequently, 150 mg of AmB was dissolved in 5 mL of DMSO, of which 1 mL was slowly added under agitation to 30 mL of solution A. The resulting solution was adjusted to pH 6 with NaOH 2N solution, thus obtaining AmB gel at a final concentration of 1000 μg/mL.

2.4. Physicochemical Characterization of the AmB gel

2.4.1. Morphological Analysis

The internal morphological structure was observed under scanning electron microscopy (SEM) using a FEI Quanta 200 (Hillsboro, OR, USA) in high-vacuum conditions. AmB gel was dried off for 14 days under a vacuum desiccator and a sample of 0.1 g was covered with carbon.

2.4.2. Swelling and Degradation Tests

Dried and fresh AmB gel were utilized to perform the swelling and degradation tests. In both studies, the AmB gel was kept in PBS (pH = 5.5) for 21 min at 32 °C. Samples (n = 5) were weighed after wiping the superficial water at determined timeslots every 3 min. The swelling ratio (SR) was calculated using the following equation:

$$\mathrm{SR} = \frac{Ws - Wd}{Wd}$$

where Ws is the weight of the swollen AmB gel at 3 min intervals and Wd is the weight of dried gel.

The degradation was expressed as the weight loss percentage (WL) and was calculated following the equation:

$$\mathrm{WL}\ (\%) = \frac{Wi - Wd}{Wi} \times 100$$

where Wi is the weight of the AmB gel at the initial point of the experiment and Wd is the gel weight every 3 min at preselected time points.

2.4.3. Porosity Study

The porosity percentage is based on the sinking of the AmB gel previously dried in absolute ethanol for 20 min and weighing it every 2 min when the excess of ethanol is blotted.

The porosity percentage (P) was calculated with the equation:

$$\mathrm{P}\ (\%) = \frac{W2 - W1}{\rho \times V} \times 100$$

where $W1$ stands for the weight of the dried AmB gel, $W2$ is the weight of the AmB gel after each immersion every 2 min, ρ is the density of ethanol and V is the volume of the AmB gel.

2.5. Stability Studies

Samples of the AmB gel were stored at different temperatures (room temperature (RT), 4 °C and 37 °C) to determine the stability of the formulation.

The pH values were registered with universal test paper (Ahlstrom-Munksjö, Helsinki, Finland) by directly spreading the samples (n = 3) and checking the visual appearance and drug loading after 1, 30 and 60 days.

The AmB content was analyzed using a previously validated High-Performance Liquid Chromatography (HPLC) methodaccording to international guidelines, with linearity, sensitivity, accuracy, precision and selectivity as described by Sosa et al. (2017) [24]. The calibration curves were prepared with freshly prepared stock solutions of AmB ranging from 0.39 to 200 µg/mL. The analytical method was precise, with coefficient of variation between 0.02% and 8.79%, a relative percent error between −1.16% and 3.46%, and linear within the range of concentrations used (0.39–200 µg/mL), with a p value corresponding to the ANOVA applied to the mean values of 0.05. AmB was determined using a Waters® 515 HPLC Pump, a 717 Plus Autosampler and a 2487 Dual λ Absorbance Detector (Waters®, Milford, MA, USA). The assay was carried out using a Kromasil® Eternity C18 (250 mm × 4.6 mm × 5 µm, Teknokroma, Barcelona, Spain). The mobile phase was a mixture of acetonitrile:acetic acid:water (52:4.3:43.7 *v*/*v*/*v*) and was pumped through the C18 column at a flow rate of 0.5 mL/min. A volume of 10 µL was injected per sample and finally the elute was analyzed at 406 nm. All measurements were performed at RT and at isocratic conditions of elution.

Destabilization phenomena were inspected by multiple light scattering and analysis of backscattering and transmission profiles using a TurbiScanLab® (Formulaction Co., L'Union, France) with a pulsed near-infrared light source (γ = 880 nm) at 25 °C, 1, 30 and 60 days after the preparation of the AmB gel.

2.6. *Rheological Studies*

A rotational rheometer (Thermo Scientific HaakeRheostress 1, Thermo Fischer Scientific, Karlsruhe, Germany) with a cone plate set-up, a fixed lower plate and a mobile upper cone Haake C60/2° Ti was used to carry out the rheological assay. Measurements were taken in duplicate at 25 °C and 4 °C 24 h after gel preparation, as the rheometer is equipped with a ThermoHaake Phoenix II + Haake C25P (Thermo Fischer Scientific, Waltham, MA, USA) to control the temperature. The shear rate ramp program encompassed a ramp-up period from 0 to 50 s^{-1} for 3 min, a constant shear rate period of 50 s^{-1} for 1 min and a ramp-down period from 50 to 0 s^{-1} for 3 min. The data acquired from flow curves ($\tau = f(\dot{\gamma})$) were fitted to different mathematical models (Newton, Bingham, Ostwald-de-Waele, Herschel-Bulkley, Casson and Cross) and the best fit was selected according to the correlation coefficient value (r). Mean viscosity curve ($\eta = f(\dot{\gamma})$) values were determined from the constant share section at 50 s^{-1} [25].

2.7. *Spreadability Test*

The spreadability (n = 3) of AmB gel was determined by placing 0.5 g of the formulation between a plate and a millimeter glass plate cover. Different weights (2, 5, 10, 20, 50, 100, 200 and 300 g) were successively placed on top for 2 min each at RT. Spread diameters were measured and fitted into mathematical models using GraphPad Prism® version 6.0 (GraphPad Software Inc., San Diego, CA, USA).

2.8. *In Vitro Release Studies*

AmB release was assessed in an 0.64 cm^2 area of Franz diffusion cells (FDC 400; Crown Glass, Somerville, NJ, USA) on nylon membranes (0.45 µm) (Sterlitech Corporation, Kent, WA, USA). Pure DMSO solution continuously stirred at 600 rpm and 32 ± 0.5 °C was used as the receptor medium to accomplish sink conditions. Then, 0.75 g of AmB gel and 0.75 mL of AmB solution were deposited in the donor compartment. The study was performed in three replicates for a period of 48 h and the AmB was determined by HPLC-UV at preselected time points.

2.9. *Ex Vivo Permeation Studies*

Human skin from a donor undergoing plastic surgery at Barcelona-SCIAS Hospital (experimental protocol reference number: BEC/001/16, Barcelona, Spain) was used to perform the permeation assays in Franz diffusion cells, as described in the previous section. Skin was sliced into 400 μm thick specimens and the integrity was checked by measuring the transepidermal water loss (TEWL) parameters [26]. To damage the tissue, the stratum corneum of healthy skin was partially removed 7 times with the tape stripping technique. Then, both healthy and damaged skin were used in the experiments. After this, 0.75 g AmB gel was deposited on the upper side of the skin, facing the stratum corneum. Transcutol P® was used as the receptor medium and was kept at 32 ± 0.5 °C in the receptor compartment. After 24 h, the amount of AmB in the receptor compartment as well as inside the skin was quantified by HPLC in three replicates. The drug retained in the skin was extracted after washing and cutting the permeation area with an ultrasound bath and cooling for 15 min.

2.10. *In Vivo Tolerance Studies*

Ten volunteers with healthy skin took part in the study, which was approved by the Ethics Committee of the University of Barcelona (reference number: IRB00003099; date: 20 March 2018), following the Declaration of Helsinki guidelines [27]. Participants were asked not to use any kind of cosmetics on the flexor side of the left forearm in the days before the test. Measurements were carried out at baseline, 30 min after the volunteers arrived in the test room, and then at 15 min, 1 h and 2 h after the application of 0.5 g of AmB gel. TEWL and the stratum corneum hydration (SCH) values were measured by a Tewameter® TM 300 (Courage-Khazaka electronic GmbH) and a Corneometer® CM 825 (Courage-Khazaka electronic GmbH), respectively, in accordance with international guidelines [28].

2.11. *In Vitro Cytotoxicity Assay*

Three different cell lines were used to establish the cytotoxic effect of the AmB gel—two macrophage cell lines (RAW 264.7 and J774A.1) and a keratinocyte cell line (HaCat). A suspension of 5×10^4 cells/mL of each cell line was seeded in 96-well plates (Costar 3596, Corning Incorporated, NY, USA) and cultured at 37 °C and 5% CO_2 atmosphere in RPMI-1640 complete medium [10% heat-inactivated fetal calf serum and 1% penicillin (100 U/mL)–streptomycin (100 mg/mL)] for 24 h. After that, serial dilutions of the AmB gel and AmB solution were added and the conditions were maintained for another 24 h. Finally, the reagent WST-1 (Roche Diagnostics GmbH) was added at a concentration of 10% to all wells and the plate was incubated for 4 h in the same conditions regarding temperature and CO_2 atmosphere. Absorbances were read at 450 nm (Multiskan EX, Thermo Electron Corporation, Shanghai, China). To determine the concentration that inhibits 50% of cell viability (CC_{50}), a linear regression analysis was performed, and the experiments were performed in triplicate [29].

2.12. *In Vitro Leishmanicidal Activity against Promastigotes*

Promastigotes were cultured in cell culture flasks. To assess their activity, serial dilutions of AmB gel and AmB solution were prepared in Schneider medium and placed in a 96-well plate (Costar 3596, Corning Incorporated, NY, USA). A suspension of 10^6 promastigotes/mL in a logarithmic phase were added to the previous dilutions and incubated at 26 °C for 48 h. Parasitic growth was evaluated using the phosphatase acid method described by Carrió et al. (2000). Briefly, the samples were lysed, and the enzymatic reaction was revealed with *p*-nitrophenyl phosphate by alkalization. The optical density was read at 405 nm (Multiskan EX, Thermo Electron Corporation, Shanghai, China). The IC_{50} (the concentration that inhibits 50% of parasite growth) was calculated by variable transformation and linear regression analysis, and the experiments were performed in triplicate [30].

2.13. *In Vitro Leishmanicidal Activity against Amastigotes*

The cell line J774A.1 was used to study the activity of the AmB gel against amastigotes. A concentration of 5×10^4 cells/mL was seeded in an 8 LabTek chamber slide system (Nunc®, Rochester, NY, USA) and incubated for 24 h at 37 °C in a 5% CO_2 atmosphere. Late stationary phase promastigotes from a 5-day growth culture were added in a ratio of 1:10 (macrophage:parasites) and incubated for 24 h in the same conditions. After the elimination of free promastigotes by washing, fresh RPMI-1640 complete medium with serial dilutions of gel or solution was added, and incubation was carried out for 48 h in the same conditions. Untreated cultures were included as a positive control. Slides were fixed and stained with Giemsa to evaluate the number of amastigotes in 300 macrophages and the percentage of infected cells was determined in triplicate. The IC_{50} was expressed as the percentage of growth inhibition with respect to the untreated controls [31].

2.14. *Statistical Analysis*

The data collected in the studies were analyzed by one-way parametric analysis of variance (ANOVA), followed by a multiple comparison Tukey test ($p < 0.05$ = statistically significant differences) using Prism® V. 5 (GraphPad Software Inc., CA).

3. Results

3.1. *Physicochemical Characterization of the AmB gel*

Figure 1 shows the homogeneous laminar disposition of undulating layers of AmB gel, with holes or cavities between the layers.

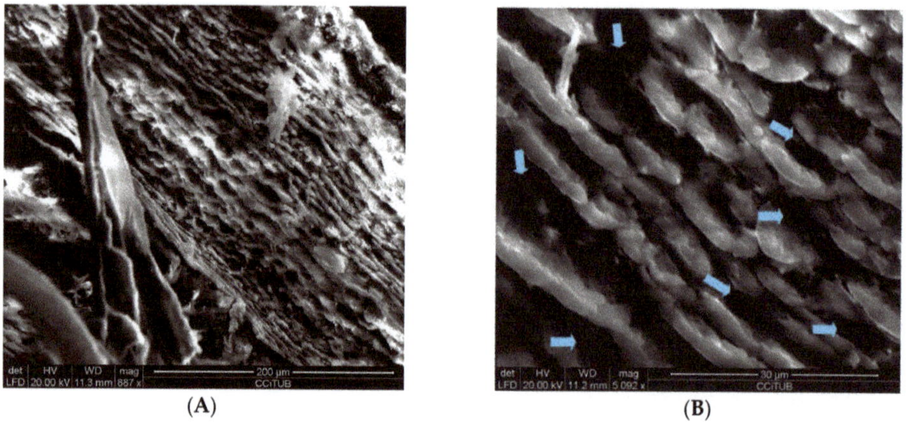

Figure 1. Images of amphotericin B (AmB) gel under SEM, (**A**) undulating layers (887×) and (**B**) detail of cavities between layers (5092×).

The AmB gel described a hyperbolic model in the swelling experiment, with a kinetic constant of k = 3.66 min ($r^2 = 0.9986$). Gel degradation was completed in 10 min and was represented by a one-phase exponential model, where the kinetic constant was k = 0.31 min^{-1} ($r^2 = 0.9992$) and the porosity percentage was ~85.47% ± 0.73%. The swelling and degradation graphs generated by the AmB gel are shown in Figure 2.

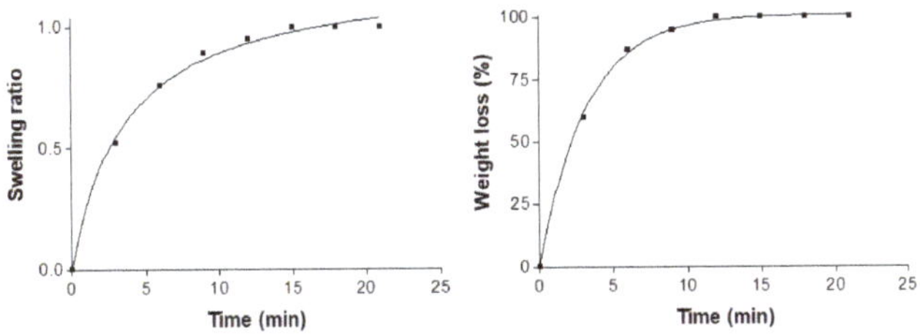

Figure 2. Swelling ratio (left) and degradation (right) of AmB gel during 21 min in PBS medium.

3.2. Stability Studies

The AmB gel presented a pH value of 5–6 throughout the experiment. The yellow colour of the AmB formulation remained unchanged at all temperatures tested in the study period. No lumps or precipitation were observed.

Figure 3 shows the backscattering profile of Amb gel at 25 °C over a period from 1 to 60 days. No sedimentation, flocculation or coalescence phenomena were detected.

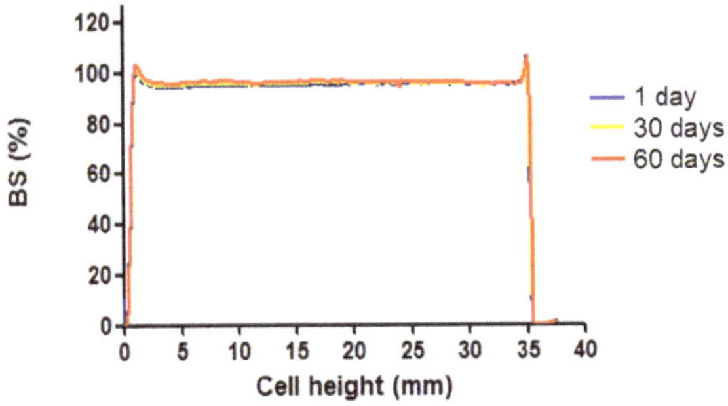

Figure 3. Laser backscattering (BS) profile of AmB gel over 60 days at 25 °C. The left side corresponds to the bottom of the vial containing the sample, whereas the right side corresponds to the sample behavior at the top.

The initial AmB content revealed the gel formulation had 95.99% entrapment efficiency. The concentration of AmB in the gel over time is summarized in Table 1. The AmB content of the gel samples did not present statistical differences ($p > 0.05$) at the tested temperatures after 60 days of storage at 4 °C, whereas a significant decrease in the AmB content of the gel was observed when it was maintained at RT and 37 °C.

Table 1. Concentration of AmB and SD at the beginning of the experiment (t_0 = initial time) and 60 days later (t_{60}) at different storage temperatures.

	AmB (µg/mL ± SD)			
	t_0	t_{60} **RT**	t_{60} **37 °C**	t_{60} **4 °C**
AmB gel	959.90 ± 84.27	199.65 ± 27.99	70.95 ± 13.59	916.70 ± 99.78

3.3. Rheological Studies

The AmB gel presented rheo-thinning (pseudoplastic) behavior at 25 °C and 4 °C (Cross model; $r^2 = 0.9996$ and $r^2 = 0.9998$, for the two temperatures, respectively). The viscosity at 50 s^{-1} was 1542.5 ± 3.49 mPa·s, and there was ahysteresis loop with an area of 194.4 Pa/s at 25 °C. The viscosity at 50 s^{-1}

was 1457 ± 4.04 mPa·s, and there was also a hysteresis loop with an area of 160.1 Pa/s at 4 °C. Figure 4 shows the rheological graphs.

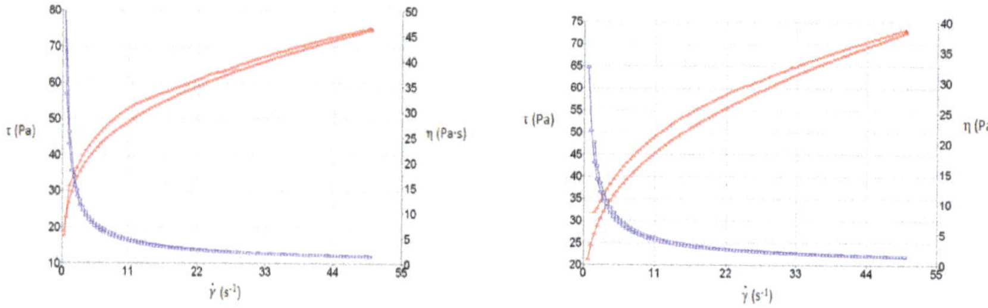

(A) **(B)**

Figure 4. Rheological behavior of AmB gel showing a hysteresis loop. (**A**) Behavior at 25 °C and (**B**) 4 °C.

3.4. Spreadability Test

The spreadability of AmB gel followed a hyperbola kinetic model:

$$[S = S_{max} \times W/(K_d + W)]$$

where S represents the extended surface in cm^2, S_{max} is the maximum extension surface in cm^2, W stands for the weight attached in g and K_d is the kinetic constant in g. Figure 5 shows the resulting graph and equation.

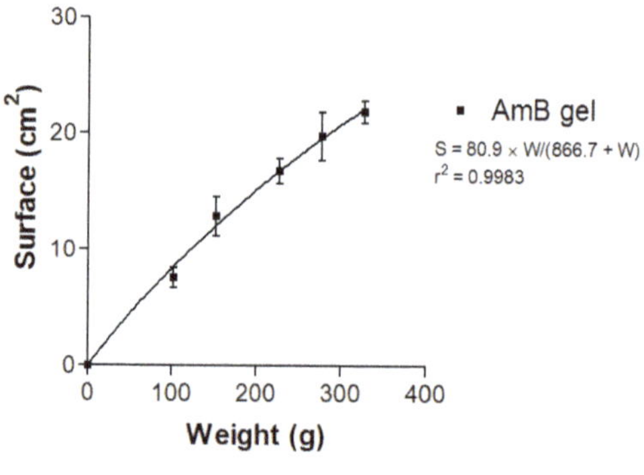

Figure 5. Graphicalhyperbolic behavior of AmB gel spreadability.

3.5. In Vitro Release Studies

The amount of AmB released from the solution and gel at 48 h of the experiment was 753.01 ± 83.43 μg/cm² and 501.02 ± 58.17 μg/cm², respectively (Figure 6), which represents an AmB release of 100.40 ± 11.13%from the solution and 66.80 ± 8.9% from the gel. The mathematical model with the best fit was one-phase exponential association.

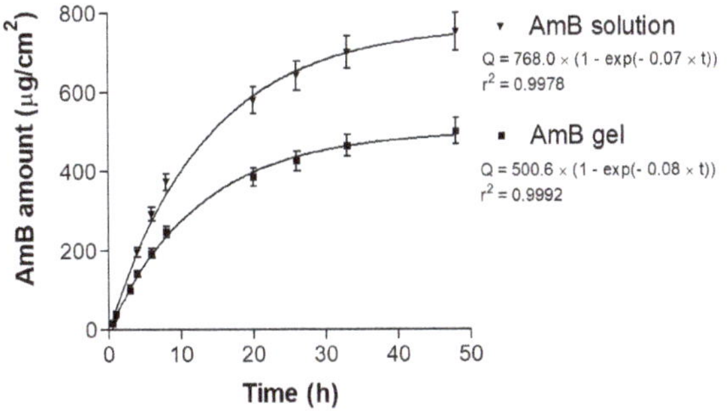

Figure 6. Released amounts (Q) of AmB from the solution and gel through nylon membranes for 48 h.

3.6. Ex Vivo Permeation Studies

Table 2 summarizes the amount of AmB obtained in the permeation studies with damaged and non-damaged skin. No AmB flux was observed across the skin barrier.

Table 2. Amounts of AmB found in the permeation studies after 24 h in damaged and non-damaged skin.

Assay	AmB gel	
	Non-Damaged Skin	**Damaged Skin**
Permeation ($\mu g/cm^2$) ± SD	Not detected	Not detected
Retention in skin ($\mu g/g/cm^2$) ± SD	2484.57 ± 439.12	1230.10 ± 331.52

3.7. In Vivo Tolerance Studies

At 15 min of AmB gel application, decreased values of TEWL were observed, as well as an increased hydration of the stratum corneum, with statistically significant differences compared with all the time points in the experiment. The graph in Figure 7 shows the variations of biomechanical properties.

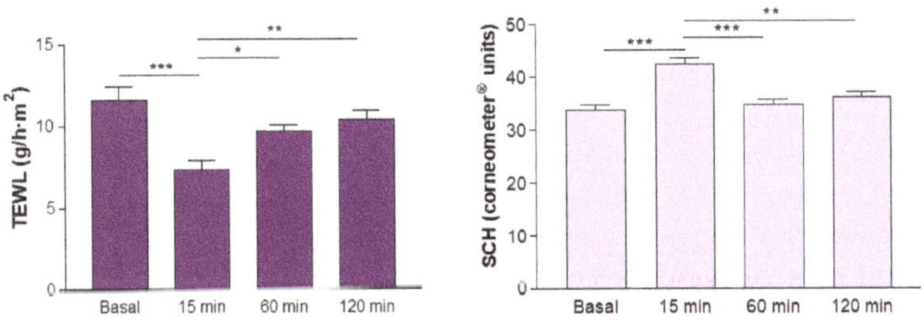

Figure 7. Biomechanical parameters: TEWL (transepidermal water loss) and SCH (stratum corneum hydration) values for 2 h after AmB gel application (* $p < 0.05$; ** $p < 0.01$; *** $p < 0.001$).

3.8. In Vitro Cytotoxicity Assay

As seen in Figure 8, the CC_{50} of Sepigel 305® in the cell lines assayed was higher than 75.0 µg/mL. The CC_{50} of the AmB gel and solution was higher than 25.0 µg/mL (Figure 9).

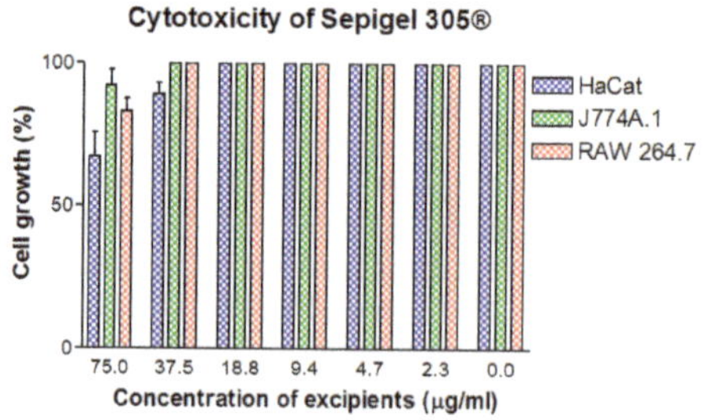

Figure 8. Cytotoxicity of the gelling excipients in cell lines HaCaT, RAW 264.7 and J774A.1.

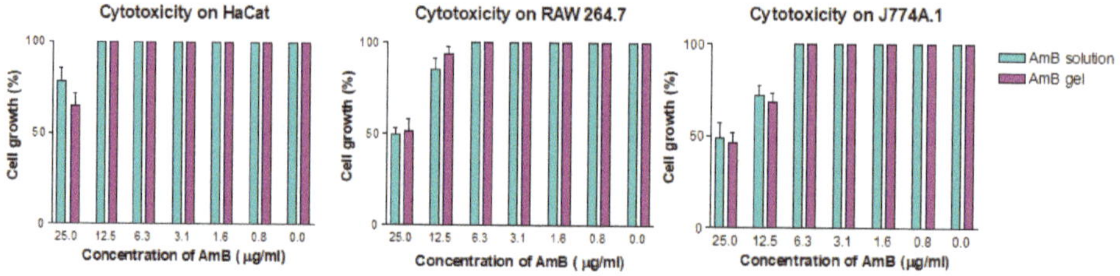

Figure 9. Cytotoxicity of AmB solution and AmB gel in cell lines HaCaT, RAW 264.7 and J774A.1.

3.9. *In Vitro Leishmanicidal Activity against Promastigotes and Amastigotes*

Table 3 summarizes the activity on promastigotes and amastigotes. The IC_{50} of the AmB solution and AmB gel was 0.35 ± 0.02 μg/mL and 0.56 ± 0.12 μg/mL against promastigotes, and 0.91 ± 0.07 μg/mL and 0.87 ± 0.10 μg/mLagainst amastigotes, respectively. The selectivity index (SI) values of AmB solution and AmB gel were higher than 25 for both macrophage cell lines.

Table 3. Activity in vitro against promastigotes and amastigotes, cytotoxicity of AmB solution and AmB gel and selectivity index (SI).

Formulations (μg/mL)	IC_{50} (μg/mL ± SD)		SI		CC_{50} (μg/mL)	
	Promastigotes	Amastigotes	SI_{RAW}	$SI_{J774A.1}$	RAW 264.7	J774A.1
AmB solution	0.35 ± 0.02	0.91 ± 0.07	27.52	27.52	>25	>25
AmB gel	0.56 ± 0.12	0.87 ± 0.10	28.74	28.74	>25	>25

4. Discussion

Although AmBisome®, an AmB liposomal formulation for intravenous administration, isvery effective for the treatment of visceral leishmaniasis, its high price limits its use in the routine treatment of CL, despite an agreement with the World Health Organization and Gilead Sciences resulting in a price reduction in developing countries [32]. A topical formulation that achieves dermal drug delivery is a goal in CL treatment, as it will allow patients to administer their own treatment, avoid the discomfort of painful injections and reduce costs.

Gels are colloidal systems used in drug delivery to the skin that may improve the distribution and stability of compounds, as well as reduce undesirable systemic effects [33]. The self-emulsifying agent Sepigel 305® allows a simple and cost-effective formulation of gels for topical use, as the emulsification process does not require any heat energy [34]. In the current study, we formulated an AmB gel made with multifunctional polymer formulation Sepigel 305® as a possible topical alternative in the CL therapy.

Drug release is affected by the degradation of the gel in a physiological environment and also the swelling ratio—the faster the swelling of the gel is accomplished, the greater its porosity.

The degradation rate of the AmB gel was constant and completed in 10 min, indicating it was not dependent on the remaining amount of polymer. The high porosity percentage of the AmB gel was corroborated by SEM images, which revealed undulating layers uniformly arranged and spaces between the layers, resembling holes or cavities. We reported similar levels of swelling, degradation and porosity in a previously characterized meglumine antimoniate Sepigel 305® [35].

Near the isoelectric point, the pH of AmB gel was 5–6, which means it is biocompatible and suitable for skin application [36]. The visual appearance of the formulation remained unchanged throughout the experiment, which was in line with the backscattering profiles used to evaluate the physical stability of the formulation over a long period of time. The superimposed graphs (Figure 3) showed variations below 10%, which is indicative of stability [37,38]. The variability in the AmB concentration at t_0 in the analysis content could be explained because different batches of AmB gel were prepared in order to dispose of fresh formulation to perform the experiments. Moreover, the AmB content in the gel remained constant over a span of 60 days at 4 °C, indicating that the drug is chemically stable when refrigerated. By contrast, at RT the stability analysis indicated that less than 20% of the main active ingredient was detectable, and it was even lower when stored at 37 °C. This could represent a limitation for the storage and clinical manipulation, as refrigeration is not always available. These stability results differ from the marketed AmB liposome formulations (AmBisome®, Abelcet®), where the stability is guaranteed for around 24–48 h at 2–8 °C once the reconstitution has been performed. Also, Rizzo et al. (2018) found rapid AmB degradation within 2 days when analyzing its stability in different combinations of AmB solutions [39]. Other studies support the use of excipients for semisolid dosage forms to increase the stability of AmB [24,38,40].

Rheological analysis provides information about aspects of the product application. The AmB gel exhibited rheo-thinning behavior (a term used by the Rheology Society to replace pseudoplastic behavior) and high viscosity, and showed a hysteresis loop in the rheograms, indicating a probable thixotropic comportment of the gel. Thixotropic behavior is an advantage in topical formulations, favoring application, as the viscosity of the formulation varies with friction and retention on skin is enhanced [41]. Friction reduces the viscosity of thixotropic fluids, which permits a good spreadability, and the initial status of the gel is recovered once the friction stops. The high spreadability of the AmB gel, as shown in Figure 5, can be explained by the dependence of the viscosity on the shear rate and shear time. When the gel was submitted to deformation (added weights), the viscosity decreased and spreadability was enhanced.

The AmB release profile was assessed to check that the gel was well formulated and permitted the AmB liberation to monitor the kinetic behavior [42]. The data obtained demonstrated a constant release for 48 h in a Fickian diffusion process. At 48 h, the amount of AmB released through the nylon membranes was 100% for the AmB solution because there were no impediments, and it confirms the suitability of the membrane, while AmB from the gel was 66.80% liberated. It is an expectable value for a modified release formulation where the excipients play an important role in the liberation of the drug. In a comparative study, Potúcková et al. (2008) reported that drug release was increased when the excipient in the marketed formulation was replaced by Sepigel 305® [43].

Permeation was studied on both damaged and non-damaged skin, as CL lesions can manifest as a nodule or a papule entirely covered with epidermis, or as an ulcer without this layer. No permeation of AmB from the gel was detected in the receptor compartment in either skin type after 24 h. In contrast, high amounts of AmB were retained in both types, with higher values in the non-damaged skin, suggesting that the stratum corneum acts as a reservoir of the drug. The reservoir effect of skin is helpful in the topical treatment of CL nodules or papules because the local depot effect potentiates the treatment duration as this kind of lesion is covered by the epidermis layer [44]. In contrast, this depot effect will not occur in ulcerated lesions. The high deposition of AmB in both kinds of skin observed in this study could indicate a long availability, as commonly required. The achieved levels of AmB retained in both kinds of skin resulted in a higher value than the IC_{50} of AmB for amastigotes, which is considered a goal for successful treatment [45].

Studies on other topical AmB formulations applied on human skin and porcine vaginal mucosa have also reported the absence of AmB in the receptor compartment and high amounts retained inside tissues [24,38]. This behavior can be explained by the high lipophilicity of AmB, which limits its ability to pass through the aqueous dermal structure. Our studies in both kinds of skin reflect that AmB is able to cross the stratum corneum to the epidermis and dermis. Our results with stripped skin ("damaged skin") are comparable to those obtained with porcine vaginal mucosa, which does not present stratum corneum layer, and AmB can reach the dermis but is not distributed in the systemic circulation. This suggests that after topical application, part of the drug would remain in the epidermis and dermis, thus avoiding systemic side effects. As well as providing a high drug concentration in the skin, an effective topical treatment of CL should target the amastigotes of *Leishmania* parasites in the phagolysosome of infected macrophages in the papillary dermis, which is found immediately below the epidermis [46].

In contrast with these results, Jaafari et al. (2019) reported an AmB flux through mouse full-thickness skin to the receptor compartment after the application of AmB liposomes and corroborated the permeation in vivo when the same liposomes were administered in a mouse model [47]. Different studies carried out with AmB nanoemulsions formulated with surfactants for topical delivery reported a high retention of the drug in rat skin and flux to the receptor compartment [40,48,49]. The surfactants in the nanoemulsions enhance AmB permeation by destabilizing the cellular bilayer lipids in the stratum corneum, increasing deformation and enhancing the permeation [50]. It is also relevant that rat skin may lead to a greater permeation of drugs [51], as observed in studies reporting the higher permeability of rat skin compared with human skin [52,53].

The biomechanical parameters of transepidermal water loss and stratum corneum hydration were monitored for 2 h after application to evaluate skin integrity. The values obtained revealed a decrease in the TEWL immediately after AmB gel application, as well as an increased hydration of the stratum corneum due to an occlusive effect of the formulation. This was probably caused by the high lipophilicity of the drug. The TEWL and hydration of the stratum corneum basal values were recovered over 1 h after application, indicating changes in the skin are reversible. Furthermore, no discomfort after the gel application was reported by the volunteers, who did not experience any burning sensation, irritation or itching.

Sepigel 305® and the AmB gel and solution did not show toxicity in the range of dilutions assayed on the three cell lines tested in the experiments. The results corroborate previous reports of safety of using Sepigel 305® in topical formulations, with the exception of one case of allergic contact dermatitis [54].

No differences in the in vitro activity against *Leishmania infantum* promastigotes and amastigotes were observed between the AmB solution and the formulation, indicating an absence of a synergistic effect between the gel excipients and the AmB.

Due to the safe usage of other AmB formulations that has been previously reported in healthy volunteers [55], and prompted by the study of López et al. (2018), who concluded that their 3% AmB cream tested in patients with uncomplicated CL needed reformulation of either the vehicle or concentration [56], we propose Sepigel 305® as a suitable vehicle for 0.1% AmB for topical treatment. Allowing a good release of the AmB with high amounts of the drug retained in excised human skin, the formulation could be a potential tool for CL treatment, as only a few doses of AmB are required to kill the parasite. Further assays in an animal model should be performed to establish the antileishmanial efficacy of the AmB gel.

5. Conclusions

The development of a topical treatment for CL is desirable, as painful intralesional treatments are widely rejected by patients. In this context, we elaborated an AmB gel with optimal sensorial and functional properties that was shown to be stable for 60 days at 4 °C. The organoleptic characteristics of the gel are compatible with usage on skin, as it has a suitable pH, good spreadability and drug release, and did not produce irritation.

Damaged and non-damaged skin were exposed to amounts of AmB considered sufficiently high to exert local action against CL. No AmB was detected in the receptor compartment due to its high molecular weight and lipophilicity. This represents an advantage as the treatment would avoid systemic toxicity.

No cytotoxic effects were observed in the macrophage or in the keratinocyte cell lines. Although the antileishmanial activity of AmB was not affected by the gel formulation in vitro, the AmB gel should undergo in vivo testing to further evaluate its activity and efficacy in the treatment of CL.

Author Contributions: D.B. carried out the experiments, analyzed the result, and wrote the original draft of the manuscript. M.M.A. collaborated in the preparation of the parasitology experiments and revised the manuscript. M.S. carried out the biopharmaceutical experiments. C.G. collaborated in the preparation of the parasitology experiments. L.H. directed the rheological tests. A.B.-M. and R.F. revised the manuscript. A.C.C.-C. validated and supervised the biopharmaceutical experiments. C.R. conceptualized the idea of the investigation, validated and supervised the parasitology experiments, reviewed and edited the manuscript. L.S. conceptualized the idea, carried out the biopharmaceutical experiments, reviewed and edited the manuscript. All authors have read and agreed to the published version of the manuscript.

Funding: This research received no external funding.

Acknowledgments: The authors would like to thank the University of Barcelona for the financial support to cover the cost of open access publication. We appreciate the contribution of Silvia Tebar in the making of culture media. Also, thanks to Lucy Brzoska for the revision of English. And we would like to thank Josefa Badia and Rodrigo Vera for helping us with the cytotoxic assay on keratinocyte cell line.

Conflicts of Interest: The authors declare no conflict of interest.

References

1. Alvar, J.; Vélez, I.D.; Bern, C.; Herrero, M.; Desjeux, P.; Cano, J.; Janin, J.; den Boer, M. WHO Leishmaniasis Control Team. Leishmaniasis worldwide and global estimates of its incidence. *PLoS ONE* **2012**, *7*, e35671. [CrossRef]
2. Garnier, T.; Croft, S.L. Topical treatment for cutaneous leishmaniasis. *Curr. Opin. Investig. Drugs* **2002**, *3*, 538–544.
3. Reithinger, R.; Dujardin, J.C.; Louzir, H.; Pirmez, C.; Alexander, B.; Brooker, S. Cutaneous leishmaniasis. *Lancet Infect. Dis.* **2007**, *7*, 581–596. [CrossRef]
4. Abu Ammar, A.; Nasereddin, A.; Ereqat, S.; Dan-Goor, M.; Jaffe, C.L.; Zussman, E.; Abdeen, Z. Amphotericin B-loaded nanoparticles for local treatment of cutaneous leihmaniasis. *Drug Deliv. Transl. Res.* **2019**, *9*, 76–84. [CrossRef]
5. Gaspari, V.; Ortalli, M.; Foschini, M.P.; Baldovinci, C.; Lanzoni, A.; Cagarelli, R.; Gaibani, P.; Rossini, G.; Vocale, C.; Tigani, R.; et al. New evidence of cutaneous leishmaniasis in north-eastern Italy. *J. Eur. Acad. Dermatol. Venereol.* **2017**, *31*, 1534–1540. [CrossRef]
6. Alcover, M.M.; Rocamora, V.; Guillén, M.C.; Berenguer, D.; Cuadrado, M.; Riera, C.; Fisa, R. Case Report: Diffuse Cutaneous Leishmaniasis by *Leishmania infantum* in a Patient Undergoing Immunosuppressive Therapy: Risk Status in an Endemic Mediterranean Area. *Am. J. Trop. Med. Hyg.* **2018**, *98*, 1313–1316. [CrossRef]
7. Aguado, M.; Espinosa, P.; Romero-Maté, A.; Tardío, J.C.; Córdoba, S.; Borbujo, J. Outbreak of cutaneous leishmaniasis in Fuenlabrada, Madrid. *Actas Dermosifiliogr.* **2013**, *104*, 334–342. [CrossRef]
8. Gupta, A.; Sardana, K.; Ahuja, A.; Gautam, R.K. Complete cure of a large complexe cutaneous leihmaniasis with a nonethanolic lipid based-amphotericin B gel. *Clin. Exp. Dermatol.* **2019**, *44*, 807–810. [CrossRef]
9. Santos, C.M.; de Oliveira, R.B.; Arantes, V.T.; Caldeira, L.R.; de Oliveira, M.C.; Egito, E.S.; Ferreira, L.A. Amphotericin B-loaded nanocarriers for topical treatment of cutaneous leishmaniasis: Development, characterization, and *in vitro* permeation studies. *J. Biomed. Nanotechnol.* **2012**, *8*, 322–329.
10. Jaafari, M.R.; Bavarsad, N.; Fazly-Bazzaz, B.S.; Samiei, A.; Soroush, D.; Ghorbani, S.; Lotfi-Heravi, M.M.; Khamesipour, A. Effect of Topical Liposomes Containing Paromomycin Sulfate in the Course of *Leishmania major* Infection in Susceptible BALB/c Mice. *Antimicrob. Agents Chemother* **2009**, *53*, 2259–2265. [CrossRef]

11. Cohen, B.E. The role of Signaling via Aqueous Pore Formation in Resistance Responses to Amphotericin B. *Antimicrob. Agents Chemother.* **2016**, *60*, 5122–5129. [CrossRef]
12. Mostafavi, M.; Sharifi, I.; Farajzadeh, S.; Khazaeli, P.; Sharifi, H.; Pourseyedi, E.; Kakooei, S.; Bamorovat, M.; Keyhani, A.; Parizi, M.H.; et al. Niosomal formulation of amphotericin B alone and in combination with glucantime: In vitro and in vivo leishmanicidal effects. *Biomed. Pharmacother.* **2019**, *116*, 108942. [CrossRef]
13. de Carvalho, R.F.; Ribeiro, I.F.; Miranda-Vilela, A.L.; de Souza Filho, J.; Martins, O.P.; Cintra e Silva Dde, O.; Tedesco, A.C.; Lacava, Z.G.; Báo, S.N.; Sampaio, R.N. Leishmanicidal activity of amphotericin B encapsulated in PLGA-DMSA nanoparticles to treat cutaneous leishmaniasis in C57BL/6 mice. *Exp. Parasitol.* **2013**, *135*, 217–222. [CrossRef]
14. Lanza, J.S.; Pomel, S.; Loiseau, P.M.; Frézard, F. Recent advances in amphotericin B delivery strategies for the treatment of leishmaniases. *Expert Opin. Drug Deliv.* **2019**, *16*, 1063–1079. [CrossRef]
15. Singh, P.K.; Jaiswal, A.K.; Pawar, V.K.; Raval, K.; Kumar, A.; Bora, H.K.; Dube, A.; Chourasia, M.K. Fabrication of 3-O-snphosphatidyl-L-serine anchored PLGA nanoparticle bearing amphotericin B for macrophage targeting. *Pharm. Res.* **2018**, *35*, 60–71. [CrossRef]
16. Rochelle Do Vale Morais, A.; Silva, A.L.; Cojean, S.; Balaraman, K.; Bories, C.; Pomel, S.; Barratt, G.; do Egito, E.S.T.; Loiseau, P.M. In-vitro and in-vivo antileishmanial activity of inexpensive Amphotericin B formulations: Heated Amphotericin B and Amphotericin B-loaded microemulsion. *Exp. Parasitol.* **2018**, *192*, 85–92. [CrossRef]
17. Wang, Y.; Ke, X.; Voo, Z.X.; Yap, S.S.L.; Yang, C.; Gao, S.; Liu, S.; Venkataraman, S.; Obuobi, S.A.O.; Khara, J.S.; et al. Biodegradable functional polycarbonate micelles for controlled release of amphotericin B. *Acta Biomater.* **2016**, *46*, 211–220. [CrossRef]
18. Sarwar, H.S.; Sohail, M.F.; Saljoughian, N.; Rehman, A.U.; Akhtar, S.; Nadhman, A.; Yasinzai, M.; Gendelman, H.E.; Satoskar, A.R.; Shahnaz, G. Design of mannosylated oral amphotericin B nanoformulation: Efficacy and safety in visceral leishmaniasis. *Artif. Cells Nanomed. Biotechnol.* **2018**, *46* (Suppl. 1), 521–531. [CrossRef]
19. Gupta, P.K.; Jaiswal, A.K.; Asthana, S.; Teja, B.V.; Shukla, M.; Sagar, N.; Dube, A.; Rath, S.K.; Mishra, P.R. Synergistic enhancement of parasiticidal activity of amphotericin B using copaiba oil in nanoemulsified carrier for oral delivery: An approach for non-toxic chemotherapy. *Br. J. Pharmacol.* **2015**, *172*, 3596–3610. [CrossRef]
20. Nguyen, A.K.; Yang, K.H.; Bryant, K.; Li, J.; Joice, A.C.; Werbovetz, K.A.; Narayan, R.J. Microneedle-based delivery of Amphotericin B for treatment of cutaneous Leishmaniasis. *Biomed. Microdevices* **2019**, *21*, 8. [CrossRef]
21. Ruiz, H.K.; Serrano, D.R.; Dea-Ayuela, M.A.; Bilbao-Ramos, P.E.; Bolás-Fernández, F.; Torrado, J.J.; Molero, G. New amphotericin B-gamma cyclodextrin formulation for topical use with synergistic activity against diverse fungal species and *Leishmania spp.*. *Int. J. Pharm.* **2014**, *473*, 148–157. [CrossRef]
22. Perez, A.P.; Altube, M.J.; Schilrreff, P.; Apezteguia, G.; Celes, F.S.; Zacchino, S.; de Oliveira, C.I.; Romero, E.L.; Morilla, M.J. Topical amphotericin B in ultradeformable liposomes: Formulation, skin penetration study, antifungal and antileishmanial activity *in vitro*. *Colloids Surf. B Biointerfaces* **2016**, *139*, 190–198. [CrossRef]
23. Cascone, S.; Lamberti, G. Hydrogel-based commercial products for biomedical applications: A review. *Int. J. Pharm.* **2019**, 118803. [CrossRef]
24. Sosa, L.; Clares, B.; Alvarado, H.L.; Bozal, N.; Domenech, O.; Calpena, A.C. Amphotericin B releasing topical nanoemulsion for the treatment of candidiasis and aspergillosis. *Nanomedicine* **2017**, *13*, 2303–2312. [CrossRef]
25. Suñer, J.; Calpena, A.C.; Clares, B.; Cañadas, C.; Halbaut, L. Development of Clotrimazole Multiple W/O/W Emulsions as Vehicles for Drug Delivery: Effects of Additives on Emulsion Stability. *AAPS PharmSciTech* **2017**, *18*, 539–550.
26. Council regulation (EC) no 440/2008 Test guideline for skin absorption: In vitro method (B45). *J. Eur. Union* **2008**, *142*, 438–443.
27. World Medical Association. World medical association declaration of Helsinki: Ethical Principles for Medical Research Involving Human Subjects. *JAMA* **2013**, *310*, 2191–2194. [CrossRef]
28. Du Plessis, J.; Stefaniak, A.; Eloff, F.; John, S.; Agner, T.; Chou, T.C.; Nixon, R.; Steiner, M.; Franken, A.; Kudla, I.; et al. International guidelines for the in vivo assessment of skin properties in non-clinical settings: Part 2. Transepidermal water loss and skin hydration. *Skin. Res. Technol.* **2013**, *19*, 265–278. [CrossRef]

29. Pujol, A.; Urbán, P.; Riera, C.; Fisa, R.; Molina, I.; Salvador, F.; Estelrich, J.; Fernández-Busquets, X. Application of Quantum Dots to the Study of Liposome Targeting in Leishmaniasis and Malaria. *Int. J. Theoret. Appl. Nanotech.* **2014**, *2*, 1–8. [CrossRef]
30. Carrió, J.; de Colmenares, M.; Riera, C.; Gállego, M.; Arboix, M.; Portús, M. Leishmania infantum: Stage-specific activity of pentavalent antimony related with the assay conditions. *Exp. Parasitol.* **2000**, *95*, 209–214. [CrossRef]
31. Carrió, J.; Riera, C.; Gállego, M.; Portús, M. In vitro activity of pentavalent antimony derivates on promastigotes and intracellular amastigotes of Leishmania infantum strains from humans and dogs in Spain. *Acta Trop.* **2001**, *79*, 179–183. [CrossRef]
32. Moon, S.; Jambert, E.; Childs, M.; von Schoen-Angerer, T. A win-win solution? A critical analysis of tiered pricing to improve access to medicines in developing countries. *Glob. Helath* **2011**, *7*, 39–49. [CrossRef]
33. Formariz, T.P.; Sarmento, V.H.; Silva-Junior, A.A.; Scarpa, M.V.; Santilli, C.V.; Oliveira, A.G. Doxorubicin biocompatible O/W microemulsion stabilized by mixed surfactant containing soya phosphatidylcholine. *Colloids Surf. B Biointerfaces* **2006**, *51*, 54–61. [CrossRef]
34. Rolim, A.; Oishi, T.; Maciel, C.P.; Zague, V.; Pinto, C.A.; Kaneko, T.M.; Consiglieri, V.O.; Velasco, M.V. Total flavonoids quantification from O/W emulsion with extract of Brazilian plants. *Int. J. Pharm.* **2006**, *308*, 107–114. [CrossRef]
35. Berenguer, D.; Sosa, L.; Alcover, M.; Sessa, M.; Halbaut, L.; Guillén, C.; Fisa, R.; Calpena-Campmany, A.C.; Riera, C. Development and Characterization of a Semi-Solid Dosage Form of Meglumine Antimoniate for Topical Treatment of Cutaneous Leishmaniasis. *Pharmaceutics* **2019**, *11*, 613. [CrossRef]
36. Sierra, A.F.; Ramirez, M.L.; Campmany, A.C.; Martinez, A.R.; Naveros, B.C. In vivo and in vitro evaluation of the use of a newly developed melatonin loaded emulsion combined with UV filters as a protective agent against skin irradiation. *J. Dermatol. Sci.* **2013**, *69*, 202–214. [CrossRef]
37. Alvarado, H.L.; Abrego, G.; Souto, E.B.; Garduño-Ramírez, M.L.; Clares, B.; García, M.L.; Calpena, A.C. Nanoemulsions for dermal controlled release of oleanolic and ursolic acids: In vitro, ex vivo and in vivocharacterization. *Colloids Surf. B Biointerfaces* **2015**, *130*, 40–47. [CrossRef]
38. Sosa, L.; Calpena, A.C.; Silva-Abreu, M.; Espinoza, L.C.; Rincón, M.; Bozal, N.; Domenech, O.; Rodríguez-Lagunas, M.J.; Clares, B. Thermoreversible Gel-Loaded Amphotericin B for the treatment of Dermal and Vaginal Candidiasis. *Pharmaceutics* **2019**, *11*, 312. [CrossRef]
39. Rizzo, J.A.; Martini, A.K.; Pruskowski, K.A.; Rowan, M.P.; Niece, K.L.; Akers, K.S. Thermal stability of mafenide and amphotericin B topical solution. *Burns* **2018**, *44*, 475–480. [CrossRef]
40. Hussain, A.; Samad, A.; Singh, S.K.; Ahsan, M.N.; Faruk, A.; Ahmed, F.J. Enhanced stability and permeation potential of nanoemulsion containing sefsol-218 oil for topical delivery of amphotericin B. *Drug Dev. Ind. Pharm.* **2015**, *41*, 780–790. [CrossRef]
41. Suñer-Carbó, J.; Calpena-Campmany, A.; Halbaut-Bellowa, L.; Clares-Naveros, B.; Rodriguez-Lagunas, M.J.; Barbolini, E.; Zamarbide-Losada, J.; Boix-Montañés, A. Biopharmaceutical Development of a Bifonazole Multiple Emulsion for Enhanced Epidermal Delivery. *Pharmaceutics* **2019**, *11*, 66. [CrossRef]
42. Martín-Villena, M.J.; Fernández-Campos, F.; Calpena-Campmany, A.C.; Bozal-de Febrer, N.; Ruiz-Martínez, M.A.; Clares-Naveros, B. Novel microparticulate systems for the vaginal delivery of nystatin: Development and characterization. *Carbohydr. Polym.* **2013**, *94*, 1–11. [CrossRef]
43. Potúckova, M.; Vitková, Z.; Tichý, E.; Simunková, V. Indometacin releae in relation to the concentration of pharmaceutical excipients. *Pharmazie* **2008**, *63*, 485–486.
44. Dar, M.J.; Khalid, S.; McElroy, C.A.; Satoskar, A.R.; Khan, G.M. Topical treatment of cutaneous leishmaniasis with novel amphotericin B-miltefosine co-incorporated second generation ultra-deformable liposomes. *Int. J. Pharm.* **2019**, 118900. [CrossRef]
45. Maes, L.; Beyers, J.; Mondelaers, A.; Van der Kerkhof, M.; Eberhardt, E.; Caljon, G.; Hendrickx, S. In vitro 'time-to-kill' assay to assess the cidal activity dynamics of current reference drugs against Leishmania donovani and Leishmania infantum. *J. Antimicrob. Chemother.* **2017**, *72*, 428–430. [CrossRef]
46. Handler, M.Z.; Patel, P.A.; Kapila, R.; Al-Qubati, Y.; Schwarts, R.A. Cutaneous and mucocutaneous leishmaniasis: Differential diagnosis, diagnosis, histopathology, and management. *J. Am. Acad. Dermatol.* **2015**, *73*, 911–926. [CrossRef]

47. Jaafari, M.R.; Hatamipour, M.; Alavizadeh, S.H.; Abbasi, A.; Saberi, Z.; Rafati, S.; Taslimi, Y.; Mohammadi, A.M.; Khamesipour, A. Development of a topical liposomal formulation of Amphotericin B for the treatment of cutaneous leishmaniasis. *Drugs Drug Resist.* **2019**, *11*, 156–165. [CrossRef]
48. Hussain, A.; Singh, V.K.; Singh, O.P.; Shafaat, K.; Kumar, S.; Ahmad, F.J. Formulation and optimization of nanoemulsion using antifungal lipid and surfactant for accentuated accentuated topical delivery of Amphotericin B. *Drug Deliv.* **2016**, *23*, 3101–3110. [CrossRef]
49. Hussain, A.; Singh, S.; Webster, T.J.; Ahmad, F.J. New perspectives in the topical delivery of optimized amphotericin B loaded nanoemulsions using excipients with innate anti-fungal activities: A mechanistic and histopathological investigation. *Nanomedicine* **2017**, *13*, 1117–1126. [CrossRef]
50. Marzulli, F.N.; Callahan, J.F.; Brown, D.W. Chemical structure and skin penetrating capacity of a short series of organic phosphates and phosphoric acid. *J. Investig. Dermatol.* **1965**, *44*, 339–344. [CrossRef]
51. Mehanna, M.M.; Motawaa, A.M.; Samaha, M.W. Nanovesicular carrier-mediated transdermal delivery of tadalafil: I-formulation and physicsochemical characterization. *Drug Dev. Ind. Pharm.* **2015**, *41*, 714–721. [CrossRef] [PubMed]
52. Van Bocxlaer, K.; Yardley, V.; Murdan, S.; Croft, S.L. Drug permeation and barrier damage in *Leishmania*-infected mouse skin. *J. Antimicrob. Chemother.* **2016**, *71*, 1578–1585. [CrossRef] [PubMed]
53. Van Ravenzwaay, B.; Leibold, E. A comparison between in vitro rat and human and in vivo rat skin absorption studies. *Hum. Exp. Toxicol.* **2004**, *23*, 421–430. [CrossRef] [PubMed]
54. Jaulent, C.; Dereure, O.; Raison-Peyron, N. Contact dermatitis caused by polyacrylamide/C13-4 isoparaffin/laureth-7 mix in an emollient cream for atopic skin. *Contact Dermat.* **2019**, *81*, 70–71. [CrossRef] [PubMed]
55. Eskandari, S.E.; Firooz, A.; Nassiri-Kashani, M.; Jaafari, M.R.; Javadi, A.; Miramin Mohammadi, A.; Khamesipour, A. Safety Evaluation of Topical Application of Nano-Liposomal Form of Amphotericin B (SinaAmpholeish) on Healthy Volunteers: Phase I Clinical Trial. *Iran J. Parasitol.* **2019**, *14*, 197–203. [CrossRef]
56. López, L.; Vélez, I.; Asela, C.; Cruz, C.; Alves, F.; Robledo, S.; Arana, B. A phase II study to evaluate the safety and efficacy of topical 3% amphotericin B cream (Anfoleish) for the treatment of uncomplicated cutaneous leishmaniasis in Colombia. *PLoS Negl. Trop. Dis.* **2018**, *12*, e0006653. [CrossRef]

pharmaceutics

MDPI

Article

A Validated IVRT Method to Assess Topical Creams Containing Metronidazole Using a Novel Approach

Seeprarani Rath [1] and Isadore Kanfer [1,2,*]

1 Division of Pharmaceutics, Faculty of Pharmacy, Rhodes University, Grahamstown 6139, South Africa; seeprarath81@gmail.com

2 Leslie Dan Faculty, University of Toronto, Toronto, ON M5S 3M2, Canada

* Correspondence: izzy.kanfer@utoronto.ca; Tel.: +1-416-568-0322

Received: 24 October 2019; Accepted: 1 December 2019; Published: 3 February 2020

Abstract: An IVRT method was developed and validated to confirm its reproducibility, precision, sensitivity, selectivity, accuracy, robustness, and reliability. A novel approach was used to demonstrate the appropriateness of the IVRT method to accurately assess "sameness" between topical products and to confirm that the methodology applied also possesses the requisite discriminatory power to detect differences should such differences exist between products. In the first instance, the reference product (Metrocreme®) containing 0.75% metronidazole (MTZ) was tested against itself as a positive control, to accurately demonstrate "sameness", where the results met the relevant acceptance criteria falling within the limits of 75–133.33% in accordance with the FDA's SUPAC-SS guidance. In addition, two specially prepared creams containing 25% less and 26% more MTZ, i.e., 0.563% and 0.945%, served as negative controls and were compared against the reference product. Neither of these creams fell within the "sameness" acceptance criteria, thereby confirming the discriminatory ability of the IVRT method to detect differences between MTZ products. Furthermore, another cream containing 0.75% MTZ tested against the reference product was shown to be pharmaceutically equivalent to the reference product. These results confirm the appropriateness of the IVRT method as a valuable tool for use in the development of topical MTZ products intended for local action and indicate the potential for general use with other topical products.

Keywords: IVRT; metronidazole; topical cream; semisolid dosage forms; sameness; FDA's SUPAC-SS guidance; acceptance criteria; positive and negative controls; discriminatory ability

1. Introduction

In vitro release testing (IVRT) entails measurement of the drug released from the vehicle into a receptor medium, separated by an inert membrane [1] and used to quantify the amount of active pharmaceutical ingredient (API) released from semisolid dosage forms and to determine its release rate [2]. The application of IVRT to assess "sameness" of semisolid dosage forms following minor changes related to an approved topical dosage form was described in the United States Food and Drug Administration's (FDA's) SUPAC-SS guidance [3]. Furthermore, IVRT is a USP compendial method used for performance testing of semisolid dosage forms [4] and is also an extremely useful tool in product development [5]. It has been proven to be useful to detect differences in qualitative (Q1) and quantitative (Q2) properties between similar products and also in the microstructure and arrangement of matter between formulations (Q3) [6]. In 2003, the experts from FIP/AAPS pointed out that there was an absence of a standard in vitro test that could be applied to semisolid dosage forms [7]. Until recently, however, amongst the numerous publications involving the application of IVRT, comprehensive validation of IVRT systems and methods have been conspicuously absent from the literature. Although various efforts [8–10] have been made by several researchers to develop a standardized method to measure in vitro drug release from a product using diffusion cells, a comprehensive validation that would be generally applicable to all topical dermatological dosage forms has only recently been published [11]. This is essential to ensure that the developed IVRT method and the associated system has the necessary discriminatory capabilities to determine "sameness" between products and also, more importantly, differences, which may affect clinical performance.

Since clinical endpoint studies have been made mandatory by most of the regulatory authorities to establish the safety and efficacy of generic topical products except in the case of topical corticosteroid products wherein a vasoconstrictor assay (VCA) or human skin blanching assay (HSBA) is accepted in accordance with the US FDA's guidance, an appropriate IVRT method could provide valuable and compelling information to justify waivers of bioequivalence studies (biowaivers) for topical semisolid products intended for local action. In this respect, it is interesting to note that the US FDA [12–15] and the European Medicines Agency (EMA) [16] have published guidances that recommend the use of IVRT for such purposes. It is interesting to note that the abovementioned FDA guidances are product-specific and the acceptance criteria are based on those recommended in the USP [4], in accordance with the FDA's SUPAC-SS guidance [3], whereas the acceptance criteria in the recent EMA draft guideline [16] are more stringent. Furthermore, the EMA draft guideline [16] describes the validation conditions and requisite discriminatory power of the method to support claims of therapeutic equivalence with a reference product instead of undertaking clinical trials.

In view of the fact that market approval of a generic topical metronidazole (MTZ) product requires a clinical endpoint study in patients to show safety and efficacy of such products, an IVRT method was developed to investigate "sameness" and differences between a test formulation and the market-approved reference product, Metrocreme®. The primary objective, therefore, was to investigate the feasibility of using a nonclinical approach, such as IVRT, for consideration as a biowaiver to obtain market approval. Consequently, an attempt was made to develop and comprehensively validate an IVRT method which has the necessary discriminatory power to detect "sameness" and differences in topical cream products containing 0.75% MTZ. A novel approach of incorporating a positive control wherein the reference product was compared to itself and two negative controls, i.e., products containing <25% or >25% potency compared to the reference product, was implemented.

2. Materials and Methods

2.1. Materials

2.1.1. Chemicals

MTZ was obtained from Sigma-Aldrich and stored in a cool, dry area that was free from light exposure. HPLC-grade methanol (200 UV ROMIL—SpSTM Super Purity Solvent) was obtained from Romil Ltd. (Waterbeach, Cambridge, UK). The water used for chromatography was prepared by reverse osmosis, followed by filtration through a Milli-Q system (Millipore, Bedford, MA, USA).

2.1.2. Formulations

Metrocreme® (Galderma Laboratorium GmbH, Dusseldorf, Germany) containing 0.75% MTZ was used as the reference MTZ cream. Creams containing 0.375%, 0.75% (T_1), and 1.125% MTZ were specially manufactured to validate the IVRT method. In addition, creams T_2 and T_3, which contained 25% less (0.563%) and 26% more (0.945%) MTZ than the reference product were used as negative controls at the lower and upper acceptance limits, respectively, in accordance with the SUPAC-SS limits [3], to establish the utility of the developed and validated IVRT method to assess inequivalence. Test cream (T_1) was also used to assess "sameness" for the purpose of marketing a generic MTZ cream.

2.1.3. Equipment

Mettler® Model AE 135 analytical balance (Mettler® Inc, Zurich, Switzerland) and MX5 Mettler® Toledo Microbalance (Mettler® Inc, Zurich, Switzerland) were used for weighing samples and standards, respectively. Micropipettes P100 and P1000 (Pipetman™, Gilson®, Villiers-le-Bel, France) were used to transfer standard and sample solutions for dilutions.

The concentration of hydrocortisone in PVT samples was analyzed on a Waters Alliance HPLC system that was equipped with a separation module (Model 2695) and a PDA detector (Model 2996) and Empower® 3 data acquisition system (Waters, CT, USA). The chromatographic separation was achieved by using a Phenomenex Luna® C18 (2) 5 µm (150 × 4.6 mm) column (Torrance, CA, USA) maintained at 25 °C. The mobile phase consisted of acetonitrile: water (30:70 *v*/*v*). A flow rate of 1 mL/min was maintained, and a detection wavelength of 254 nm was used. Samples were injected at ambient temperature during analysis.

The concentrations of MTZ were determined by using a Waters Acquity UPLC system equipped with a photo diode array detector (PDA), Empower® 3 data acquisition system (Waters, Milford, MA, USA). The chromatographic separation was achieved by using an Acquity UPLC BEH C18 1.7 µm (2.1 × 100 mm). A mobile phase of methanol/water (40/60 *v*/*v*) was pumped at a flow rate of 0.2 mL/min, and the eluate was monitored at a wavelength of 318 nm. Samples (2 µL) were injected at ambient temperature during analysis.

In vitro release studies were performed by using a Hanson VDC system (Hanson Research Corporation, Chatsworth, CA, USA) consisting of six vertical diffusion cells (Volume: 7.9 mL, orifice: 15 mm) with closed cell tops, mounted on a six-station LGA platform and a magnetic stirrer (Variomag®, Berkley, CA, USA), and a Control Unit (Telemodul 40S H+P Labortechnik GmbH, Munich, Germany), connected to a PolyScience circulating water bath (Niles, IL, USA). The diffusion cells and apparatus were assembled with donor and receptor chambers that were separated by a chosen membrane. The receptor chamber was filled with 7.9 mL of SABAX Pour Saline (0.9% NaCl solution, Adcock Ingram Critical Care (Pty) Ltd., Midrand, South Africa), which served as the receptor fluid and maintained at 32 °C (to mimic the physiological temperature). The receptor medium was continuously stirred, using individual magnetic stirrer bars, coupled with helical mixer springs, in each of the VDCs. One-milliliter syringes (Terumo® (Philippines) Corporation, Laguna, Philippines) with sampling needles (21G x 3.5″ Terumo® Spinal Needle, Terumo® Corporation, Tokyo, Japan) were purchased from local pharmacies.

2.2. Methods

2.2.1. UPLC Method Validation

The UPLC method was validated according to ICH guidelines and relevant criteria, as described by Tiffner et al. [11].

2.2.2. Apparatus Qualification

Factors that can influence the drug release were assessed to comply with the requirements of an apparatus qualification test in accordance with the USP procedures for apparatus qualification for the VDC system [4,17]. Environmental factors such as suitable working area, workbench levelness, no direct exposure to sunlight and/or direct cooling vents, and failure-resistant power supply to all the electronic components were ensured. The system was placed on a dedicated sturdy wooden workbench with a free distance of more than 76 cm above the system. Additionally, the orifice diameters and capacities of each of the VDCs, the temperature of the receptor medium, stirrer speed, and the dispensed sample volume were validated.

2.2.3. Performance Verification Test (PVT)

The PVT was performed by using 1% hydrocortisone cream (Emo-Cort®, GlaxoSmithKline Inc., Mississauga, ON, Canada) applied on Tuffryn membranes [17,18]. Two IVRT runs were performed, each with six VDCs in parallel, by stirring the receptor medium at 600 rpm and maintaining the receptor medium temperature at 32 ± 1 °C. Prior to the commencement of the experiment, the receptor chambers were filled with degassed receptor medium consisting of ethanol: water (30:70 *v*/*v*) and VDC system were allowed to equilibrate at 32 ± 1 °C for approximately 30 min. The cream was accurately weighed (~300 mg) and applied evenly onto the relevant membranes, which had been presoaked in the receptor medium for 30 min. Aliquots of 200 µL were withdrawn from the receptor chambers of each of the 6 VDCs at 1, 2, 3, 4, 5, and 6 h, and the VDCs were subsequently replenished with 200 µL of receptor medium after each withdrawal.

2.2.4. MTZ Solubility and Receptor-Fluid Selection

Various receptor fluids such as SABAX Pour Saline (0.9% NaCl solution, Adcock Ingram Critical Care (Pty) Ltd., Midrand, South Africa), lactate buffer pH 4.5, phosphate buffer pH 4.5, phosphate buffer pH 6.8, water/ethanol (50:50 *v*/*v*), phosphate buffer pH 4.5: ethanol (50:50 *v*/*v*), and 0.9% NaCl solution/ethanol (50:50 *v*/*v*) were investigated. The solubility of MTZ in these receptor fluids was evaluated in triplicate by placing 200 mg MTZ in 10 mL of receptor fluid to yield a saturated solution. The solution was stirred for 6 h at 600 rpm and 32 ± 1 °C and allowed to stand at 32 ± 1 °C overnight [11]. Aliquots of the supernatant were withdrawn, filtered, diluted, and then analyzed on a UPLC, to determine the concentration of dissolved MTZ. The receptor medium should be able to dissolve >10-fold maximum expected concentration of the drug.

2.2.5. Membrane Screening

Membrane screening was carried out by using various synthetic membranes: Magna Nylon (0.45 µm, 25 mm, GVS Life Sciences, Sanford, ME, USA); Tuffryn (0.45 µm, 25 mm, Pall Corporation, Ann Arbor, MN, USA); HVLP (0.45 µm, 47 mm, Merck Millipore Ltd., Ireland); Cellulose acetate (0.45 µm, 25 mm, Sartorius, Göttingen, Germany); Mixed Cellulose Ester (0.45 µm, 47 mm, Advantec MFS, Inc., Pleasanton, CA, USA), and Strat-M® (25 mm, Millipore, MA, USA). Binding of MTZ to the membranes was investigated by immersing individual membranes ($n = 3$) in 10 mL of 0.9% sodium chloride solution containing MTZ at 32 ± 1 °C, for 6 h. The test solution without any immersed membrane, prepared in triplicate, was allowed to equilibrate for 6 h at 32 ± 1 °C and was used as a control. The MTZ concentrations in all the solutions were determined by using the UPLC method described above. Recoveries were calculated for each of the test solutions containing the membranes by comparing them with the control solution. The mean percent recovery for each membrane should be within ±5% [11].

2.2.6. Sampling Duration

IVRT runs were performed by varying the duration of the runs and the sampling intervals. Three runs were performed—6 h IVRT run with sampling at every 30 min; a 3 h run with sampling at every 15 min; and a 1.5 h run with sampling at every 15 min. The sampling duration with desired linearity ($R^2 > 0.95$) and recovery (≤30%) was considered based on Higuchi's assumptions [19,20]. At least 6 sampling intervals were used.

2.2.7. IVRT Method

Each of the IVRT runs was conducted by using six VDCs in parallel, and the receptor medium was stirred at 600 rpm, while maintaining the temperature at 32 ± 1 °C. Prior to the commencement of the experiment, the receptor chambers were filled with degassed 0.9% NaCl solution, and the VDC system was allowed to equilibrate at 32 ± 1 °C, for approximately 30 min. The cream was accurately weighed (~300 mg) and applied evenly onto the Nylon membranes, which had been presoaked in the receptor medium for 30 min. Aliquots of 200 µL were withdrawn from the receptor chambers of each of the 6 VDCs every 15 min for 90 min, and the VDCs were subsequently replenished with 200 µL of receptor medium after each withdrawal. The stirring was stopped during sample withdrawal and immediately resumed once the aliquots were withdrawn and receptor media replenished in all the VDCs. Care was taken that the duration between the stopping and resumption of the stirring was less than 1.5 min. The aliquots were analyzed by using the UPLC method described above.

2.2.8. Calculation of Release Rates

The periodical concentrations of MTZ measured using a UPLC method were used to determine the amount of API released. The Higuchi model, which assumes the existence of perfect sink conditions, was used to determine the release rates, using Equation (1). Dilution of the receptor medium due to replacement of the sampled amount was taken into account, and the concentrations of MTZ in the receptor medium (C_n) at different sampling times were calculated, using Equation (1).

$$Q_n = C_n \frac{V_c}{A_c} + \frac{V_s}{A_c} \sum_{i=1}^{n} C_{i-1} \quad (1)$$

where

Q_n = amount released at time (n) per unit area in µg/cm^2;
C_n = concentration of drug in receptor medium at different sampling times (n) in µg/cm^3;
V_s = volume of the sample in cm^3;
V_c = volume of the cell in cm^3;
A_c = area of the orifice of the cell in cm^2.

In accordance with Higuchi's square root approximations [20] given by Equation (2), a plot of Q vs. $\sqrt{t}$ will be linear with a slope of $\sqrt{2ADC_s}$.

$$Q = \sqrt{2ADC_s t} \quad (2)$$

where

Q = the amount absorbed at time t per unit area of exposure µg/cm^2;
A = the concentration of drug expressed in µg/cm^3;
C_s = the solubility of the drug in µg/cm^3;
D = the diffusion constant of the drug molecule.

Hence, the release rate corresponds to the slope of the regression line of the plot of Q_n vs. $\sqrt{t}$. Q_n is affected by sample volume, VDC volume, and by the diameter of the orifice of the VDC. Hence, these parameters were carefully evaluated during apparatus qualification [11,17].

2.2.9. Validation of the IVRT Method

The IVRT system was validated in accordance with the method described by Tiffner et al. [11]. Metrocreme® (Galderma Laboratorium GmbH, Düsseldorf, Germany) containing 0.75% MTZ, being an RLD, was used as the reference MTZ cream. Cream products containing 0.375%, 0.75%, and 1.125% MTZ were used to establish the sensitivity, selectivity, and specificity of the IVRT method.

Differences in release rates between the creams containing different concentrations of MTZ were evaluated to determine the sensitivity of the method.

Specificity of the method was assessed by investigating proportionality of the MTZ release rate to the MTZ concentration in the test creams. A box and whisker plot was prepared to estimate the coefficient of determination (R^2). The specificity of the method can be confirmed if a specifically proportional linear relationship can be established between the formulations of different strengths, i.e., $R^2 > 0.9$.

The statistical approach for product "sameness" testing described in the USP general chapter <1724> [4] was applied to analyze all results. The selectivity of the IVRT method was investigated by determining the release rates of the lower and higher strengths of MTZ test creams (i.e., 0.375% and 1.125%, respectively) and compared with the release rates of the 0.75% MTZ test cream. Pairwise comparisons of MTZ release rates in three IVRT runs performed as a part of linearity, precision, and reproducibility investigations were evaluated in order to establish whether the reference, Metrocreme®, 0.75% MTZ was equivalent to itself.

The effect of two temperature variations (−2 and +2 °C) relative to the nominal temperature of 32 °C (at 32 ± 1 °C) and also two stirring-rate variations (−60 rpm and +60 rpm) relative to the nominal stirring rate of 600 rpm were investigated in order to determine the robustness of the method to minor perturbations, using the reference product, Metrocreme®, 0.75% MTZ.

Dose depletion was assessed by determining the amounts of MTZ released from the cream during the IVRT runs and recovered in the receptor solution. The recovery was calculated by dividing the average cumulative amount released at the last time point (t = 90 min) by the amount of MTZ present in the applied dose (~2.25 mg) by using data from each of the 18 VDCs within the 3 IVRT runs.

2.2.10. Comparative IVRT of MTZ Cream Products

In order to confirm the utility of the developed and validated IVRT method for assessment of "sameness" and differences between MTZ creams, comparative IVRT runs were conducted with the test (T_1, T_2, and T_3) and the reference cream. The testing was carried out in accordance with the FDA's SUPAC-SS guidance [3]. Initially, two IVRT runs were carried out to compare T_1 and the reference, such that the arrangement enabled the measurement of drug release from each of the creams in all six cells at the end of the experiment. Following this, three IVRT runs were carried out to compare creams T_2 and T_3 with the reference, to serve as negative controls in such a way that the drug release from each of the creams was measured in all six cells at the end of the experiment. Additionally, the two IVRT runs conducted as a part of IVRT validation served to determine whether the method can accurately detect "sameness", wherein the reference product was compared to itself to serve as a positive control.

The cumulative amount of MTZ released per unit area was plotted against the square root of time and the release rates were determined. A total of six release rates per cream were obtained. Pairwise comparison was carried out by computing the ratios of release rates (T/R ratios) and establishing the 90% confidence interval (CI), using the Mann–Whitney U Test, where the 90% CI should lie within the limits of 75–133.33% to confirm "sameness" between products, in accordance with the FDA's SUPAC-SS guidance [3].

3. Results

3.1. Validation of the UPLC Method and Qualification of the IVRT System

The developed UPLC method was validated for the analysis of MTZ in IVRT samples, and the results are summarized in Table 1, according to the acceptance criteria defined in the ICH guidelines. The results for qualification of the IVRT system are described in Table 2.

Table 1. Predefined acceptance criteria and the results obtained from the UPLC validation for IVRT method [11].

Parameter	Acceptance Criteria	Results	Pass
Selectivity and specificity	$\overline{RT_p} - \overline{RT_{pm}} < 10\%$ $IC_n = 0$ μg/mL, $IC_{nm} = 0$ μg/mL	0.063% $IC_n = 0$ μg/mL, $IC_{nm} = 0$ μg/mL	Yes
Linearity	75% of the standards meet the following criteria: For 5–100 μg/mL: $IC_{meas,lin} \in [IC_{nom} \pm 15\%]$ For 0.5 μg/mL: $IC_{meas,lin} \in [IC_{nom} \pm 20\%]$ $R^2 \geq 0.950$	30 out of 30 standards (100%) met the acceptance criteria $R^2 \geq 0.999$	Yes
Accuracy	For IS_{100} and IS_{50}: $\overline{IS_{meas,ac}} \in [IS_{nom} \pm 15\%]$ For IS_5: $\overline{IS_{meas,ac}} \in [IS_{nom} \pm 20\%]$	0.69% and 1.48% for IS_{100} and IS_{50} 2.08% for IS_5	Yes
Precision	Intra-day CV < 15% for IS_{100} to IS_{50} Intra-day CV < 20% for IS_5	1.30%, 0.63%, and 0.66% for IS_{100} 1.03%, 0.93%, and 0.11% for IS_{50} 1.07%, 6.29%, and 7.35% forIS_5	Yes
	Inter-day CV < 15% for IS_{100} to IS_{50} Inter-day CV < 20% for IS_5	6.00% for IS_{100} 0.72% for IS_{50} 1.07% for IS_5	Yes
Robustness	Inter-run CV < 15% for IS_{100} to IS_{50} Inter-run CV < 20% for IS_5	10.03% for IS_{100} 9.05% for IS_{50} 9.27% for IS_5	Yes
Stability	For IS_{100} and IS_{50}: $\overline{IS_{meas,ac}} \in [IS_{nom} \pm 15\%]$ For IS_5: $\overline{IS_{meas,ac}} \in [IS_{nom} \pm 20\%]$	Bench-top after 7 days: 0.22% for IS_{100} 0.36% for IS_{50} 5.01% for IS_5 UPLC machine after 7 days: 0.23% for IS_{100} 0.29% for IS_{50} 0.45% for IS_5 Refrigerator after 7 days: 0.34% for IS_{100} 0.11% for IS_{50} 0.49% for IS_5	Yes
LLOQ, LOD	-	LLOQ: 0.5 μg/mL LOD: 0.167 μg/mL	

RT_p = retention time of MTZ in positive control (min). RT_{pm} = retention time of MTZ in matrix positive control (min). IC_n = concentration in negative control (μg/mL). IC_{nm} = concentration in matrix negative control (μg/mL). $IC_{meas,lin}$ = measured concentration during the linearity run (μg/mL). IC_{nom} = nominal concentration (μg/mL). $IS_{meas,ac}$ = measured average concentration of the spiked solutions in the accuracy run (μg/mL). IS_{nom} = nominal concentration of the spiked solutions (μg/mL). IS_x = concentration of the spiked samples where x is concentration in μg/mL.

Table 2. Predefined acceptance criteria and the results obtained from apparatus qualification for the VDC system.

Parameter	Acceptance Criteria		Results		Pass
	Mean ± Tolerance	Range of Variation	Mean	Range of Variation	
Capacity of the cells	7.00 ± 0.35 mL	≤0.21 mL	7.92 mL	0.02 mL	No
Diameter of the orifice	15.00 ± 0.75 mm	≤0.45 mm	14.98 mm	0.10 mm	Yes
Temperature of the receptor medium	32 ± 1 °C	-	32.07 °C	0.05 °C	Yes
Speed of the magnetic stirrer	600 ± 60 rpm	≤12 rpm	601.67 rpm	2.53 rpm	Yes
Dispensed sampling volume	200 ± 10 μL	-	203.67 μL	4.58 μL	Yes
Bench top levelness	Not more than 1°		<1°		Yes

3.2. *Performance Verification Test*

The results obtained from the PVT runs are summarized in Table 3.

Table 3. Predefined acceptance criteria and results of the performance verification test (PVT).

Parameter	Acceptance Criteria	Results
Intra-run variability	Intra-run CV for the first run (*n* = 6 VDCs) < 15%	8.13%
	Intra-run CV for the second run (*n* = 6 VDCs) < 15%	12.85%
Inter-run variability	Inter-run CV for both runs (*n* = 12 VDCs) < 15%	10.30%
Product "sameness" testing	The 90% CI should fall within the limits of 75–133.33%	Lower limit: 87.82% Upper limit: 116.52%

3.3. *Receptor-Fluid Selection*

The observed solubilities of MTZ were >2848.10 μg/mL in all the receptor fluids, which is >10 times the maximum expected concentration.

3.4. *Membrane Screening*

Average percentage recoveries of 98.47 ± 0.81, 98.07 ± 2.09, 97.84 ± 1.27, 97.70 ± 1.63, 96.80 ± 1.97, and 91.04 ± 3.28 for Nylon, Tuffryn, Cellulose acetate, Strat-M, HVLP, and Mixed Cellulose Ester, respectively, were obtained.

3.5. *Sampling Duration*

The release rates and coefficients of determination (R^2) for different times are shown in Table 4. Significant differences between release rates by using different sampling durations were observed by using the F-test, which generated p-values > 0.05.

Table 4. Differences in parameters observed by using various sampling duration (mean ± SD).

Time (min)	Release Rate (μg/cm^2/min$^{1/2}$)	R^2 Value	Recovery (%)
90	39.47 ± 2.30	0.998 ± 0.003	29.90 ± 1.20
180	34.19 ± 1.97	0.988 ± 0.006	38.32 ± 1.19
360	27.58 ± 2.09	0.994 ± 0.002	42.75 ± 3.57

3.6. *Validation of the IVRT Method*

The results obtained from the three IVRT runs of 0.75% MTZ cream confirmed a linear relationship ($R^2 \geq 0.99$) between the amount of drug released and the square root of time.

The mean release rates for 0.375%, 0.75%, and 1.125% MTZ creams were 19.17 μg/cm^2/min$^{1/2}$, 40.04 μg/cm^2/min$^{1/2}$, and 66.28 μg/cm^2/min$^{1/2}$, respectively, and a linear relationship ($R^2 = 0.9994$) was observed between the release rates of the different strengths of MTZ cream (Figure 1).

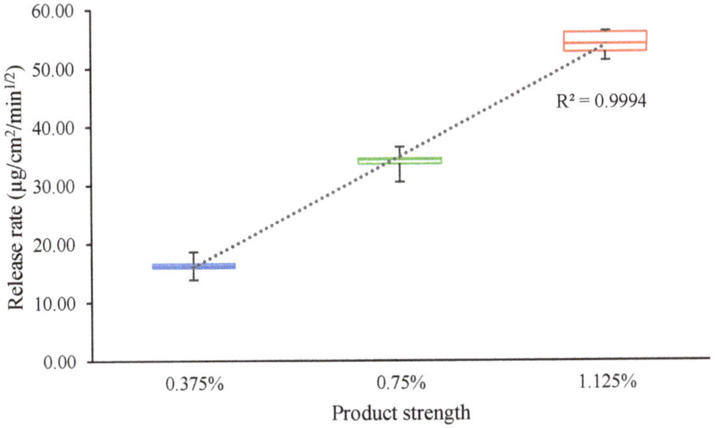

Figure 1. Box and whisker plot of the measured release rates for the three test MTZ creams, with concentrations of 0.5% (blue), 1% (green), and 1.5% (red).

The data to assess selectivity are depicted in Table 5, where the 90% CI for the reference product, Metrocreme®, 0.75% MTZ, against itself, fell within the acceptance criteria of 75–133.33% [3], whereas that for the 0.75% MTZ cream against the 0.375% and 1.125% MTZ creams fell completely outside the 75–133.33% limits.

Table 5. Computed 90% CI to assess the selectivity of the IVRT method.

Pairwise Comparison *	Computed 90% CI	
	Lower Limit	Upper Limit
0.375% MTZ cream vs. 0.75% MTZ cream	45.10	52.47
1.125% MTZ cream vs. 0.75% MTZ cream	152.04	167.79
Metrocreme®, 0.75% MTZ (run 1) vs. Metrocreme®, 0.75% MTZ (run 2)	93.61	100.22
Metrocreme®, 0.75% MTZ (run 1) vs. Metrocreme®, 0.75% MTZ (run 3)	87.40	97.66
Metrocreme®, 0.75% MTZ (run 2) vs. Metrocreme®, 0.75% MTZ (run 3)	93.06	99.76

* The release rates used for pairwise comparison are provided under supplementary materials in Tables S1–S5.

The mean release rates obtained for the robustness runs were 45.67 µg/cm^2/min$^{1/2}$ for 30 °C, 600 rpm; 47.83 µg/cm^2/min$^{1/2}$ for 34 °C, 600 rpm; 47.02 µg/cm^2/min$^{1/2}$ for 32 °C, 540 rpm; and 48.19 µg/cm^2/min$^{1/2}$ for 32 °C, 660 rpm.

The mean recoveries for IVRT runs conducted as a part of linearity, precision, and reproducibility were found to be 30.27 ± 0.52%, 29.00 ± 0.60%, and 29.98 ± 0.81% respectively, confirming that the dose depletion was within the specified range of ≤30%.

3.7. Comparative IVRT of MTZ Topical Cream Products

A comparison between the reference and test product T_1 is depicted in Figure 2. The mean release rates were 37.80 ± 2.01 µg/cm^2/min$^{1/2}$ and 32.89 ± 1.60 µg/cm^2/min$^{1/2}$ for the reference and T_1, respectively. The calculated upper and lower limits for the pairwise comparison were 81.72% and 91.24%, which fell within the CI limits of 75–133.33% (supplementary materials, Table S6).

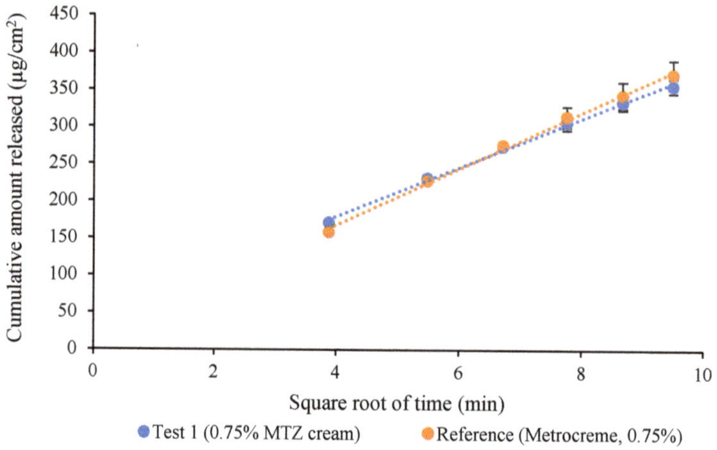

Figure 2. Release-rate curves from 0.75% MTZ cream (T_1) vs. Metrocreme®, 0.75% MTZ (R).

The comparison between the reference and the test products T_2 and T_3 is depicted in Figure 3. The mean release rates were 38.47 ± 1.35 μg/cm^2/min$^{1/2}$ for the reference and 27.42 ± 0.99 μg/cm^2/min$^{1/2}$ and 51.20 ± 0.60 μg/cm^2/min$^{1/2}$ for the test creams T_2 and T_3, respectively.

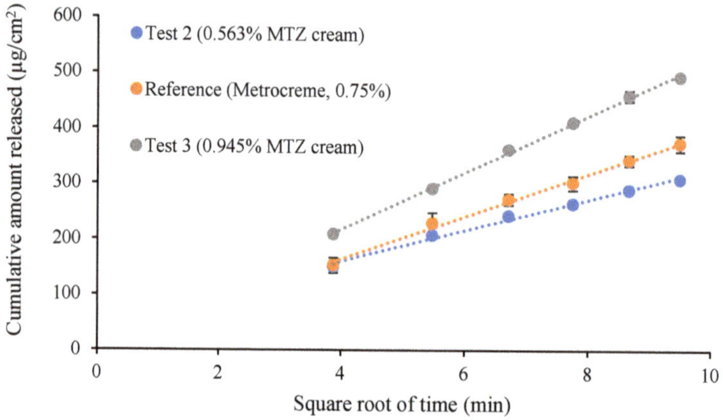

Figure 3. Release-rate curves from 0.563% and 0.945% MTZ cream (T_2 and T_3) vs. Metrocreme®, 0.75% MTZ (R) (n = 6).

The calculated upper and lower limits for the pairwise comparisons were outside the CI limits of 75–133.33% for both test creams (Table 6). The CI limits for the positive control were well within the acceptance criteria (75–133.33%), as shown in Table 6.

Table 6. Computed 90% CI for negative and positive controls used to assess discriminatory power of the IVRT method.

Pairwise Comparison *	Computed 90% CI		Decision
	Lower Limit	Upper Limit	
Positive control			
Metrocreme®, 0.75% MTZ vs. Metrocreme®, 0.75% MTZ	93.61	100.22	Pass
Negative controls			
0.563% MTZ cream vs. Metrocreme®, 0.75% MTZ	68.25	74.21	Fail
0.945% MTZ cream vs. Metrocreme®, 0.75% MTZ	128.36	137.11	Fail

* The release rates used for pairwise comparison are provided under supplementary materials in Tables S7–S9.

4. Discussion

The developed UPLC method, validated for the analysis of MTZ in IVRT samples in accordance with the ICH guidelines, met the acceptance criteria for all the validation parameters described by Tiffner et al. [11]. It was found to be selective, linear over a range of 0.5–100 μg/mL, accurate, precise, robust, sensitive with an LLOQ of 0.5 μg/mL, and offering sample stability for seven days. All the parameters essential for qualification of the IVRT system met the predefined acceptance criteria as described by Tiffner et al. [11], with an exception of the VDC volume. The mean capacity of the VDCs did not conform to the specifications provided by the manufacturer. However, it was precise and suitable for conducting IVRT experiments. Hence, the subsequent IVRT experiments were conducted by using these cells, and the calculations were tailored accordingly.

The results obtained from the PVT runs duly complied with the predefined acceptance criteria, and the low variabilities observed during the runs confirm the suitability and reproducibility of the IVRT system for its relevant application.

Although the observed solubilities of MTZ were >10 times the maximum expected concentration, as recommended [9], 0.9% NaCl solution was chosen as the receptor medium for subsequent studies, as it more appropriately reflects physiological conditions and is inexpensive and readily available. All the membranes except the Mixed Cellulose Ester membrane showed an acceptable recovery, indicating low MTZ binding. The membranes were therefore confirmed to be inert and would not act as a rate-limiting barrier for MTZ. Because of its higher-percentage recovery and availability, Nylon was chosen as the membrane of choice for this study.

The release profiles obtained from the IVRT runs with different sampling durations and intervals showed significant differences in MTZ release rates. It was observed that the release rates decreased considerably with time, whereas the recovery increased, resulting in curvature in the release profile. The profiles showed a deviation from linearity after 90 min. This is in agreement and closely correlated with the Higuchi's square root approximations [19,20]. Deviation from linearity of release of API from different semisolid dosage forms may be due to differences in physicochemical properties of such formulations. This can be explained by considering the square root approximations developed by Higuchi, which presumes that the percent of API released from the applied dose is ≤30%. The Higuchi equation describes the initial 30% release from topical formulations under perfect sink conditions as linear. Since the ultimate objective of this study was not to evaluate complete release from the cream but to assess the "sameness" between two creams containing 0.75% MTZ, an IVRT method spanning over a duration of 90 min, with a sampling interval of 15 min, was chosen in accordance with the Higuchi's approximation (recovery ≤30%).

The inter-run and intra-run variabilities were <15%, confirming that the IVRT method was precise and reproducible. The mean release rate for 0.75% MTZ cream was higher than that of 0.375% MTZ cream and lower than that of 1.125% MTZ cream, indicating that the method was sensitive to the changes in MTZ concentrations. The linear relationship (Figure 1) indicated that the release rate proportionately increased with the increase in MTZ concentration, demonstrating the specificity of the developed IVRT method. The IVRT method has the necessary ability to determine "sameness" as the 90% CI for the reference product, Metrocreme®, 0.75% MTZ, against itself, fell within the acceptance criteria of 75–133.33% [3]. Furthermore, the ability of the method to assess differences was confirmed as the 90% CI for the 0.75% MTZ cream against the 0.375% and 1.125% MTZ creams fell completely outside the 75–133.33% limits. From the results obtained, it is evident that the method also has the discriminatory ability to detect differences in MTZ concentrations between the respective products. This outcome was expected, as the creams (0.375%, 0.75%, and 1.125%) differed only in terms of Q2 properties (i.e., the amount of MTZ) and contained the same ingredients and also were manufactured using the same process. Q1 and Q3 properties were therefore constant for all the creams. The developed IVRT method is thus sensitive to the changes in the formulations specifically related to differences in Q2. Minor differences in stirring rates (±60 rpm) or temperature (±2 °C) did not significantly affect MTZ release rates, i.e., they did not deviate from the nominal values by more than 15%. These results suggest that the developed IVRT method possesses the necessary properties to confirm robustness.

Since it is important to confirm the discriminatory ability of the IVRT method, both positive and negative controls were included to indicate "sameness" and differences, if any, in terms of the FDA's SUPAC-SS acceptance criteria [3]. Interestingly, acceptance criteria of 90–111% with a 90% CI was recommended in the recent EMA draft guideline [16]. This increased stringency is somewhat questionable. The reference product was used as a positive control when compared to itself during validation studies, whereas, for different strengths of the MTZ creams at concentrations below (T_2) and above (T_3) the acceptance limits were used as negative controls. Accordingly, a comparison between the reference and test product T_1 indicated "sameness" between the two creams, thereby confirming that the IVRT method has the requisite properties.

Based on the results from the positive control studies, the ability of the IVRT method to indicate "sameness" was confirmed. Furthermore, data using negative controls indicated the capability of the IVRT method to detect inequivalence between MTZ creams.

5. Conclusions

The apparatus qualification and PVT of the IVRT system duly complied with the necessary requirements to assess the release of API from topical cream products. The low variabilities observed during the PVT runs confirm the suitability and reproducibility of the IVRT system for its relevant application. An IVRT method was carefully developed and comprehensively validated to assess the release of MTZ from cream products, taking into account the various parameters that may affect the API release rate. The validation procedures were carried out in accordance with the recommendations in both the FDA guidance [3,4] and EMA draft guideline [16]. It was then successfully applied to assess "sameness" for the purpose of marketing a generic MTZ cream, wherein a 0.75% MTZ cream was compared with the reference, Metrocreme®, 0.75% MTZ. Furthermore, the inclusion of a positive and negative controls was a novel approach to demonstrate the discriminatory power of the IVRT method. The positive and negative controls complied with the necessary acceptance criteria for equivalence and inequivalence, respectively, confirming the discriminatory power of the IVRT method. This is in accordance with the SUPAC-SS acceptance criteria [3] for a biowaiver, where generic products containing <25% or >25% potency compared to the reference product are deemed inequivalent. The resulting data indicate that the developed IVRT method can be applied to accurately and precisely assess "sameness" and differences (Q2) between MTZ cream products as a valuable procedure in formulation development. Furthermore, this method has potential for use as a tool to obtain a biowaiver for MTZ creams.

Supplementary Materials: The following are available online at http://www.mdpi.com/1999-4923/12/2/119/s1, Table S1: 0.375% MTZ cream vs 0.75% MTZ cream, Table S2: 1.125% MTZ cream vs 0.75% MTZ cream, Table S3: Metrocreme®, 0.75% MTZ (run 1) vs Metrocreme®, 0.75% MTZ (run 2), Table S4: Metrocreme®, 0.75% MTZ (run 1) vs Metrocreme®, 0.75% MTZ (run 3), Table S5: Metrocreme®, 0.75% MTZ (run 2) vs Metrocreme®, 0.75% MTZ (run 3), Table S6: 0.75% MTZ cream vs Metrocreme®, 0.75% MTZ, Table S7: Metrocreme®, 0.75% MTZ vs

Metrocreme®, 0.75% MTZ, Table S8: 0.563% MTZ cream vs Metrocreme®, 0.75% MTZ, Table S9: 0.945% MTZ cream vs Metrocreme®, 0.75% MTZ.

Author Contributions: Conceptualization, I.K.; Formal analysis, S.R.; Funding acquisition, I.K.; Investigation, S.R.; Methodology, S.R. and I.K.; Resources, I.K.; Software, S.R.; Supervision, I.K.; Validation, S.R.; Writing—original draft, S.R.; Writing—review & editing, I.K. All authors have read and agreed to the published version of the manuscript.

Funding: This research was funded by the Biopharmaceutics Research Institute, Rhodes University, Grahamstown, South Africa. BRI Grant No. 01012019.

Acknowledgments: GALENpharma GmbH, Kiel, Germany, is gratefully acknowledged for providing the test creams.

Conflicts of Interest: The authors declare no conflict of interest.

References

1. Shah, V.P. Progress in Methodologies for Evaluating Bioequivalence of Topical Formulations. *Am. J. Clin. Dermatol.* **2001**, *2*, 275–280. [CrossRef] [PubMed]
2. Olejnik, A.; Goscianska, J.; Nowak, I. Active Compounds Release from Semisolid Dosage Forms. *J. Food Drug Anal.* **2012**, *101*, 4032–4045. [CrossRef] [PubMed]
3. US Food and Drug Administration. *Guidance for Industry: Nonsterile Semisolid Dosage Forms, Scale-up and Post Approval Changes, Chemistry, Manufacturing, and Control;* In vitro Release Testing and In vivo Bioequivalence Documentation (SUPAC-SS); Center for Drug Evaluation and Research: Rockville, MD, USA, 1997.
4. USP General Chapter <1724> Semisolid Drug Products—Performance Tests. In *United States Pharmacopeia and National Formulary (USP 41-NF 36);* The United States Pharmacopeial Convention: Rockville, MD, USA, 2018; pp. 7944–7956.
5. Bashaw, E.D.; Benfeldt, E.; Davit, B.; Ganes, D.; Ghosh, T.; Kanfer, I.; Lionberger, R. Current Challenges in Bioequivalence, Quality, and Novel Assessment Technologies for Topical Products. *Pharm. Res.* **2014**, *31*, 837–846.
6. Ilić, T.; Pantelić, I.; Lunter, D.; Đorđević, S.; Marković, B.; Ranković, D.; Savić, S. Critical quality attributes, in vitro release and correlated in vitro skin permeation—in vivo tape stripping collective data for demonstrating therapeutic (non)equivalence of topical semisolids: A case study of "ready-to-use" vehicles. *Int. J. Pharm.* **2017**, *528*, 253–267. [CrossRef] [PubMed]
7. Aiache, J.; Aoyagi, N.; Bashaw, D.; Brown, C.; Brown, W.; Burgess, D.; Crison, J. FIP/AAPS Guidelines to Dissolution/In Vitro Release Testing of Novel/Special Dosage Forms. *AAPS PharmSciTech.* **2003**, *4*, 1–10.
8. Shah, V.P.; Elkins, J.S.; Williams, R.L. Evaluation of the Test System Used for In Vitro Release of Drugs for Topical Dermatological Drug Products. *Pharm. Dev. Technol.* **1999**, *4*, 377–385. [CrossRef] [PubMed]
9. Klein, R.R.; Heckart, J.L.; Thakker, K.D. In vitro release testing methodology and variability with the vertical diffusion cell (VDC). *Dissolution Technol.* **2018**, *25*, 52–61. [CrossRef]
10. Thakker, K.D.; Chern, W.H. Development and validation of in vitro release tests for semisolid dosage forms—Case study. *Dissolution Technol.* **2003**, *10*, 10–15. [CrossRef]
11. Tiffner, K.I.; Kanfer, I.; Augustin, T.; Raml, R.; Raney, S.G.; Sinner, F. A comprehensive approach to qualify and validate the essential parameters of an in vitro release test (IVRT) method for acyclovir cream, 5%. *Int. J. Pharm.* **2018**, *535*, 217–227. [CrossRef] [PubMed]
12. US Food and Drug Administration. Draft Guidance on Acyclovir. Available online: https://www.accessdata.fda.gov/drugsatfda_docs/psg/Acyclovir_oint_18604_RC03-12.pdf (accessed on 20 October 2019).
13. US Food and Drug Administration. Draft Guidance on Acyclovir Cream. Available online: https://www.accessdata.fda.gov/drugsatfda_docs/psg/Acyclovir_topical%20cream_RLD%2021478_RV12-16.pdf (accessed on 20 October 2019).
14. US Food and Drug Administration. Draft Guidance on Docosanol Topical Cream. Available online: https://www.accessdata.fda.gov/drugsatfda_docs/psg/Docosanol_topical%20cream_NDA%20020941_RC08-17.pdf (accessed on 20 October 2019).
15. US Food and Drug Administration. Draft Guidance on Dapsone Gel. Available online: https://www.accessdata.fda.gov/drugsatfda_docs/psg/Dapsone_Topical%20gel_NDA%20207154_RV%20Nov%202018.pdf (accessed on 20 October 2019).

16. European Medicines Agency; Committee for Medicinal Products for Human Use. Draft Guideline on Quality and Equivalence of Topical Products. London, UK, 2018. Available online: https://www.ema.europa.eu/en/documents/scientific-guideline/draft-guideline-quality-equivalence-topical-products_en.pdf (accessed on 20 October 2019).
17. Ueda, C.T.; Shah, V.P.; Derdzinski, K.; Ewing, G.; Flynn, G.; Maibach, H.; Yacobi, A. Topical and transdermal drug products. *Pharmacop. Forum.* **2009**, *35*, 750–764. [CrossRef]
18. Klein, R.R.; Bechtel, J.L.; Burchett, K.; Thakker, K.D. Hydrocortisone as a Standard for In Vitro Release Testing Hydrocortisone as a Standard for In Vitro Release Testing. *Dissolution Technol.* **2010**, *17*, 37–38. [CrossRef]
19. Higuchi, W.I. Analysis of data on the medicament release from ointments. *J. Pharm. Sci.* **1962**, *51*, 802–804. [CrossRef] [PubMed]
20. Higuchi, T. Rate of Release of Medicaments from Ointment Bases Containing Drugs in Suspension. *J. Pharm. Sci.* **1961**, *50*, 874–875. [CrossRef] [PubMed]

pharmaceutics

MDPI

Article

Curcumin-In-Deformable Liposomes-In-Chitosan-Hydrogel as a Novel Wound Dressing

Selenia Ternullo †, Laura Victoria Schulte Werning †, Ann Mari Holsæter and Nataša Škalko-Basnet *

Drug Transport and Delivery Research Group, Department of Pharmacy, University of Tromsø The Arctic University of Norway, Universitetsveien 57, 9037 Tromsø, Norway; selenia89.ternullo@gmail.com (S.T.); laura.v.schulte-werning@uit.no (L.V.S.W.); ann-mari.holsater@uit.no (A.M.H.)

* Correspondence: natasa.skalko-basnet@uit.no; Tel.: +47-776-46640; Fax: +47-776-46151

† These authors contributed equally to this work.

Received: 30 November 2019; Accepted: 18 December 2019; Published: 20 December 2019

Abstract: A liposomes-in-hydrogel system as an advanced wound dressing for dermal delivery of curcumin was proposed for improved chronic wound therapy. Curcumin, a multitargeting poorly soluble active substance with known beneficial properties for improved wound healing, was incorporated in deformable liposomes to overcome its poor solubility. Chitosan hydrogel served as a vehicle providing superior wound healing properties. The novel system should assure sustained skin delivery of curcumin, and increase its retention at the skin site, utilizing both curcumin and chitosan to improve the therapy outcome. To optimize the properties of the formulation and determine the effect of the liposomal charge on the hydrogel properties, curcumin-containing deformable liposomes (DLs) with neutral (NDLs), cationic (CDLs), and anionic (ADLs) surface properties were incorporated in chitosan hydrogel. The charged DLs affected the hydrogel's hardness, cohesiveness, and adhesiveness. Importantly, the incorporation of DLs, regardless of their surface charge, in chitosan hydrogel did not decrease the system's bioadhesion to human skin. Stability testing revealed that the incorporation of CDLs in hydrogel preserved hydrogel's bioadhesiveness to a higher degree than both NDLs and ADLs. In addition, CDLs-in-hydrogel enabled the most sustained skin penetration of curcumin. The proposed formulation should be further evaluated in a chronic wound model.

Keywords: curcumin; deformable liposomes; liposome surface charge; hydrogel; chitosan; wound therapy

1. Introduction

The treatment of chronic wounds is one of the most important global health care issues in the aging society. Chronic wounds are challenging to treat due to the diversity of factors contributing to slow/impaired healing. The hostile environment of the wound comprising degradative enzymes and elevated pH, as well as the complexity of physiological processes, requires an effective advanced drug delivery system as a wound dressing [1,2]. An ideal wound dressing should reduce infection, moisturize the wound, stimulate the healing mechanism, accelerate the wound closure, and reduce/control scar formation [3].

Recently, the incessant release of free radicals has been proposed as one of the key factors responsible for activation of the inflammatory system, leading to impaired repair of the wound [4]. Therefore, the effective control of free radical levels in the wound and subsequent inflammation could assist in enhanced wound healing and scar control. Various antioxidants could be utilized to control free radicals during wound healing.

Curcumin has been proposed as one of the most promising [5]. Moreover, curcumin is a molecule able to active multiple pathways, contributing to improved wound healing [6]. The antioxidant, anti-inflammatory, and anti-bacterial properties of this pleiotropic molecule need to be more utilized [7,8]. Although curcumin is a very promising molecule to be included in wound dressings, its hydrophobicity, extensive metabolism, and limited skin penetration often hamper its wider use [9]. We have recently proven that curcumin, a multitargeting active substance, exhibits superior anti-inflammatory properties when incorporated in tailored deformable liposomes [10]. In this work, we went a step further in the development of curcumin-based wound dressings and combined the beneficial properties of curcumin as an active moiety and chitosan hydrogel as a superior vehicle to form a bioactive wound dressing targeting the treatment of chronic wounds.

An ideal dressing should assure an enhanced therapeutic outcome and reduction of pain accompanied with wound dressing changes [11]. Among the possible material to be used in the manufacturing of bioactive dressings, natural polymer-based wound dressings, such as hydrogels, represent promising advanced delivery systems with a low risk of toxicity and side effects due to their biodegradability and biocompatibility [12,13]. Hydrogels mimic the biochemical, biomechanical, and structural features of the extracellular matrix (ECM), serving as superior matrices for wound treatment [13,14]. Hydrogels additionally possess good bioadhesiveness that can contribute to a prolonged retention time of the incorporated drug/active substance at the wounded skin site. This, together with the sustained drug release via hydrogel, can result in higher drug/active substances' concentrations at the skin site while reducing possible systemic absorption and consequent adverse effects [15].

Chitosan represents one of the most studied natural polymers for the development of effective hydrogel-based wound dressings due to its numerous intrinsic biological properties. Its biocompatibility and bioadhesiveness, together with intrinsic bacteriostatic effect, make this biopolymer effective in promoting wound healing while also preventing biofilm formation [16,17]. In spite of the numerous advantages of chitosan hydrogels, the hydrophilic environment provided by chitosan hydrogel limits the incorporation of lipophilic drugs/active compounds and remains a pharmaceutical challenge.

Liposomes as carriers for poorly soluble drugs/active molecules assist in overcoming this hydrogel limitation; the combination of these two delivery systems is a promising approach to achieve controlled dermal drug delivery and effective localized skin therapy [18–20]. The liposomal phospholipid bilayers allow the incorporation of lipophilic substances, improving their solubilization and enabling their inclusion into the hydrophilic chitosan hydrogel. Moreover, the ability of liposomes to assure sustained drug/substance release might improve targeted drug delivery to the specific skin layer(s) [19,21]. Liposomes also benefit from their incorporation in the hydrogel vehicle. The hydrogel can prevent rapid liposome clearance from the skin site and additionally protect from rapid degradation by preserving their membrane integrity [22]. Moreover, incorporation of liposomes in hydrogel will confer adequate viscosity to the liposomal dispersions to be topically administered [23].

The drug/substance release from a liposomes-in-hydrogel system is determined by the hydrogel properties, such as the polymer composition, mesh size, and porosity, combined with the liposomal physicochemical characteristics, namely the liposomal composition, size, and surface charge. In addition, the lipophilicity of the incorporated drug needs to be considered [24]. To the best of our knowledge, relatively little has been published on the incorporation of deformable liposomes (DLs) in chitosan hydrogel. DLs have shown superior ability in promoting drug penetration into the deeper skin layers in comparison to conventional liposomes [10,25]. In this study, we designed the DLs-in-chitosan hydrogel as a combined advanced delivery system, targeting the treatment of chronic wounds. Considering that chitosan has lateral amino groups conferring positive charge to its chains, the incorporation of charged liposomes could trigger interactions between the two delivery systems, affecting the hydrogel's texture properties, liposomes' integrity, and drug release [24]. We therefore focused on the effect of the liposomal surface charge on the hydrogel's properties, such as the texture properties and bioadhesiveness; neutral (NDLs), cationic (CDLs), and anionic (ADLs) DLs were individually incorporated in chitosan hydrogel.

The effect of the liposomal surface charge on curcumin penetration from DLs-in-hydrogel systems through the ex vivo full thickness human skin was also evaluated.

2. Materials and Methods

2.1. Materials

Curcumin (≥94% curcuminoid content; ≥80% curcumin) was purchased from Sigma-Aldrich (St. Louis, MO, USA). Lipoid S 100 (>94% soybean phosphatidylcholine, PC) was a generous gift from Lipoid GmbH (Ludwigshafen, Germany). High molecular weight (MW) chitosan (Brookfield viscosity 800.000 cps and degree of deacetylation of 77%), polysorbate 20, stearylamine (SA), sodium deoxycholate (SDCh), methanol, disodium hydrogen phosphate dihydrate, monobasic potassium phosphate, sodium chloride, propylene glycol (PG), glycerol, and acetic acid were all purchased from Sigma-Aldrich (St. Louis, MO, USA). Albunorm® (human serum albumin, 200 mg/mL) was produced by Octapharma AG (Lachen, Switzerland).

2.2. Preparation and Characterization of Deformable Liposomes

Curcumin-containing DLs bearing different surface charges were prepared by the film hydration method as previously described [26]. NDLs comprised PC and polysorbate 20 (total 200 mg), in a weight ratio of 85:15. CDLs comprised the same lipid and surfactant composition as NDLs, in addition to SA (weight ratio to PC 1:9). ADLs were composed of PC and SDCh (total 200 mg) in a ratio of 85:15 (*w*/*w*) (Table 1). All DLs were prepared by dissolving curcumin (20 mg), PC, and, when applicable, the different surfactants, in methanol. The organic solvent was evaporated under vacuum (55 mbar) at 55 °C (Büchi Rotavapor R-124 with Büchi Vacuum Pump V-700, Büchi Labortechnik AG, Flawil, Switzerland) and the obtained film was hydrated with 10 mL of phosphate buffer saline (PBS). PBS (pH 7.4) contained the following salts composition: 2.98 g/L $Na_2HPO_4{\cdot}2H_2O$, 0.19 g/L KH_2PO_4, 8 g/L NaCl. The liposomal dispersions were kept at 4 °C for 24 h prior to size reduction.

Table 1. Liposomal composition.

Liposomes	Curcumin (mg/mL)	Lipoid S 100 (mg/mL)	Sodium Deoxycholate (mg/mL)	Stearylamine (mg/mL)	Polysorbate 20 (mg/mL)
NDLs	2.0	17.0	-	-	3.0
CDLs	2.0	15.3	-	1.7	3.0
ADLs	2.0	17.0	3.0	-	-

All DLs were reduced to a vesicle size of 200 × 300 nm by hand extrusion through the polycarbonate membrane (Nuclepore® Track-Etched Membranes, Whatman House, Maidstone, UK). In brief, all DLs were extruded five times through 800-nm pore size membrane. NDLs were further extruded four times through 400-nm pore size membrane, whereas CDLs and ADLs were extruded through the same pore size membrane two and seven times, respectively. All liposomal dispersions were characterized in terms of vesicle size by photon correlation spectroscopy using a NICOMP Submicron Particle Sizer Model 370 (NICOMP Particle Sizing system, Santa Barbara, CA, USA) and zeta potential using Malvern Zetasizer Nano—ZS (Malvern, Oxford, UK) [26].

The entrapment efficiency of curcumin in DLs was determined after the centrifugation of the liposomal dispersion at 3000 *g* for 10 min using a Biofuge stratos centrifuge (Heraeus instruments GmbH, Hanau, Germany) to remove unentrapped curcumin. Liposomes were subsequently dissolved in methanol and the entrapped curcumin determined spectophotometrically at 425 nm (SpectraMax 190 Microplate Reader, Molecular Devices, San Jose, CA, USA). The entrapment efficiency was expressed as curcumin/lipid ratio (μg/mg), after quantification of the PC content in all DLs formulations (data not shown).

2.3. Preparation of Chitosan Hydrogels

Chitosan hydrogels were prepared according to a method described earlier [27]. In short, glycerol (10%, *w*/*w*) was mixed with an aqueous solution of acetic acid (2.5%, *w*/*w*). High MW chitosan

(2.5%, *w/w*) was introduced into the mixture by hand stirring. To remove entrapped air, the mixture was bath-sonicated for 30 min. The prepared hydrogels were stored in a sealed container at room temperature for 48 h to allow complete swelling.

2.4. Preparation of DLs-In-Hydrogels

To prepare 10 g of liposomes-in-hydrogel formulation, 1.5 g of the different DLs (15%, *w/w*) were individually incorporated in the freshly prepared chitosan hydrogel after it was allowed to swell for 48 h at room temperature (Section 2.3) by hand-stirring [28]. The final concentration of curcumin in the liposomal hydrogel was 135 μg/g. As a control, free curcumin was incorporated in the hydrogel in the same concentration after dissolving in PG and subsequent incorporation in chitosan hydrogel by hand stirring. The DLs-in-hydrogel formulations were kept at room temperature for 2 h prior to further handling. The homogeneity test was performed to assure that liposomes were well dispersed within the liposomes-in-hydrogel formulation by sampling (5 aliquots were sampled from various places within hydrogel) and the curcumin concentration was determined in each aliquot.

2.5. Texture Analysis

All liposomes-in-hydrogel formulations were characterized in terms of the hardness, cohesiveness, and adhesiveness using a Texture Analyzer TA.XT Plus (Stable Micro Systems Ltd., Surrey, UK) [27]. The hydrogel (25 g) was placed in a beaker and a disc (35 mm in diameter) pushed down into the gel (distance of 10 mm) and withdrawn at a speed of 4 mm/s. The starting position of the disc was below the hydrogel surface. The hardness was calculated as the maximal force achieved when the disc was pushed down into the gel. The cohesiveness was expressed as the work necessary to push down the disc into the hydrogel while the adhesiveness as the work required during the upwards movement of the disc. Each formulation was tested five times and the measurements performed in triplicates.

2.6. Bioadhesion Test

The bioadhesion of hydrogels to the skin was tested as described earlier [28]. The full thickness human skin originated from the abdomen of female patients after plastic surgery. A written consent was obtained from the patients prior the surgery. No ethical approval was required from the Norwegian Ethical Committee, since we used skin to be disposed of after the surgery; the experiments were conducted according to the Declaration of Helsinki principles. The skin was cleared from the subcutaneous fatty tissue and rinsed with PBS prior the storage at −20 °C. The skin was thawed in PBS ca. 30 min prior to the experiment and subsequently fixed on a rig for Texture Analyzer TA.XT Plus (Stable micro systems, Surrey, UK). The bioadhesion test was performed by filling a die with the hydrogel formulation (150 μL), which was consequently pinched onto the skin for 10 s applying a force of 25 g. The bioadhesion was determined by measuring the force required to detach the die from the skin (detachment speed of 0.1 mm/s). Moreover, the die was weighed before and after each bioadhesion test to determine the amount of formulation retained onto the skin surface at the end of the test. Each formulation was tested five times and the human skin rinsed with ethanol between each measurement. Tests were conducted in triplicates.

2.7. Hydrogel Stability Testing

To evaluate the chitosan hydrogel stability and the influences of the liposomal surface charge on the stability of DLs-in-hydrogel, the stability testing was performed after the storage of the DLs-in-chitosan hydrogels for one month at room temperature (23–24 °C). The texture properties (Section 2.5) and bioadhesiveness (Section 2.6) of the chitosan hydrogel were determined before (one day after the formulation was prepared) and after the storage (day 30).

2.8. Ex Vivo Skin Penetration Studies

Ex vivo curcumin penetration from the different DLs-in-chitosan hydrogels was evaluated using the full thickness human skin in Franz diffusion cells (diffusion area of 1.77 cm^2, PermeGear, Bethlehem, PA, USA) [26]. The human skin originated from the excised skin panni obtained from female patients who underwent abdominoplasty, after they gave written consent (see Section 2.6). The experiments were conducted in agreement with the Declaration of Helsinki principles. The human skin for the ex vivo penetration studies was prepared as described in Section 2.6. The slices of human skin used in the skin penetration studies had a thickness of 1.10 to 1.30 mm. All DLs-in-chitosan hydrogel formulations (1.2 mL) were added in the donor chamber, whereas the receptor chamber was filled with 12.0 mL of Albunorm (5%, *v*/*v*) solution in PBS. As a control, curcumin in PG-in-hydrogel served as a control. The experiments were conducted for 8 h and sampling of the receptor medium (500 µL) was performed every hour. To maintain the sink conditions, the withdrawn receptor medium was replaced by an equal volume of fresh Albunorm® (5%, *v*/*v*) solution in PBS. The penetrated curcumin was quantified as described in Section 2.2 using a standard curve of curcumin in Albunorm®/PBS (1:1, *v*/*v*). Experiments were performed in three replicates.

2.9. Statistical Analyses

To determine the level of significance ($p < 0.05$), statistical analyses were performed using one-way ANOVA test followed by Bonferroni's multiple comparisons test performed on GraphPad Prism version 7.00 for Windows (GraphPad Software, La Jolla, CA, USA).

3. Results and Discussion

Chronic wounds exhibit severe molecular and cellular deficiencies and are heterogenous across the patient population; therefore, they are difficult to treat. At present, no wound dressing can be considered as "one size fits all"; however, there is a consensus in the field that chronic wound treatment should shift from conventional dressings towards precision medicine approaches [14]. It is known that the remodeling phase of wound healing comprises the deposition of extracellular matrix (ECM) in a well-defined network prior to wound contraction [3]. Chitosan promotes wound healing via stimulation of ECM formation as well as facilitating the mobilization, adhesion, and accumulation of red blood cells and platelets forming blood clots at the wound site [14]. Chitosan hydrogel could therefore be a perfect vehicle to incorporate bioactive molecules within nanoformulations. The combination of liposomal curcumin, assuring anti-inflammatory activity, and chitosan, providing wound healing and antimicrobial activities, could assure a synergistic effect and superior performance. The therapeutic potential of the novel dressing will be dependent on the characteristics of each component as well as their interplay.

3.1. Liposomal Characteristics

Considering the liposomes-in-hydrogel formulation, the liposomal size is known to influence both the hydrogel properties and the release of lipophilic compounds from liposomes-in-hydrogel systems [24]. Therefore, focusing on exploring the effect of the liposomal surface charge on both hydrogel properties and curcumin penetration through human skin, we aimed to prepare DLs of a similar vesicle size. The chosen vesicle size range was 200 to 300 nm, which has been suggested as appropriate for assuring dermal delivery via liposomes by offering the reservoir of the liposome-associated drug in the skin [29]. The extrusion method, utilized to reduce the vesicle size, allows the manufacturing of rather homogeneously distributed vesicles in the desired size range, as reported earlier [26]. For each liposomal dispersion, we adjusted both the number of extrusion cycles and membrane pore size, obtaining curcumin-containing DLs within the size range of 200 to 300 nm (Table 2), as targeted. Moreover, the vesicle size distribution was rather homogeneous for all DLs, as indicated by the rather low polydispersity.

Table 2. Liposomal characteristics.

Liposomes	Diameter (nm)	Polydispersity Index	Zeta Potential (mV)	Curcumin/Lipid Ratio (μg/mg)	Entrapment Efficiency (%)
NDLs	288.73 ± 2.46	0.17 ± 0.02	−3.03 ± 0.24	51.54 [a] ± 0.99	43.97 ± 0.85
CDLs	252.24 ± 51.63	0.17 ± 0.01	34.01 ± 0.56	71.94 ± 2.32	55.04 ± 1.78
ADLs	291.54 ± 26.48	0.17 ± 0.01	−34.83 ± 0.64	89.67 ± 14.03	76.40 ± 11.96

Results are presented as mean (n = 3) ± SD. [a] Significantly lower vs. ADLs ($p < 0.05$).

DLs bearing different surface charges (Table 2) were obtained by including the selected surfactant in the liposomal phospholipid bilayers. NDLs comprised polysorbate 20 as a non-ionic surfactant, which conferred a neutral surface to DLs, as well as the neutral lipid, namely PC. Ionic surfactants were employed to obtain CDLs and ADLs, respectively. SA was responsible for the positive charge of CDLs, whereas SDCh conferred the negative charge to ADLs surface, both in agreement with the literature [30,31].

The entrapment efficiency of curcumin in the different DLs varied according to the liposomal composition (Table 2). The presence of surfactant might contribute to a lower entrapment of lipophilic compounds, such as curcumin; both substances are competing for accommodation within the liposomal phospholipid bilayer. Moreover, it is known that the drug/active substance incorporation capacity is additionally dependent on the type of employed surfactant [32]. In our case, ADLs exhibited the highest entrapment efficiency for curcumin. A possible explanation might be the higher lipophilicity of SDCh compared to polysorbate 20, thus improving the curcumin solubility and therefore enhancing the curcumin loading capacity for ADLs [32]. The presence of SA in CDLs has been shown to alter the lipid packing of liposomes by causing a charge repulsion [33]. This can therefore affect curcumin's accommodation within the CDLs bilayer, as previously reported for the drugs of a similar lipophilicity as curcumin, such as celecoxib [34].

3.2. *Effect of the Liposomal Surface Charge on the Texture Properties of Liposomes-In-Hydrogel*

The development of effective hydrogel-based wound dressings requires their optimization in terms of hydrogel's texture properties. For hydrogels as wound dressings, the hydrogel's hardness can determine the ease of its application onto the skin, whereas the adhesiveness influences the hydrogel's contact time with the skin. These factors consequently contribute to the efficacy of the treatment and assure patient compliance by reducing the frequencies of administration and the related pain caused by wound dressing changes [11]. While optimizing liposomes-in-hydrogel formulations, an evaluation of the texture properties of the hydrogel is required considering that the incorporation of DLs bearing different surface charges can affect the hydrogel texture properties [24]. Possible interactions between charged DLs and positive chitosan chains might change/affect the chitosan network, thus modifying its texture characteristics. The effect of the liposomal surface charge of curcumin-containing DLs on the hydrogel properties is presented in Table 3.

Table 3. The effect of the liposomal surface charge on the texture properties of liposomes-in-hydrogel.

Chitosan Hydrogel Composition	Hardness (g)	Cohesiveness (g*s)	Adhesiveness (g*s)
Plain hydrogel	164.8 ± 11.1	359.6 ± 10.6	346.8 ± 8.0
CUR-in-hydrogel	148.7 ± 20.1	262.2 ± 17.0	248.5 ± 20.1
CUR-NDL-in-hydrogel	107.0 [a] ± 4.2	226.5 [a,b] ± 1.7	216.5 [a] ± 2.8
CUR-CDL-in-hydrogel	116.8 [a] ± 6.7	212.3 [a,b] ± 5.5	200.9 [a,b] ± 9.4
CUR-ADL-in-hydrogel	124.6 ± 21.0	204.0 [a,b] ± 13.5	190.7 [a,b] ± 8.6

Results are presented as mean (n = 3) ± SD. CUR: curcumin. [a] Significantly lower vs. plain hydrogel ($p < 0.05$); [b] significantly lower vs. CUR-in-hydrogel ($p < 0.05$).

The incorporation of DLs negatively affected the original hydrogel texture properties (plain hydrogel). The incorporation of deformable liposomes weakened the hydrogel properties to a higher extent than the incorporation of free curcumin (CUR-in-hydrogel, Table 3). Due to the hydrophobic nature of curcumin, its incorporation in chitosan hydrogel in the form of free curcumin (not incorporated in DLs) was achieved by prior dispersion of curcumin in PG. The presence of PG has been shown to exert a positive effect on the viscoelastic properties of hydrogels by triggering hydrogen bonding between chitosan, water, and the solvent [35]. This might explain the positive effect of free curcumin in PG on the hydrogel properties compared to DLs. Vanić and co-workers [36] observed changes in the hydrogel texture properties when deformable propylene glycol liposomes were incorporated in Carbopol hydrogel; as in our case, the hydrogel texture properties were reduced. The incorporation of DLs in Carbopol hydrogel also affected the hydrogel texture when compared to a marketed gel product, although the authors did not focus on the effect of the liposomal surface charge [37]. Similar to our findings, Hurler and collaborators [24] also observed weakened chitosan hydrogel properties due to the incorporation of conventional liposomes bearing different surface charges. The charged DLs enhanced the hydrogel hardness while weakening both the cohesiveness and adhesiveness, as compared to NDLs (Table 3).

3.3. *Effect of Liposomal Surface Charge on Hydrogel Bioadhesion to Human Skin*

Bioadhesiveness represents an important feature responsible for the effectiveness of hydrogel-based wound dressings. Good hydrogel bioadhesion to human skin can prolong the retention time of the incorporated drug/active substance at the skin site, thus resulting in an enhanced therapeutic effect. Considering the presence of the exudate in chronic wounds/burns, the contact time of the hydrogel to the skin might be reduced by a loss of the original hydrogel texture characteristics due to the high water content in the wounded area of exudating wounds [11]. Improved hydrogel bioadhesion to human skin might overcome this limitation. We therefore evaluated a possible effect of the liposomal surface charge on the chitosan hydrogel bioadhesiveness. Based on the method developed earlier in our laboratory [28], we evaluated the hydrogel bioadhesion to human skin by determining the force required to remove the hydrogel formulation from the skin (Figure 1a) and the amount of hydrogel formulations retained onto the skin surface at the end of the bioadhesion test (Figure 1b).

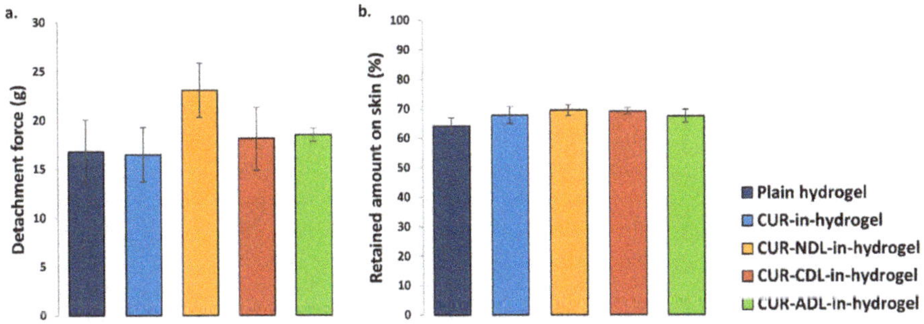

Figure 1. Effect of the liposomal surface charge on liposomes-in-hydrogel bioadhesiveness, expressed as the (**a**) detachment force and (**b**) amount of formulation retained onto the human skin surface. Results are expressed as mean ($n = 3$) ± SD.

The bioadhesiveness expressed as the detachment force was not affected by the incorporation of curcumin-containing DLs, regardless of the liposomal surface charge. Both CDLs- and ADLs-in-hydrogel exhibited a similar bioadhesiveness as plain hydrogel, whereas NDLs-in-hydrogel showed the strongest bioadhesion to human skin. As observed for the texture properties, NDLs with a neutral surface seemed to stabilize the chitosan network to a higher extent compared to the charged DLs. Their neutral liposomal surface assures minimal interactions with the polymer, thus leaving unaltered the intrinsic bioadhesive properties of chitosan hydrogel.

The amount of the hydrogel retained on the skin was similar for all tested DLs-in-hydrogel systems. Moreover, the high amount of hydrogel retained onto the skin (approximately 70%) observed for all DLs-in-hydrogel is encouraging considering the need to potentially overcome the challenge of hydrogel exposure to wound exudate and reduced retention time when hydrogel is applied on exudate-rich wounded area. The high water content associated to those wound types is responsible for the limited adhesion of the wound dressing at the skin site. Therefore, the good bioadhesive properties of DLs-in-hydrogel systems confirmed herewith are promising in prolonging the retention time of novel dressing, including curcumin, at the wounded area rich in exudate, potentially enhancing its therapeutic outcome. Further studies involving the exposure to wound exudate are required to confirm these preliminary findings.

3.4. *Stability of Hydrogel*

The incorporation of charged DLs in chitosan hydrogel has shown to influence, to a higher extent, the hydrogel's texture properties (Table 2) and, to a lesser extent, the bioadhesiveness (Figure 1), possibly attributable to triggered interactions between charged DLs and chitosan. We therefore further explored the effect of the liposomal surface charge on the stability of liposomes-in-hydrogel. Wound dressings that can maintain their original properties when stored at room temperature would enable easier administration both by the patient itself or a caretaker. The liposomes-in-hydrogel formulations were stored at room temperature (23–24 °C) for one month and both the texture properties and bioadhesiveness of formulations were determined and compared with the properties of the original formulations. As expected, the original texture properties were preserved to a higher extent when NDLs were incorporated in the hydrogel compared to both CDLs and ADLs (Figure 2). The minimal interaction between neutral DLs and chitosan network seems to maintain the original hydrogel texture properties whereas the charged DLs weakened the texture properties due to electrostatic interactions. However, the findings were still considered acceptable, considering that the testing was performed at room temperature.

Interestingly, the evaluation of the hydrogel's stability in terms of its bioadhesiveness showed that the original bioadhesion to human skin was better preserved when CDLs were incorporated in the hydrogel (Figure 3). Both the detachment force (Figure 3a) and the amount of formulation retained onto the skin surface (Figure 3b) for CDLs-in-hydrogel moderately increased compared to both NDLs- and ADLs-in-chitosan hydrogel. However, the differences were not significant, and more experiments would be required to confirm the observed trend.

Although the original bioadhesiveness of liposomes-in-hydrogel was enhanced by the presence of NDLs, suggesting that the neutral surface of NDLs might exert a positive effect on hydrogel bioadhesiveness (Figure 1), the results from the hydrogel stability testing indicate that the positively charged DLs can better preserve hydrogel bioadhesiveness for a longer time as compared to NDLs. Considering the variability of human skin in respect to the source, the differences were not significant. The repulsion between positive CDLs and chitosan chains might stabilize the liposomes in the hydrogel matrix, thus preserving chitosan bioadhesion to human skin.

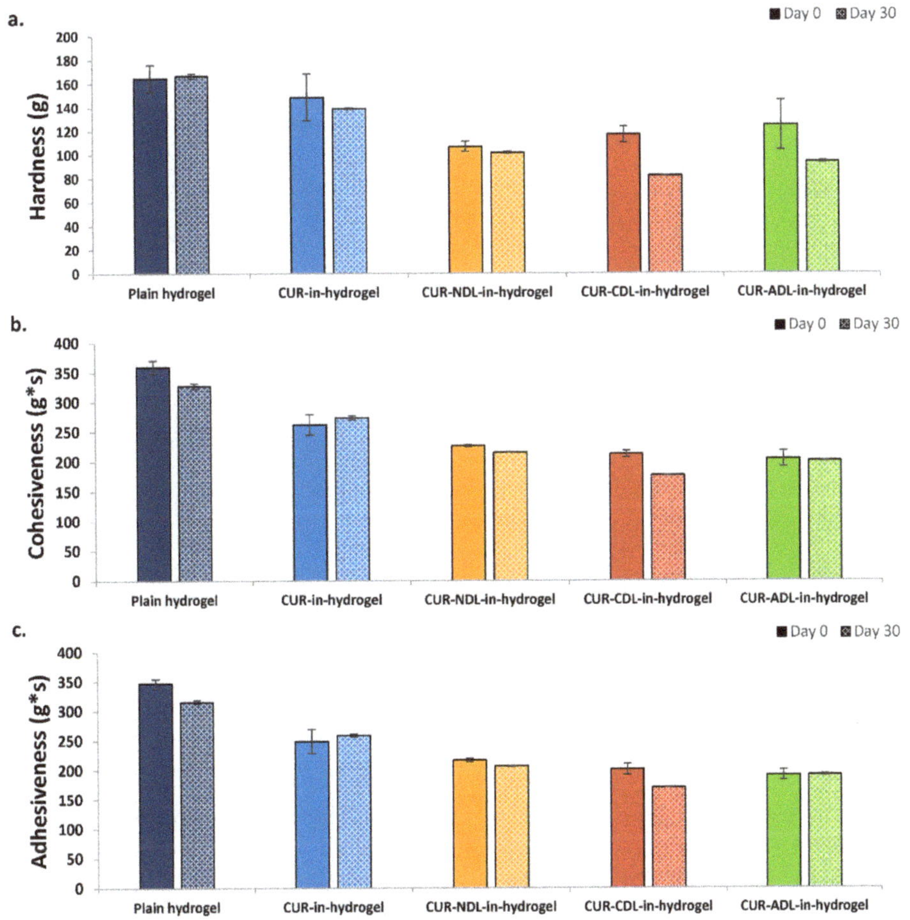

Figure 2. The effect of the liposomal surface charge on liposomes-in-hydrogel texture properties: stability testing. (**a**) hardness, (**b**) cohesiveness, and (**c**) adhesiveness, determined on day 0 and after storage at 23 to 24 °C for 30 days. Results are expressed as mean (n = 3) ± SD.

The bioadhesiveness of the dressing is one of the main factors determining the time curcumin is retained at the skin site. Despite the rather negative effect of charged liposomes on the texture properties of DLs-in-hydrogel, the incorporation of CDLs in hydrogel might increase hydrogel bioadhesiveness, thus assuring a longer time for curcumin to exert its biological activities. The significance of the superiority of CDLs in hydrogels needs to be confirmed. For comparison, visual evaluation of the hydrogels stored for one month indicated that the control, namely curcumin-in-hydrogel (non-liposomal curcumin in hydrogel), exhibited clear curcumin precipitation (data not shown). This was additional conformation that to deliver curcumin at the wounded site, combined formulations comprising liposomes and hydrogel are highly advantageous.

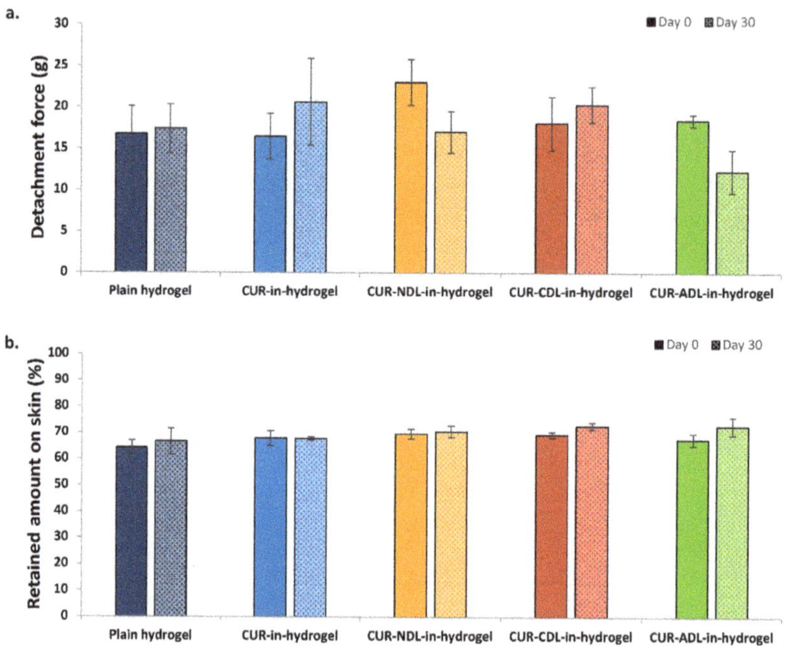

Figure 3. The effect of the liposomal surface charge on liposomes-in-hydrogel bioadhesiveness: stability testing. (**a**) Detachment force and (**b**) amount of formulation retained onto the skin surface, determined on day 0 and after the storage at 23 to 24 °C for 30 days. Results are expressed as mean (n = 3) ± SD.

3.5. Ex Vivo Curcumin Penetration from DLs-In-Hydrogel into Human Skin

As dermal delivery systems, both DLs and chitosan hydrogel have shown ability to assure controlled and sustained skin penetration of the associated drug. When used in combination, this action can be enhanced and, together with the prolonged retention time at the targeted skin site, might lead to improved localized wound therapy [18,19]. Moreover, this can result in a reduction in frequency of wound dressings' changes, improving patient compliance and the easiness of dressing administration. The incorporation of curcumin-DLs in the hydrogel introduces additional barriers that curcumin has to face and cross before reaching the targeted site. Therefore, curcumin release from the DLs-in-hydrogel followed by its skin penetration is a complex process and depends on several factors. The lipophilicity of curcumin will influence this process, especially its partitioning into the hydrogel, whereas its aqueous solubility will determine the diffusion rate through the hydrophilic hydrogel matrix, as reported for other lipophilic compounds [38]. The liposomal surface charge represents an additional factor that can affect curcumin penetration through/into the skin [39]. Moreover, due to the positively charged chitosan chains, the liposomal surface charge can determine possible interaction between DLs and chitosan [24]. This can affect the integrity of the liposomal bilayer when embedded into the hydrogel, thus influencing the release of curcumin. By exploring the abovementioned factors, the development of liposomes-in-hydrogel formulations for controlled dermal delivery of curcumin can be tailored and effective therapy assured.

Figure 4 presents the skin penetration profiles of curcumin from the different curcumin-DLs-in-hydrogel systems. A minimal amount of penetrated curcumin was detected, regardless of the liposomal surface charge. This can be contributed to the slow diffusion of curcumin when released into the hydrophilic hydrogel due to its poor water solubility. In agreement with our findings, Jain and collaborators [25] also reported a rather slow in vitro release of curcumin from lipospheres embedded in hydroxyl propyl methyl cellulose-based gel.

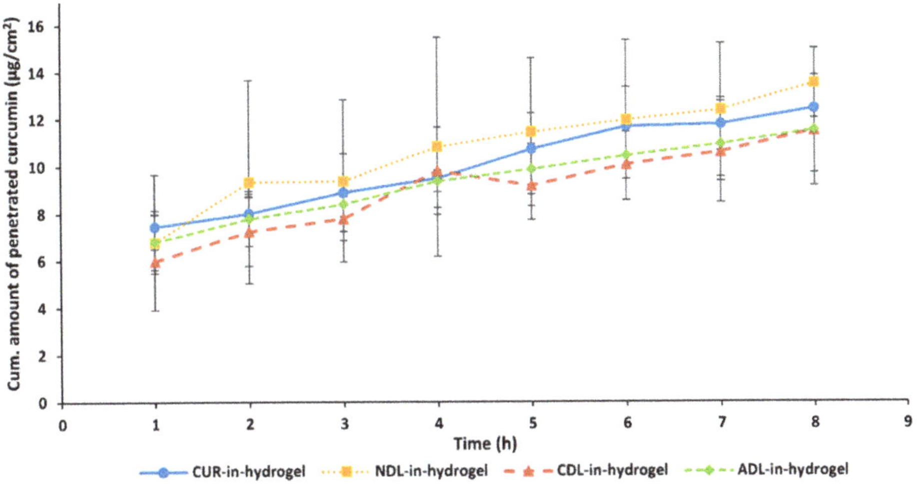

Figure 4. Ex vivo curcumin penetration from different DLs-in-hydrogel through full thickness human skin ($n = 3 \pm$ SD).

As a control, curcumin-in-hydrogel was used; curcumin was incorporated in the hydrogel in a form of solution in PG in the same concentration as in DLs.

The NDLs-in-hydrogel release profile exhibited the highest amount of penetrated curcumin, even in comparison to curcumin-in-hydrogel (Figure 4). However, the differences were not statistically different and can only be considered as a trend. It is important to point out that the experiments were performed using human skin of different donors, adding to larger SD. NDLs with their neutral surface are not expected to interact with the chitosan chains. The minimal interaction between NDLs and chitosan chains might also marginally interfere with NDLs' mobility within the polymer matrix, allowing faster curcumin delivery into/through the skin via NDLs. Thomas and collaborators [40] reported the enhancement of curcumin skin penetration from nanosystems-in-chitosan hydrogel compared to free curcumin-in-hydrogel. They incorporated curcumin in nanoemulsions further incorporated in chitosan hydrogel and observed a higher rat skin penetration of curcumin as compared to free curcumin-in-hydrogel. Sun and co-workers [41] reported higher penetration of curcumin from PLGA nanoparticles-loaded in Carbopol gel compared to free curcumin-in-gel, although they tested the formulations on mouse skin.

The charged DLs-in-hydrogel exhibited more sustained, although not significant, skin penetration of curcumin compared to NDLs-in-hydrogel and control (curcumin-in-hydrogel). Considering the possible electrostatic interactions that can be triggered when charged DLs are embedded into the chitosan network, the liposomal membrane might be more preserved, thus limiting curcumin partitioning into the hydrogel. The electrostatic interactions between negative DLs and positive chitosan chains can cause immobilization of ADLs within the hydrogel matrix, thus limiting initial curcumin diffusion into the hydrogel prior to reaching the skin. El Kechai and collaborators [42] proposed low mobility of liposomes bearing opposite charge to the hydrogel chains; the authors observed that positive liposomes were highly immobilized in the negative hyaluronic acid hydrogel. On the other hand, the higher repulsion occurring between CDLs and chitosan, both positively charged, might stabilize the CDLs membrane and limit curcumin partitioning into the chitosan hydrogel. Hurler and collaborators [24] also observed a similar release pattern when testing the in vitro release of a lipophilic compound from positively charged liposomes embedded in chitosan hydrogel, in agreement with our findings.

In our previous work [10], we showed a successful inhibition of *S. aureus* and *S. pyogenes* growth when testing curcumin in deformable liposomes in a curcumin concentration of 100 and 200 µg/mL.

Furthermore, the curcumin-containing liposomes (even at a curcumin concentration of 2.5 μg/mL) successfully inhibited nitric oxide production. The concentrations used in the current study are in the same range as the ones in the aforementioned study, indicating that the delivery rate is compatible with the working concentration of curcumin in this type of carrier. Compared to Ternullo et al. [10], the ex vivo release through full thickness human skin exhibited a more sustained release when the DLs were incorporated into a hydrogel, as expected. Recently, Nguyen and coauthors [43] reported improved wound healing when utilizing a curcumin–oligochitosan nanoparticle complex and oligochitosan-coated curcumin-loaded liposomes with a curcumin concentration of 100 μg/mL. The hydrogel prepared in the current study contains curcumin in a concentration of 135 μg/g and is therefore similar to the concentration used by Nguen et al. (2019). The curcumin concentration in the novel dressing is sufficient to achieve the desired biological response.

Considering the prolonged retention time of curcumin assured by chitosan hydrogel and sustained delivery provided by liposomes-in-hydrogel, we can postulate that curcumin will have a sufficient time and required concentration at the skin site to exert its therapeutic effect. However, the findings should be further explored in a suitable wound model.

4. Conclusions

To utilize the wound healing potential of both curcumin and chitosan, we developed a novel wound dressing comprising curcumin-in-liposomes-in-chitosan hydrogel. Curcumin was incorporated in deformable liposomes of various surface charges and the effect of the liposomal surface charge on the performance of chitosan hydrogels was evaluated. Although the original texture properties were changed to a certain degree upon inclusion of the charged liposomes, the incorporation of DLS in the chitosan hydrogel did not affect its bioadhesiveness. Neutral deformable liposomes-in-hydrogel exhibited the strongest bioadhesiveness; however, their neutral surface did not preserve the hydrogels´s bioadhesion to human skin over longer storage times. The positively charged deformable liposomes exhibited an ability to stabilize the formulation's bioadhesiveness and additionally assured sustained penetration of curcumin through the ex vivo full human skin. The developed advanced dermal delivery system is therefore promising as a wound dressing.

Author Contributions: N.Š.-B. designed the study and supervised the research fellows. S.T. and L.V.S.W. performed the experiments and statistical analyses. All authors were involved in data interpretation and discussions. S.T., L.V.S.W., A.M.H. and N.Š.-B. contributed to manuscript generation. All authors read, reviewed and approved the final manuscript. All authors have read and agreed to the published version of the manuscript.

Funding: The research received no external funding. The publication charges for this article have been funded by a grant from the publication fund of UiT The Arctic University of Norway.

Acknowledgments: The authors are grateful to Lipoid GmbH, Germany, for providing the lipids.

Conflicts of Interest: The authors declare no conflict of interest.

References

1. Hamdan, S.; Pastar, I.; Drakulich, S.; Dikici, E.; Tomic-Canic, M.; Deo, S.; Daunert, S. Nanotechnology-Driven Therapeutic Interventions in Wound Healing: Potential Uses and Applications. *ACS Cent. Sci.* **2017**, *3*, 163–175. [CrossRef] [PubMed]
2. Saghazadeh, S.; Rinoldi, C.; Achot, M.; Kashaf, S.S.; Sharifi, F.; Jalilian, E.; Nuutila, K.; Giatsidis, G.; Mostafalu, P.; Derakhshandeh, H.; et al. Drug delivery systems and materials for wound healing applications. *Adv. Drug Deliv. Rev.* **2018**, *127*, 138–166. [CrossRef] [PubMed]
3. Kalashnikova, I.; Das, S.; Seal, S. Nanomaterials for wound healing: Scope and advancement. *Nanomedicine* **2015**, *10*, 2593–2612. [CrossRef] [PubMed]
4. Puertas-Bartolomé, M.; Benito-Garzón, L.; Fung, S.; Kohn, J.; Vázquez-Lasa, B.; San Román, J. Bioadhesive functional hydrogels: Controlled release of catechol species with antioxidant and antiinflammatory behaviour. *Mater. Sci. Eng. C* **2019**, *105*, 110040. [CrossRef]

5. Kamar, S.S.; Abdel-Kader, D.H.; Rasshed, L.A. Beneficial effect of curcumin nanoparticle.hydrogel on excisional skin wound helaing in type-1 diabetic rat; Histological and immunohistochemical studies. *Ann. Anat.* **2019**, *222*, 94–102. [CrossRef]
6. Bhattacharya, D.; Tiwari, R.; Bhatia, T.; Purohit, M.P.; Pal, A.; Jagdale, P.; Reddy Mudiam, M.K.; Chaudhari, B.P.; Shukla, Y.; Ansari, K.M.; et al. Accelerated and scarless wound repair by a multicomponet hydrogel through siumulataneous activation of multiple pathways. *Drug Deliv. Transl. Res.* **2019**, *9*, 1143–1158. [CrossRef]
7. Mehanny, M.; Hathout, R.M.; Geneidi, A.S.; Mansour, S. Exploring the use of nanocarrier systems to deliver the magical molecule; Curcumin and its derivatives. *J. Control. Release* **2016**, *225*, 1–30. [CrossRef]
8. Amini-Nik, S.; Yousuf, Y.; Jeschke, M.G. Scar management in burn injuries using drug delivery and molecular signalling: Current treatments and future directions. *Adv. Drug Deliv. Rev.* **2018**, *123*, 135–154. [CrossRef]
9. El-Refai, W.M.; Elnagger, Y.S.R.; El-Massik, M.A.; Abdallah, O.Y. Novel curcumin-loaded gel-core hyaluosomes with promising burn-wound healing potential: Development, in-vitro appraisal and in-vivo studies. *Int. J. Pharm.* **2015**, *486*, 88–98. [CrossRef]
10. Ternullo, S.; Gagnat, E.; Julin, K.; Johannessen, M.; Basnet, P.; Vanić, Ž.; Škalko-Basnet, N. Liposomes augment biological benefits of curcumin for multitargeted skin therapy. *Eur. J. Pharm. Biopharm.* **2019**, *144*, 154–164. [CrossRef]
11. Boateng, J.; Catanzano, O. Advanced therapeutic dressings for effective wound healing—A review. *J. Pharm. Sci.* **2015**, *104*, 3653–3680. [CrossRef] [PubMed]
12. Bhattarai, N.; Gunn, J.; Zhang, M. Chitosan-based hydrogels for controlled, localized drug delivery. *Adv. Drug Deliv. Rev.* **2010**, *62*, 83–99. [CrossRef] [PubMed]
13. Stern, D.; Cui, H. Crafting polymeric and peptidic hydrogels for improved wound healing. *Adv. Healthc. Mater.* **2019**, *8*, 1900104. [CrossRef] [PubMed]
14. Dickinson, L.E.; Gerecht, S. Engineered biopolymeric scaffolds for chronic wound healing. *Front. Physiol.* **2016**, *7*, 341. [CrossRef] [PubMed]
15. Pitorre, M.; Gondé, H.; Haury, C.; Messous, M.; Poilane, J.; Boudaud, D.; Kanber, E.; Rossemond Ndombina, G.A.; Benoit, J.-P.; Bastiat, G. Recent advances in nanocarrier-loaded gels: Which drug delivery technologies against which diseases? *J. Control. Release* **2017**, *266*, 140–155. [CrossRef]
16. Ng, V.W.; Chan, J.M.; Sardon, H.; Ono, R.J.; García, J.M.; Yang, Y.Y.; Hedrick, J.L. Antimicrobial hydrogels: A new weapon in the arsenal against multidrug-resistant infections. *Adv. Drug Deliv. Rev.* **2014**, *78*, 46–62. [CrossRef]
17. Pérez-Díaz, M.; Alvarado-Gomez, E.; Magaña-Aquino, M.; Sánchez-Sánchez, R.; Velasquillo, C.; Gonzalez, C.; Ganem-Rondero, A.; Martínez-Castañon, G.; Zavala-Alonso, N.; Martinez-Gutierrez, F. Anti-biofilm activity of chitosan gels formulated with silver nanoparticles and their cytotoxic effect on human fibroblasts. *Mater. Sci. Eng. C* **2016**, *60*, 317–323. [CrossRef]
18. Hurler, J.; Sørensen, K.K.; Fallarero, A.; Vuorela, P.; Škalko-Basnet, N. Liposomes-in-hydrogel delivery system with mupirocin: In vitro antibiofilm studies and in vivo evaluation in mice burn model. *BioMed Res. Int.* **2013**, *2013*, 1–8.
19. Billard, A.; Pourchet, L.; Malaise, S.; Alcouffe, P.; Montembault, A.; Ladavière, C. Liposome-loaded chitosan physical hydrogel: Toward a promising delayed-release biosystem. *Carbohydr. Polym.* **2015**, *115*, 651–657. [CrossRef]
20. Grijalvo, S.; Mayr, J.; Eritja, R.; Díaz, D. Biodegradable liposome-encapsulated hydrogels for biomedical applications: A marriage of convenience. *Biomater. Sci.* **2016**, *4*, 555–574. [CrossRef]
21. Banerjee, R. Overcoming the stratum corneum barrier: A nano approach. *Drug Deliv. Transl. Res.* **2013**, *3*, 205–208. [CrossRef] [PubMed]
22. Gao, W.; Vecchio, D.; Li, J.; Zhu, J.; Zhang, Q.; Fu, V.; Li, J.; Thamphiwatana, S.; Lu, D.; Zhang, L. Hydrogel containing nanoparticle-stabilized liposomes for topical antimicrobial delivery. *ACS Nano* **2014**, *8*, 2900–2907. [CrossRef] [PubMed]
23. Pavelić, Ž.; Škalko-Basnet, N.; Schubert, R. Liposomal gels for vaginal drug delivery. *Int. J. Pharm.* **2001**, *219*, 139–149. [CrossRef]
24. Hurler, J.; Žakelj, S.; Mravljak, J.; Pajk, S.; Kristl, A.; Schubert, R.; Škalko-Basnet, N. The effect of lipid composition and liposome size on the release properties of liposomes-in-hydrogel. *Int. J. Pharm.* **2013**, *456*, 49–57. [CrossRef]

25. Jain, A.; Doppalapudi, S.; Domb, A.J.; Khan, W. Tacrolimus and curcumin co-loaded liposphere gel: Synergistic combination towards management of psoriasis. *J. Control. Release* **2016**, *243*, 132–145. [CrossRef]
26. Ternullo, S.; de Weerd, L.; Holsæter, A.M.; Flaten, G.E.; Škalko-Basnet, N. Going skin deep: A direct comparison of penetration potential of lipid-based nanovesicles on the isolated perfused human skin flap model. *Eur. J. Pharm. Biopharm.* **2017**, *121*, 14–23. [CrossRef]
27. Hurler, J.; Engesland, A.; Poorahmary Kermany, B.; Škalko-Basnet, N. Improved texture analysis for hydrogel characterization: Gel cohesiveness, adhesiveness, and hardness. *J. Appl. Polym. Sci.* **2012**, *125*, 180–188. [CrossRef]
28. Hurler, J.; Škalko-Basnet, N. Potentials of chitosan-based delivery systems in wound therapy: Bioadhesion study. *J. Funct. Biomater.* **2012**, *3*, 37–48. [CrossRef]
29. Du Plessis, J.; Ramachandran, C.; Weiner, N.; Müller, D.G. The influence of particle size of liposomes on the deposition of drug into the skin. *Int. J. Pharm.* **1994**, *103*, 277–282. [CrossRef]
30. Dragicevic-Curic, N.; Gräfe, S.; Gitter, B.; Winter, S.; Fahr, A. Surface charged temoporfin-loaded flexible vesicles: In vitro skin penetration studies and stability. *Int. J. Pharm.* **2010**, *384*, 100–108. [CrossRef]
31. Al Shuwaili, A.H.; Rasool, B.K.A.; Abdulrasool, A.A. Optimization of elastic transfersomes formulations for transdermal delivery of pentoxifylline. *Eur. J. Pharm. Biopharm.* **2016**, *102*, 101–114. [CrossRef] [PubMed]
32. Bnyan, R.; Khan, I.; Ehtezazi, T.; Saleem, I.; Gordon, S.; O'Neill, F.; Roberts, M. Surfactant effects on lipid-based vesicles properties. *J. Pharm. Sci.* **2018**, *107*, 1237–1246. [CrossRef] [PubMed]
33. El Zaafarany, G.M.; Awad, G.A.S.; Holayel, S.M.; Mortada, N.D. Role of edge activators and surface charge in developing ultradeformable vesicles with enhanced skin delivery. *Int. J. Pharm.* **2010**, *397*, 164–172. [CrossRef] [PubMed]
34. Bragagni, M.; Mennini, N.; Maestrelli, F.; Cirri, M.; Mura, P. Comparative study of liposomes, transfersomes and ethosomes as carriers for improving topical delivery of celecoxib. *Drug Deliv.* **2012**, *19*, 354–361. [CrossRef] [PubMed]
35. Islam, M.T.; Rodríguez-Hornedo, N.; Ciotti, S.; Ackermann, C. Rheological characterization of topical carbomer gels neutralized to different pH. *Pharm. Res.* **2004**, *21*, 1192–1199. [CrossRef]
36. Vanić, Ž.; Hurler, J.; Ferderber, K.; Golja Gašparović, P.; Škalko-Basnet, N.; Filipović-Grčić, J. Novel vaginal drug delivery system: Deformable propylene glycol liposomes-in-hydrogel. *J. Liposome Res.* **2014**, *24*, 27–36. [CrossRef]
37. Garg, V.; Singh, H.; Bhatia, A.; Raza, K.; Singh, S.K.; Singh, B.; Beg, S. Systematic development of transethosomal gel system of piroxicam: Formulation optimization, in vitro evaluation, and ex vivo assessment. *AAPS PharmSciTech* **2017**, *18*, 58–71. [CrossRef]
38. Mourtas, S.; Fotopoulou, S.; Duraj, S.; Sfika, V.; Tsakiroglou, C.; Antimisiaris, S.G. Liposomal drugs dispersed in hydrogels. Effect of liposome, drug and gel properties on drug release kinetics. *Colloids Surf. B Biointerfaces* **2007**, *55*, 212–221. [CrossRef]
39. Jain, S.; Patel, N.; Shah, M.K.; Khatri, P.; Vora, N. Recent advances in lipid-based vesicles and particulate carriers for topical and transdermal application. *J. Pharm. Sci.* **2017**, *106*, 423–445. [CrossRef]
40. Thomas, L.; Zakir, F.; Mirza, M.A.; Anwer, M.K.; Ahmad, F.J.; Iqbal, Z. Development of Curcumin loaded chitosan polymer based nanoemulsion gel: In vitro, ex vivo evaluation and in vivo wound healing studies. *Int. J. Biol. Macromol.* **2017**, *101*, 569–579. [CrossRef]
41. Sun, L.; Liu, Z.; Wang, L.; Cun, D.; Tong, H.H.Y.; Yan, R.; Chen, X.; Wang, R.; Zheng, Y. Enhanced topical penetration, system exposure and anti-psoriasis activity of two particle-sized, curcumin-loaded PLGA nanoparticles in hydrogel. *J. Control. Release* **2017**, *254*, 44–54. [CrossRef] [PubMed]
42. El Kechai, N.; Geiger, S.; Fallacara, A.; Cañero Infante, I.; Nicolas, V.; Ferrary, E.; Huang, N.; Bochot, A.; Agnely, F. Mixtures of hyaluronic acid and liposomes for drug delivery: Phase behavior, microstructure and mobility of liposomes. *Int. J. Pharm.* **2017**, *523*, 246–259. [CrossRef] [PubMed]
43. Nguyen, M.-H.; Vu, N.-B.-D.; Nguyen, N.-B.-D.; Le, H.-S.; Le, H.-T.; Tran, T.-T.; Le, X.-C.; Le, V.-T.; Nguyen, T.-T.; Bui, C.-B.; et al. In vivo comparison of wound healing and scar treatment effect between curcumin–oligochitosan nanoparticle complex and oligochitosan-coated curcumin-loaded-liposome. *J. Microencapsul.* **2019**, *36*, 156–168. [CrossRef] [PubMed]

pharmaceutics

MDPI

Article

Topical Delivery of Niacinamide: Influence of Binary and Ternary Solvent Systems

Yanling Zhang [1,*], Chin-Ping Kung [1], Bruno C. Sil [2], Majella E. Lane [1], Jonathan Hadgraft [1], Michael Heinrich [1] and Balint Sinko [3]

1 Department of Pharmaceutics, UCL School of Pharmacy, 29-39 Brunswick Square, London WC1N 1AX, UK; c.kung@ucl.ac.uk (C.-P.K.); majella.lane@btinternet.com (M.E.L.); jonathan.hadgraft@btinternet.com (J.H.); m.heinrich@ucl.ac.uk (M.H.)

2 School of Human Sciences, London Metropolitan University, 166-220 Holloway Road, London N7 8DB, UK; b.dasilvasildossantos@londonmet.ac.uk

3 Pion Inc., 10 Cook Street, Billerica, MA 01821, USA; balint.sinko@googlemail.com

* Correspondence: yanling.zhang.15@ucl.ac.uk

Received: 15 November 2019; Accepted: 9 December 2019; Published: 10 December 2019

Abstract: Niacinamide (NIA) is the amide form of vitamin B3 and has been widely used in pharmaceutical and personal care formulations. Previously, we reported a comparative study of NIA permeation from neat solvents using the Skin Parallel Artificial Membrane Permeability Assay (PAMPA) and mammalian skin. A good correlation between NIA permeation in the different models was found. In the present work, ten binary and ternary systems were evaluated for their ability to promote NIA delivery in the Skin PAMPA model, porcine skin and human epidermis. Penetration enhancement was evident for binary systems composed of propylene glycol and fatty acids in human skin studies. However, propylene glycol and oleic acid did not promote enhancement of NIA compared with other systems in the Skin PAMPA model. A good correlation was obtained for permeation data from Skin PAMPA and porcine skin. However, data from the Skin PAMPA model and from human skin could only be correlated when the PG-fatty acid systems were excluded. These findings add to our knowledge of the potential applications of Skin PAMPA for screening dermal/transdermal preparations.

Keywords: in vitro; permeation; niacinamide; solvent; PAMPA; skin

1. Introduction

Niacinamide (NIA) is the water-soluble form of vitamin B3 (Figure 1). Since its discovery as a "pellagra-preventing" agent, this molecule has been widely used in personal care and cosmetic products [1,2]. NIA has been demonstrated to have a number of anti-inflammatory and photo-protective effects following topical application. The therapeutic benefits of NIA in the management of acne and atopic dermatitis and promotion of the up-regulation of epidermal lipid synthesis have also been reported [3,4]. Mohammed, et al. [5] investigated the influence of NIA on the molecular properties of the human stratum corneum (SC) in vivo. The authors assessed the corneocyte maturity and surface area from NIA treated and untreated (control) areas, as well as trans-epidermal water loss (TEWL). The thickness of the SC before and after the application of NIA was determined using confocal Raman spectroscopy (CRS). The NIA treatment decreased TEWL values, increased the thickness of the SC, and larger and more mature corneocytes were found in the treated versus control sites. More recently, evidence from a phase 3 randomized clinical trial points to NIA having a role in the prevention of non-melanoma skin cancer [6,7].

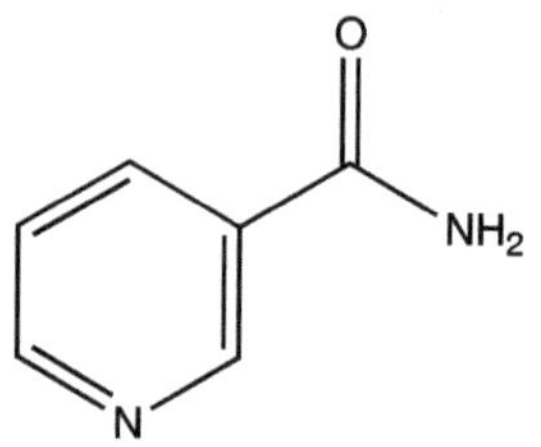

Figure 1. The 2D structure of niacinamide.

The discovery and development of robust and accessible human skin surrogates continues to be an area of considerable interest to industry and regulatory authorities. Recently, we reported the use of the Skin Parallel Arterial Membrane Permeability Assay (PAMPA) model to assess in vitro permeation of NIA from a number of solvents, namely, propylene glycol (PG), dimethyl isosorbide (DMI), Transcutol® P (TC), *t*-butyl alcohol (T-BA), PEG 400, PEG 600, and a commercial product containing NIA [8]. In vitro permeation studies were also performed using porcine skin and heat-separated human epidermis. The permeation studies were conducted under finite dose conditions, namely, 5 μL/cm^2 for human/pig skin and 3 μL/cm^2 for the Skin PAMPA model. When the permeation data for the models were compared, a correlation coefficient (R^2) of 0.71 for human skin and PAMPA was obtained and the corresponding correlation coefficient for porcine skin and PAMPA was 0.88.

A number of studies have reported that combinations of vehicles and/or chemical penetration enhancers may improve skin uptake and the permeation of actives in a synergistic manner [9,10]. PG is one of the most commonly used glycols in skin preparations [11]. The synergistic enhancement of drug delivery to the skin was reported when PG was employed as a co-solvent in delivery systems [12]. In our previous work, a range of neat solvents were evaluated for NIA skin delivery; both PG and TC were identified as the most promising vehicles for this active [8]. The primary aim of the present work was to examine the efficacy of combinations of PG or TC with other solvents on the skin uptake of NIA. The solvents selected were T-BA, DMI, oleic acid (OA), linolenic acid (LA) and caprylic/capric triglyceride (CCT). These solvents were selected as they encompass varying physicochemical properties and, where known, different mechanisms of skin penetration enhancement [11,13]. A secondary aim was to further explore the feasibility of the Skin PAMPA for screening multi-component formulations.

2. Materials and Methods

2.1. Materials

NIA, PG, T-BA, OA, LA, high-performance liquid chromatography (HPLC) grade water and methanol, were purchased from Sigma-Aldrich, Dorset, UK. DMI and IPM were supplied from Croda Ltd., Goole, UK. TC and CCT were kind donations from Gattefossé, St. Priest, France. Phosphate buffered saline (PBS) (pH 7.3 ± 0.2 at 25 °C) tablets was supplied by Oxoid, Cheshire, UK. Pre-coated PAMPA Plates (Pion Inc. PN120657), hydration solution, stirring disks and a Gut-Box™ device were obtained from pION Inc. Billerica, MA, USA.

2.2. Miscibility and Stability Studies

Miscibility studies of all vehicles were conducted to identify appropriate combinations of solvents for binary and ternary systems. The stability of NIA at a concentration of 5% (*w*/*v*) in PG:T-BA (90:10), PG:OA (10:90), PG:TC (50:50), PG:DMI (50:50), PG:LA (50:50), PG:TC:DMI (50:25:25), TC: T-BA (90:10) and TC:DMI (50:50), TC:CCT:DMI (50:25:25) and TC:PG:DMI (50:25:25) was examined at 32 ± 1 °C up to 72 h [14]. The concentration of NIA was determined at 0, 24, 48 and 72 h. Samples were analyzed using the HPLC method validated earlier with a Kinetix® 5 mm Phenyl-Hexyl 250 × 4.6 mm reversed column (Phenomenex, Macclesfield, UK) with water:methanol (80:20) as the mobile phase.

The injection volume was set at 10 μL, and the flow rate of the mobile phase was set to 1 mL/min. The column temperature was set to 30 °C and the UV detection wavelength was 263 nm [8].

2.3. The Skin PAMPA Permeation Studies

The influence of binary and ternary solvent systems on the permeation of NIA was initially screened using the Skin PAMPA model. The Skin PAMPA model was hydrated and prepared following the procedure described by Luo, et al. [15]. The permeation studies were conducted using a modified protocol described previously [8]. A dose of 1 μL (corresponding to 3 μL/cm^2) was used, as it was shown to represent a finite dose of NIA formulations in previous Skin PAMPA studies. To maintain the temperature of the membrane at 32 ± 1 °C, the Skin PAMPA apparatus was incubated in a "Gut-Box™" chamber during the course of permeation studies. Freshly prepared and degassed phosphate buffered saline (PBS, pH 7.3 ± 0.2) solution served as the receptor medium. Samples were collected at 0.1, 0.2, 0.3, 0.7 1, 1.5, 2 and 2.5 h. The concentration of NIA in the receptor medium at each interval was quantified using the HPLC method validated previously [8].

2.4. Permeation Studies in Porcine and Human Skin

Vertical glass Franz diffusion cells were used to conduct in vitro permeation studies of NIA in full thickness porcine and heat-separated human skin, as reported previously [16,17]. All permeation studies were conducted under finite dose conditions (5 μL/cm^2). Porcine tissue was obtained from a local abattoir. The human (female, Caucasian) abdominal tissue from three donors following plastic surgery was obtained from a tissue bank with institutional approval (Research Ethics Committee reference 07/H1306/98). Porcine and human tissue membranes with a diffusion area of around 1 cm^2 were prepared following the procedures described earlier, and the membrane integrity was examined by a measurement of electrical resistance [8]. The Franz cells were placed into a thermostatically controlled water bath (JB Nova, Grant, Cambridge, UK) set at 36 ± 1 °C during the course of the permeation studies. The NIA formulations were applied to the skin when the temperature of the skin surface had equilibrated to 32 ± 1 °C (TM-22 Digitron digital thermometer, RS Components, Corby, UK). A total of 200 μL of receptor medium was withdrawn and replaced with an equal volume of PBS solution at each sampling interval: 0, 1, 2, 4, 6, 8, 10, 12 and 24 h. At the end of the permeation studies, the receptor phase was removed, and mass balance evaluation was performed following a procedure validated previously [18]. The mass balance method is described in the Supplementary Materials.

2.5. Data Analysis

Data were recorded using Microsoft® Excel and analyzed using SPSS® Statistics version 24 (IBM, Feltham, UK) using the procedure described previously [8]. One-way ANOVA with a post hoc Tukey Test was performed for data that met the assumption of normality and homogeneity of variance. The Kruskal–Wallis H Test was used for non-parametric data. A p-value of <0.05 was considered as a statistically significant difference. The correlation between the cumulative amounts of NIA that permeated in the Skin PAMPA model and mammalian skin was calculated using the Pearson Product–moment correlation coefficient (R^2) in Microsoft® Excel.

3. Results and Discussion

3.1. Stability Determination

The stability of NIA in the seven binary and three ternary systems was confirmed. After 72 h, the recovery values of NIA in all tested systems were greater than 91.0%. The stability of NIA in the receptor medium, PBS solution, was confirmed in our earlier work [8]. Stability results are reported in the Supplementary Materials (Figure S1).

3.2. Skin PAMPA Permeation Studies

Figure 2A shows the permeation profiles of NIA for PG:T-BA (90:10), PG:OA (10:90), PG:TC (50:50), PG:DMI (50:50), PG:LA (50:50) and PG:TC:DMI (50:25:25) in the Skin PAMPA model. At 2.5 h, the cumulative amounts of NIA that permeated through the membrane ranged from 44.2 to 177.4 μg/cm^2. PG:T-BA was the most efficient system for NIA delivery compared with all other PG binary or ternary systems ($p < 0.05$). The cumulative amount of NIA delivered through the Skin PAMPA model from neat PG was determined as 163.1 μg/cm^2 [8]. No difference was evident when comparing NIA permeation from PG:T-BA (90:10) and neat PG ($p > 0.05$). The amount of NIA delivered by PG:OA (10:90), 140.2 ± 18.9 μg/cm^2, was significantly greater than corresponding values for PG:TC (50:50), PG:DMI (50:50) and PG:LA (50:50) ($p < 0.05$). The ternary system composed of PG, TC and DMI did not enhance the permeation of NIA in Skin PAMPA compared with PG:DMI (50:50) and PG:TC (50:50) ($p > 0.05$). A significantly lower permeation of NIA was observed for PG:LA (50:50), 44.2 ± 9.4 μg/cm^2, compared with all other binary and ternary systems and neat PG ($p < 0.05$). Formulations containing TC and other solvents were subsequently assessed in the Skin PAMPA model under finite dose conditions (Figure 2B). At 2.5 h, the cumulative amounts of NIA that permeated from TC:T-BA (90:10) and TC:DMI (50:50) were 160.0 ± 8.5 and 159.9 ± 5.4 μg/cm^2, respectively ($p > 0.05$). The amounts of NIA that permeated from TC:T-BA (90:10) and TC:DMI (50:50) were significantly higher compared with corresponding values for TC:CCT:DMI (50:25:25) and TC:PG:DMI (50:25:25) ($p < 0.05$).

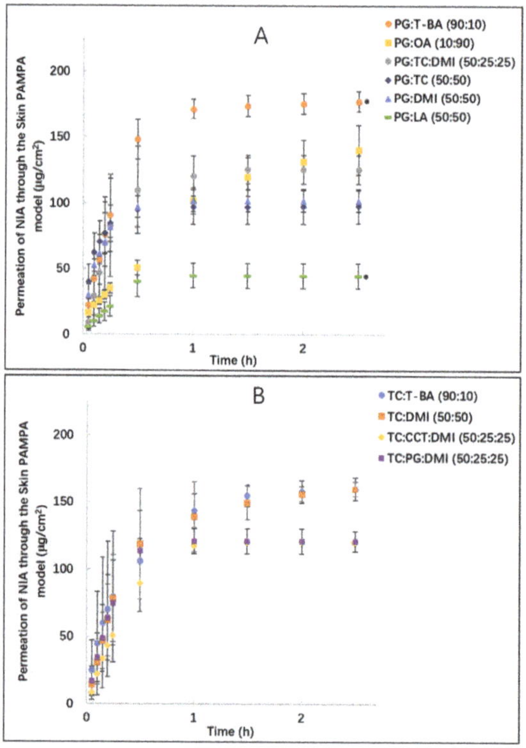

Figure 2. Cumulative permeation of niacinamide (NIA) from binary and ternary solvent systems composed of propylene glycol (PG): *t*-butyl alcohol (T-BA) (●), PG: oleic acid (OA) (■), PG: Transcutol® P (TC) (◆), PG: dimethyl isosorbide (DMI) (▲), PG: linolenic acid (LA) (▬), PG:TC:DMI (50:25:25, ●) (**A**), TC:T-BA(●), TC:DMI(■), TC:PG:DMI (50:25:25, ■) and TC: caprylic/capric triglyceride (CCT):DMI (50:25:25, ◆) (**B**) in the Skin PAMPA model following the application of 1 μL per well (corresponding to 3 μL/cm^2) of formulations. Each data point represents the mean ± SD, $n = 4$. * $p < 0.05$.

Table 1 summarizes the percentages of NIA permeation from the binary and ternary systems. At 2.5 h, for PG:OA (10:90), PG:T-BA (90:10), PG:TC:DMI (50:25:25), TC:DMI (50:50) and TC:T-BA (90:10), more than 80% of the applied active was delivered into the receptor phase ($p > 0.05$). In the previous study, the cumulative amounts of NIA that permeated for neat TC and PG in the Skin PAMPA model were 184.7 ± 8.9 and 163.1 ± 1.1 μg/cm^2, accounting for 97% and 95% of the applied amounts, respectively [8]. Compared with neat TC, the TC binary systems did not enhance the permeation of NIA in the Skin PAMPA model ($p > 0.05$). Interestingly, compared with neat PG, the permeation of NIA was enhanced for PG:T-BA (90:10) ($p < 0.05$). However, the permeation of NIA from PG:LA (50:50) was significantly lower than NIA permeation from neat PG ($p < 0.05$).

Table 1. Percentage permeation of NIA from the binary systems in the Skin PAMPA model (n = 4, mean ± SD).

Formulation	Percentage Permeation (%) at 2.5 h
PG:LA (50:50)	26.9 ± 5.7
PG:DMI (50:50)	66.0 ± 6.9
PG:TC (50:50)	68.0 ± 12.3
PG:OA (10:90)	95.2 ± 13.8
PG:T-BA (90:10)	103.7 ± 0.5
TC:T-BA (90:10)	97.3 ± 5.1
TC:DMI (50:50)	97.2 ± 3.3
TC:PG:DMI (50:25:25)	77.5 ± 8.2
TC:CCT:DMI (50:25:25)	75.3 ± 4.9
TC:CCT:DMI (50:25:25)	81.2 ± 3.2

3.3. Porcine Skin Permeation and Mass Balance Studies

The various binary and ternary solvent systems were examined for their influence on NIA permeation using porcine skin under finite dose conditions (5 μL/cm^2). Figure 3A,B show the permeation profiles for the binary formulations composed of PG or TC. For PG:T-BA (90:10), NIA permeation was detected after 1 h and this system delivered a significantly higher amount of NIA through the tissue compared with other formulations, namely, 150.3 ± 26.5 μg/cm^2 at 24 h ($p < 0.05$). The cumulative amounts of NIA that permeated from PG:OA (10:90) and PG:TC:DMI (50:25:25) were 70.2 ± 18.1 and 58.4 ± 7.0 μg/cm^2, respectively ($p > 0.05$). The cumulative permeation of NIA from PG: LA (50:50) was 19.3 ± 13.7 μg/cm^2, a value that was significantly lower than PG:T-BA (90:10). The amounts of NIA that permeated through porcine skin from binary and ternary formulations of TC ranged from 34.1 to 178.0 μg/cm^2 (Figure 3B). The cumulative amounts of NIA that permeated from neat TC and PG were previously reported as 95.1 and 46.0 μg/cm^2 in pig skin, respectively [8]. At 24 h, a higher cumulative permeation of NIA was evident for TC:T-BA (90:10) compared with neat TC or other assessed binary and ternary systems containing TC ($p < 0.05$).

The overall recoveries in the mass balance studies for PG:OA (10:90), PG:DMI (50:50), PG:TC (50:50), TC:DMI (50:50) and PG:TC:DMI were <85% (Table 2). These results are consistent with the findings of Haque et al. [18]. As the stability of NIA in all formulations was confirmed, it is possible that the lower recovery might be attributed to the chemical derivatization of this molecule during the permeation process [19]. The higher total recovery in binary TC-T-BA systems may reflect the potential of TC:T-BA (90:10) to prevent the chemical derivatization of NIA. However, this hypothesis needs to be probed further. For PG:T-BA (90:10) and TC:T-BA (90:10), lower percentages of NIA were recovered from the skin surface compared with all other binary and ternary systems, accounting for 3.5% and 6.1% of applied NIA amounts, respectively ($p < 0.05$). After 24 h, for all formulations, skin extraction values ranged from 3.2% to 32.9% of the applied amounts. PG:TC (50:50) significantly increased the percentage of NIA deposited in porcine skin compared with neat PG ($p < 0.05$), while no difference was detected when compared with TC ($p > 0.05$). The skin retention values observed for the three tested ternary systems were not significantly different ($p > 0.05$). Interestingly, comparing the distribution of

NIA in the tissue for binary and ternary systems, a higher skin retention was evident for TC:CCT:DMI (50:25:25) than for TC:DMI (50:50) ($p < 0.05$). CCT is a triglyceride comprising a mixture of caprylic and capric acid esters and has been widely used in cosmetic products as an emollient [20]. Leopold and Lippold [21] investigated the mechanism of the penetration enhancing effects of several lipophilic vehicles including CCT using Differential Scanning Calorimetry (DSC). These authors suggested that any penetration enhancement effects of CCT are probably caused by the dissolution or extraction of the stratum corneum lipids. The systems composed of CCT examined here appear promising for the dermal delivery of NIA, and these formulations were further evaluated using human skin.

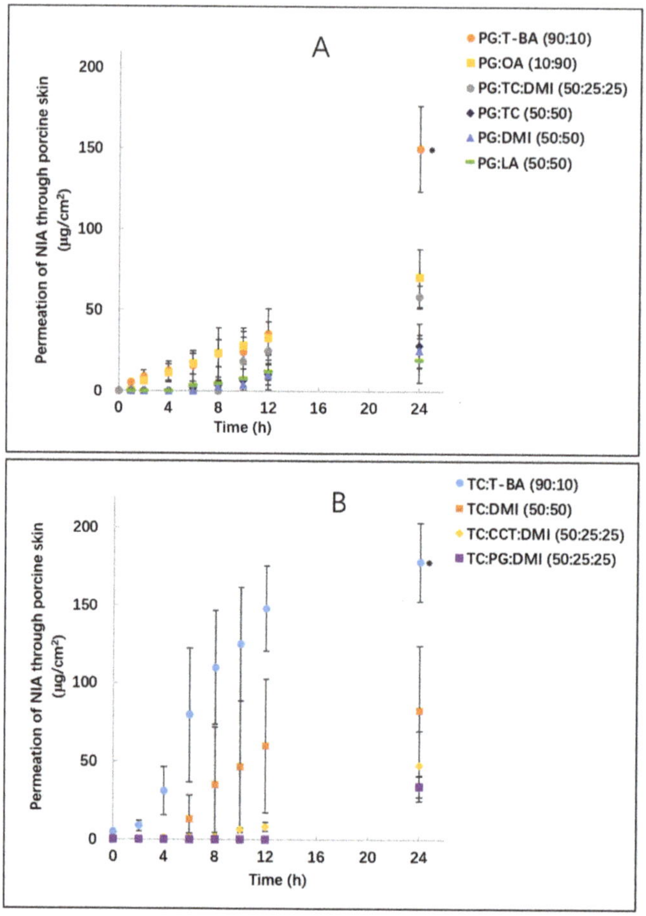

Figure 3. Cumulative permeation of NIA from binary and ternary solvent systems in porcine skin following the application of 5 µL/cm^2 of formulations. (**A**) shows the permeation profiles of PG:T-BA(●), PG:OA(■), PG:TC(◆), PG:DMI(▲), PG:LA(▬), PG:TC:DMI (50:25:25, ●); (**B**) shows the permeation profiles of TC:T-BA(●), TC:DMI(■), TC:PG:DMI (50:25:25, ■) and TC:CCT:DMI (50:25:25, ◆). Each data point represents the mean ± SD, $n = 4$. * $p < 0.05$.

Table 2. The results of the mass balance studies after the permeation studies using porcine skin under finite dose conditions (n = 4, mean ± SD).

Formulation	Washing %	Extraction %	Permeation %	Total %
PG:DMI (50:50)	47.1 ± 5.4	22.9 ± 13.2	11.5 ± 3.9	81.5 ± 5.6
PG:OA (10:90)	37.1 ± 5.4	9.6 ± 1.0	30.2 ± 7.2	76.8 ± 5.9
PG:TC (50:50)	43.4 ± 3.9	23.4 ± 5.6	13.4 ± 6.9	80.2 ± 6.7
PG:LA (50:50)	55.6 ± 12.3	20.6 ± 4.4	9.2 ± 6.6	85.4 ± 7.9
PG:T-BA (90:10)	3.5 ± 0.8	10.1 ± 7.6	71.3 ± 12.6	84.9 ± 7.1
TC:T-BA (90:10)	6.1 ± 5.2	15.3 ± 11.9	79.5 ± 12.0	100.9 ± 13.8
TC:DMI (50:50)	35.3 ± 13.6	10.7 ± 3.5	35.2 ± 16.0	81.2 ± 1.8
PG:TC:DMI (50:25:25)	36.1 ± 8.5	18.8 ± 8.8	25.1 ± 3.8	80.1 ± 9.7
TC:CCT:DMI (50:25:25)	39.8 ± 15.1	28.0 ± 12.8	18.2 ± 7.6	86.0 ± 8.9
TC:PG:DMI (50:25:25)	43.2 ± 4.0	32.9 ± 13.8	13.2 ± 1.9	89.2 ± 16.8

As shown in Figure 4, 19.3–178.0 μg/cm^2 of NIA penetrated through porcine skin at 24 h, while 44.2–177.4 μg/cm^2 was delivered in the Skin PAMPA model at 2.5 h. A correlation coefficient (R^2) of 0.63 was determined for the linear regression of the data (Figure 4). The value was lower compared with the correlation coefficient determined between the permeation data in Skin PAMPA and porcine skin for the single solvents under finite dose conditions, R^2 = 0.88 [8]. This may reflect the different interactions of the more complex vehicles studied here in the Skin PAMPA lipids compared with the single solvents studied previously.

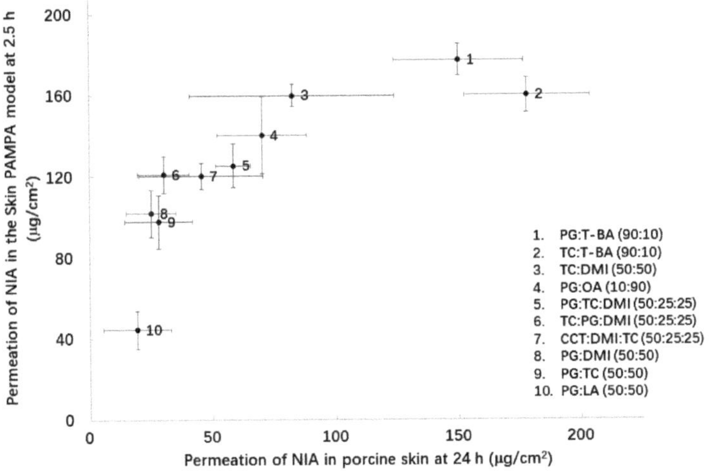

Figure 4. Cumulative amounts of NIA that permeated from assessed binary and ternary solvent systems in the Skin PAMPA model at 2.5 h plotted against the corresponding values observed in porcine skin at 24 h. Each data point represents the mean ± SD, n = 4.

3.4. Human Skin Permeation and Mass Balance Studies

NIA permeation was further investigated using heat-separated human epidermis. The permeation profiles of NIA for these experiments are shown in Figure 5. For the two binary systems, PG:LA (50:50) and PG:OA (10:90), permeation of NIA was detected 2 h after application. At 24 h, significantly higher amounts of NIA were delivered from PG:LA (50:50) and PG:OA (10:90) compared with all other binary and ternary systems ($p < 0.05$), with cumulative permeation values of 100.4 ± 2.4 and 93.3 ±2.4 μg/cm^2, respectively. The cumulative amounts of NIA that permeated in human skin for neat T-BA, DMI, PG or TC were reported previously as 50.8, 15.0, 1.8 and 16.4 μg/cm^2 [8]. A more efficient skin penetration enhancement of NIA is clearly evident for PG:LA and PG:OA compared with these neat solvents ($p < 0.05$). No significant increase was observed for NIA permeation from TC binary and ternary systems compared with neat TC ($p > 0.05$).

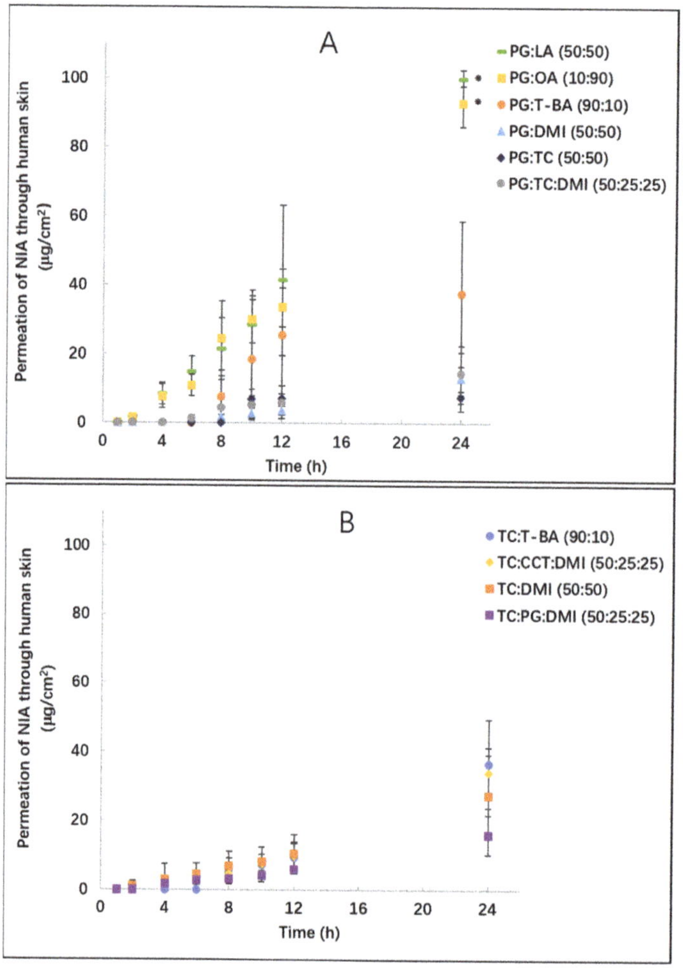

Figure 5. Cumulative permeation of NIA from binary and ternary solvent systems in human skin following the application of 5 μL/cm^2 of formulation. (**A**) shows the permeation profiles of PG:T-BA(●), PG:OA(■), PG:TC(◆), PG:DMI(▲), PG:LA(▬), PG:TC:DMI (50:25:25, ●); (**B**) shows the permeation profiles of TC:T-BA(●), TC:DMI(■) TC:PG:DMI (50:25:25, ■) and TC:CCT:DMI (50:25:25, ◆). Each data point represents the mean ± SD, $n = 4$. * $p < 0.05$.

Table 3 summarizes the mass balance results of NIA for the human skin studies. The amounts of NIA remaining on the skin surface range from 27% to 75% of the amounts applied, respectively. No difference was detected comparing the percentage of NIA recovered from the skin surface for the different formulations ($p > 0.05$). The skin retention of NIA for PG:LA (50:50) was determined as 3.4% of the applied dose. This value was significantly lower ($p < 0.05$) compared with the skin extraction values for TC:T-BA (34.7%) and TC:CCT:DMI (29.7%). The percentage of NIA extracted from human epidermis for neat TC was 32.9% [8]. The corresponding value for TC:T-BA (90:10) was comparable to the value for neat TC ($p > 0.05$). As for the percentage permeation, higher values were observed for

PG:LA (50:50) (46.1%) and PG:OA (10:90) (40.7%) compared to all other binary and ternary systems ($p < 0.05$). There was no significant increase in the percentage permeation of NIA from TC binary systems compared with neat TC ($p > 0.05$). Statistical analysis confirmed the penetration enhancement of NIA for the PG/fatty acids (LA and OA) compared with neat PG [8] ($p < 0.05$). However, in porcine skin studies, the percentage permeation of NIA for PG:LA (50:50) was significantly lower than for neat PG and PG:OA (10:90) ($p < 0.05$).

Table 3. The results of mass balance studies after permeation studies using human skin under finite dose conditions ($n = 4$, mean ± SD).

Formulations	Washing%	Extraction%	Permeation%	Total%
PG:DMI (50:50)	59.6 ± 7.1	17.4 ± 3.9	5.6 ± 4.0	82.6 ± 7.8
PG:OA (10:90)	37.7 ± 6.7	9.2 ± 0.6	40.7 ± 6.5	87.6 ± 0.8
PG:TC (50:50)	69.8 ± 7.8	29.0 ± 18.5	4.4 ± 2.3	103.1 ± 13.4
PG:LA (50:50)	27.1 ± 5.6	3.4 ± 2.0	46.1 ± 5.1	76.5 ± 5.1
PG:T-BA (90:10)	52.8 ± 9.0	20.1 ± 6.0	12.3 ± 4.2	85.2 ± 10.9
TC:T-BA (90:10)	39.8 ± 16.5	34.7 ± 10.5	15.6 ± 5.6	90.1 ± 5.2
TC:DMI (50:50)	75.1 ± 11.7	13.2 ± 4.7	10.2 ± 4.4	98.5 ± 11.7
PG:TC:DMI (50:25:25)	64.6 ± 4.5	12.2 ± 2.0	6.2 ± 2.3	83.0 ± 4.2
TC:CCT:DMI (50:25:25)	44.9 ± 6.0	29.7 ± 4.9	12.9 ± 3.3	87.5 ± 4.9
TC:PG:DMI (50:25:25)	66.5 ± 9.1	14.6 ± 3.4	6.6 ± 2.5	87.8 ± 6.7

Fatty acids have been reported to be skin permeation enhancers for a range of substances possessing varying physicochemical properties [11,22,23]. Recently, Pham, et al. [24] applied ^{13}C polarization transfer solid-state nuclear magnetic resonance (NMR) to investigate the effects of OA on SC molecular components. The authors mixed 30 mg of dry SC powder with 5% of OA and then hydrated the mixture with water. The samples were incubated at 32 °C for 24 h before NMR measurement. It was suggested that OA promoted increased mobility of both stratum corneum protein components and the cholesterol chain segments in the intercellular lipid domains. However, the exact synergistic mechanism of PG and fatty acids remains unclear. It may also be hypothesized that the fatty acid first penetrates into the stratum corneum and contributes to increased lipid fluidity, which allows the diffusion of PG with dissolved NIA.

In the present study, there was no significant difference between the permeation in human skin and porcine skin for NIA in TC:DMI (50:50) PG:DMI (50:50), TC:CCT:DMI (50:25:25) ($p > 0.05$). A higher permeation of NIA in porcine skin compared to human skin was evident for PG:T-BA (90:10), PG:DMI (50:50), PG:TC (50:50), PG:TC:DMI (50:25:25), TC:T-BA (90:10) and TC:PG:DMI (50:25:25) ($p < 0.05$). However, a lower permeation of NIA in porcine skin compared to human tissue was evident for PG:LA (50:50) and PG:OA (10:90) ($p < 0.05$). Similar results have been reported by other researchers for other actives. Shin, et al. [25] noted higher flux values of fentanyl for human skin compared with porcine skin. Although pig skin has generally been considered to be more permeable than human skin [26–28], the permeability may be dependent on the molecule of interest. Jung and Maibach [29] reviewed 46 studies which evaluated the permeation of 77 chemicals using both porcine and human skin; for 16 chemicals, permeation was greater in human skin permeation compared with porcine skin.

The cumulative permeation of NIA in human skin ranged from 14.5 to 100.4 μg/cm^2; the corresponding values determined in the Skin PAMPA model ranged from 44.2 to 177.4 μg/cm^2. Higher NIA permeation was observed in the artificial membrane compared with human epidermis for PG:T-BA (90:10), TC:T-BA (90:10), TC:DMI (50:50), PG:OA (10:90), PG:TC:DMI (50:25:25), TC:CCT:DMI (50:25:25), PG:DMI (50:50) and PG:TC (50:50) ($p < 0.05$). Attempts to fit all the permeation data from the Skin PAMPA model and human epidermis were not successful. However, excluding results for PG:LA (50:50) and PG:OA (10:90), an R^2 value of 0.68 was obtained for the linear regression of the data (Figure 6). The higher permeability of the Skin PAMPA studies observed in this study is consistent with findings reported by others. Luo et al. [15] investigated the permeation of ibuprofen from PG,

PEG 300, commercial gel and spray formulations in the Skin PAMPA model, porcine and human skin. The authors reported the more permeable nature of the Skin PAMPA model compared to human skin. Although the authors did not correlate the permeation data obtained from different models, they reported formulations that delivered a higher amount of ibuprofen in the Skin PAMPA model were also more efficient in human skin. In our previous work, NIA permeation from neat T-BA, DMI, TC, PG, PEG 400 and PEG 600 and one commercial product in the Skin PAMPA model were correlated with porcine/human skin [8]. A correlation coefficient (R^2) of 0.71 was established for the Skin PAMPA with human skin under finite dose conditions. The corresponding correlation between PAMPA model and porcine skin was determined as 0.88. In this work, a correlation of NIA permeation data in human skin and PAMPA model could only be obtained when the permeation data for PG-OA and PG-LA were excluded. Statistical analysis confirmed that the permeation of NIA from PG:LA (50:50) was significantly lower than neat PG ($p < 0.05$) in the Skin PAMPA. Additionally, in the Skin PAMPA model, the permeation of NIA from PG:OA (10:90) was significantly higher compared with PG:LA (50:50) ($p < 0.05$), while no difference was observed between these two systems in human epidermis ($p > 0.05$).

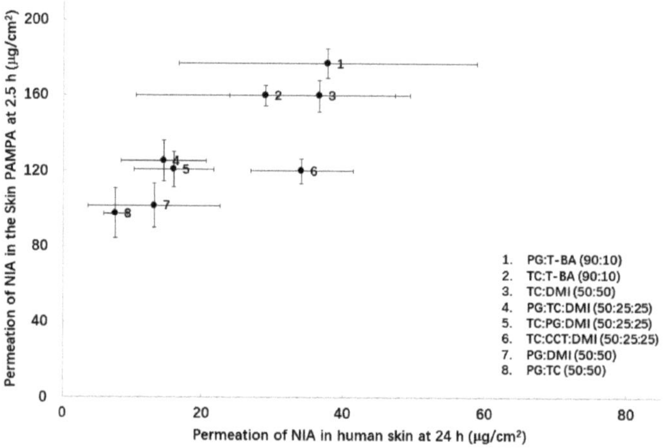

Figure 6. Cumulative permeation data of NIA from assessed binary and ternary solvent systems in the Skin PAMPA model at 2.5 h, plotted against the corresponding values observed in human skin at 24 h. Each data point represents the mean ± SD, $n = 4$.

To our knowledge, this is the first study that has investigated the permeation enhancement of fatty acids with PG in the Skin PAMPA model. The results obtained in this study suggested that the Skin PAMPA model is not a suitable model for screening such combinations. The Skin PAMPA model uses a homogeneous filter-impregnated lipid mixture membrane, containing ~50% of synthesized ceramides (Certramide), 25% of stearic acid and 25% of cholesterol [30]. The lower permeation of binary solvent systems composed of PG and fatty acid may reflect the interaction of the lipid components with those formulations. Both OA and LA are unsaturated C_{18} fatty acids [31]. These two fatty acids have a double bond in the conformation [32]. It is possible that OA and LA integrated into the PAMPA membrane and modified the lateral chain packing in the lipid matrix. This may lead to changes in the physicochemical properties and permeability of this artificial model. Further studies are needed to probe this theory.

4. Conclusions

Previous work investigated the dermal delivery of NIA from a series of single solvents. In the present work, the influence of binary and ternary solvents on the in vitro permeation of NIA was assessed in the Skin PAMPA model, porcine skin and heat separated human epidermis. The higher skin penetration of NIA was evident in human skin for the binary systems composed of PG with fatty acids (PG-OA, PG-LA) compared with neat solvents investigated previously. A correlation of 0.63 was determined for the permeation data of binary and ternary systems in Skin PAMPA and in porcine skin. Excluding the PG-OA and PG-LA systems, a correlation of 0.68 (R^2) was also evident between the permeation data obtained in the Skin PAMPA model and human epidermis. Further studies to investigate the interactions between the Skin PAMPA model and the fatty acids OA and LA are needed to better understand the potential of this model in the assessment of transdermal/dermal products. Ultimately, a robust, efficient, accessible artificial skin permeability assay would benefit the regulatory authorities, the pharmaceutical industry and the patients.

Supplementary Materials: The following are available online at http://www.mdpi.com/1999-4923/11/12/668/s1, Figure S1: Results of stability studies. Percentage of NIA recovered from tested binary and ternary solvent systems at 24, 48 and 72 h at 32 ± 1 °C (n = 3, mean ± SD).

Author Contributions: Conceptualization, M.E.L.; Methodology, M.E.L., Y.Z. and C.-P.K.; Software, Y.Z., C.-P.K.; Validation, M.E.L. and Y.Z.; Formal Analysis, M.E.L. and Y.Z.; Investigation, Y.Z.; Resources, M.E.L., Y.Z. and B.S.; Data Curation, Y.Z.; Writing—Original Draft Preparation, Y.Z.; Writing—Review and Editing, M.E.L., J.H., Y.Z., B.C.S., M.H., B.S., C.-P.K.; Visualization, Y.Z., C.-P.K., M.E.L., J.H.; Supervision, M.E.L., M.H. and J.H.; Project Administration, M.E.L.; Funding Acquisition, Y.Z.

Funding: This research received no external funding.

Acknowledgments: We thank our colleagues from the UCL Skin Research Group who provided insight and expertise that greatly assisted the research.

Conflicts of Interest: The authors declare no conflict of interest. This company (Pion Inc.) had no role in the design of the study; in the collection, analyses, or interpretation of data; in the writing of the manuscript, and in the decision to publish the results.

List of Abbreviations

NIA	Niacinamide
PAMPA	Parallel Artificial Membrane Permeability Assay
ANOVA	One-way analysis of variance
PG	Propylene glycol
DMI	Dimethyl isosorbide
OA	Oleic acid
LA	Linolenic acid
T-BA	*t*-butyl alcohol
TC	Transcutol® P
CCT	Caprylic/capric triglyceride
PEG	Polyethylene glycol
CIRP	Cosmetic Ingredient Review Panel
SD	Standard deviation
SC	Stratum corneum
NMR	Nuclear magnetic resonance
FTIR	Fourier transform infrared spectroscopy

References

1. Matts, P.; Oblong, J.; Bissett, D.L. A Review of the range of effects of niacinamide in human skin. *Int. Fed. Soc. Cosmet. Chem. Mag.* **2002**, *5*, 285–289.
2. Wohlrab, J.; Kreft, D. Niacinamide-mechanisms of action and its topical use in dermatology. *Ski. Pharmacol. Physiol.* **2014**, *27*, 311–315. [CrossRef] [PubMed]
3. Lee, M.-H.; Lee, K.-K.; Park, M.-H.; Hyun, S.-S.; Kahn, S.-Y.; Joo, K.-S.; Kang, H.-C.; Kwon, W.-T. In vivo anti-melanogenesis activity and in vitro skin permeability of niacinamide-loaded flexible liposomes (Bounsphere™). *J. Drug Deliv. Sci. Technol.* **2016**, *31*, 147–152. [CrossRef]
4. Papich, M.G. Niacinamide. In *Saunders Handbook of Veterinary Drugs*, 4th ed.; Saunders: St. Louis, MO, USA, 2016; pp. 562–563. [CrossRef]

5. Mohammed, D.; Crowther, J.M.; Matts, P.J.; Hadgraft, J.; Lane, M.E. Influence of niacinamide containing formulations on the molecular and biophysical properties of the stratum corneum. *Int. J. Pharm.* **2013**, *441*, 192–201. [CrossRef]
6. Chen, A.C.; Martin, A.J.; Choy, B.; Fernández-Peñas, P.; Dalziell, R.A.; McKenzie, C.A.; Scolyer, R.A.; Dhillon, H.M.; Vardy, J.L.; Kricker, A. A phase 3 randomized trial of nicotinamide for skin-cancer chemoprevention. *N. Engl. J. Med.* **2015**, *373*, 1618–1626. [CrossRef]
7. Snaidr, V.A.; Damian, D.L.; Halliday, G.M. Nicotinamide for photoprotection and skin cancer chemoprevention: A review of efficacy and safety. *Exp. Dermatol.* **2019**, *28*, 15–22. [CrossRef]
8. Zhang, Y.; Lane, M.E.; Hadgraft, J.; Heinrich, M.; Chen, T.; Lian, G.; Sinko, B. A comparison of the in vitro permeation of niacinamide in mammalian skin and in the Parallel Artificial Membrane Permeation Assay (PAMPA) model. *Int. J. Pharm.* **2019**, *556*, 142–149. [CrossRef]
9. Oliveira, G.; Hadgraft, J.; Lane, M.E. The influence of volatile solvents on transport across model membranes and human skin. *Int. J. Pharm.* **2012**, *435*, 38–49. [CrossRef]
10. Parisi, N.; Matts, P.J.; Lever, R.; Hadgraft, J.; Lane, M.E. Preparation and characterisation of hexamidine salts. *Int. J. Pharm.* **2015**, *493*, 404–411. [CrossRef]
11. Lane, M.E. Skin penetration enhancers. *Int. J. Pharm.* **2013**, *447*, 12–21. [CrossRef]
12. Karande, P.; Mitragotri, S. Enhancement of transdermal drug delivery via synergistic action of chemicals. *Biochim. Biophys. Acta—Biomembr.* **2009**, *1788*, 2362–2373. [CrossRef] [PubMed]
13. Hadgraft, J.; Lane, M.E. Advanced topical formulations (ATF). *Int. J. Pharm.* **2016**, *514*, 52–57. [CrossRef] [PubMed]
14. Haque, T.; Rahman, K.M.; Thurston, D.E.; Hadgraft, J.; Lane, M.E. Topical delivery of anthramycin II. Influence of binary and ternary solvent systems. *Eur. J. Pharm. Sci.* **2018**. [CrossRef] [PubMed]
15. Luo, L.; Patel, A.; Sinko, B.; Bell, M.; Wibawa, J.; Hadgraft, J.; Lane, M.E. A comparative study of the in vitro permeation of ibuprofen in mammalian skin, the PAMPA model and silicone membrane. *Int. J. Pharm.* **2016**, *505*, 14–19. [CrossRef] [PubMed]
16. Santos, P.; Watkinson, A.C.; Hadgraft, J.; Lane, M.E. Oxybutynin permeation in skin: The influence of drug and solvent activity. *Int. J. Pharm.* **2010**, *384*, 67–72. [CrossRef]
17. Kung, C.-P.; Sil, B.C.; Hadgraft, J.; Lane, M.E.; Patel, B.; McCulloch, R. Preparation, Characterization and Dermal Delivery of Methadone. *Pharmaceutics* **2019**, *11*, 509. [CrossRef]
18. Haque, T.; Lane, M.E.; Sil, B.C.; Crowther, J.M.; Moore, D.J. In vitro permeation and disposition of niacinamide in silicone and porcine skin of skin barrier-mimetic formulations. *Int. J. Pharm.* **2017**, *520*, 158–162. [CrossRef]
19. Sil, B.C.; Moore, D.J.; Lane, M.E. Use of LC-MS analysis to elucidate by-products of niacinamide transformation following in vitro skin permeation studies. *Int. J. Cosmet. Sci.* **2018**, *40*, 525–529. [CrossRef]
20. CIRP. Caprylic/Capric Triglyceride. *Int. J. Toxicol.* **2003**, *22*, 4–5. [CrossRef]
21. Leopold, C.S.; Lippold, B.C. An attempt to clarify the mechanism of the penetration enhancing effects of lipophilic vehicles with differential scanning calorimetry (DSC). *J. Pharm. Pharmacol.* **1995**, *47*, 276–281. [CrossRef]
22. Ng, K.W.; Lau, W.M.; Williams, A. Synergy Between Chemical Penetration Enhancers. In *Percutaneous Penetration Enhancers Chemical Methods in Penetration Enhancement*; Springer: Berlin/Heidelberg, Germany, 2015; pp. 373–385. [CrossRef]
23. van Zyl, L.; du Preez, J.; Gerber, M.; du Plessis, J.; Viljoen, J. Essential Fatty Acids as Transdermal Penetration Enhancers. *J. Pharm. Sci.* **2016**, *105*, 188–193. [CrossRef] [PubMed]
24. Pham, Q.D.; Björklund, S.; Engblom, J.; Topgaard, D.; Sparr, E. Chemical penetration enhancers in stratum corneum—Relation between molecular effects and barrier function. *J. Control. Release* **2016**, *232*, 175–187. [CrossRef] [PubMed]
25. Shin, S.H.; Srivilai, J.; Ibrahim, S.A.; Strasinger, C.; Hammell, D.C.; Hassan, H.E.; Stinchcomb, A.L. The Sensitivity of In Vitro Permeation Tests to Chemical Penetration Enhancer Concentration Changes in Fentanyl Transdermal Delivery Systems. *AAPS Pharmscitech* **2018**, *19*, 2778–2786. [CrossRef] [PubMed]
26. Dick, I.P.; Scott, R.C. Pig ear skin as an in-vitro model for human skin permeability. *J. Pharm. Pharmacol.* **1992**, *44*, 640–645. [CrossRef] [PubMed]
27. Singh, S.; Zhao, K.; Singh, J. In vitro permeability and binding of hydrocarbons in pig ear and huamn abdominal skin. *Drug Chem. Toxicol.* **2002**, *25*, 83–92. [CrossRef]

28. Barbero, A.M.; Frasch, H.F. Pig and guinea pig skin as surrogates for human in vitro penetration studies: A quantitative review. *Toxicol. Vitr.* **2009**, *23*, 1–13. [CrossRef]
29. Jung, E.C.; Maibach, H.I. Animal Models for Percutaneous Absorption. *J. Appl. Toxicol.* **2014**, *35*, 1–10. [CrossRef]
30. Sinkó, B.; Garrigues, T.M.; Balogh, G.T.; Nagy, Z.K.; Tsinman, O.; Avdeef, A.; Takács-Novák, K. Skin–PAMPA: A new method for fast prediction of skin penetration. *Eur. J. Pharm. Sci.* **2012**, *45*, 698–707. [CrossRef]
31. Ibrahim, S.A.; Li, S.K. Efficiency of Fatty Acids as Chemical Penetration Enhancers: Mechanisms and Structure Enhancement Relationship. *Pharm. Res.* **2010**, *27*, 115–125. [CrossRef]
32. Small, D.M. Lateral chain packing in lipids and membranes. *J. Lipid Res.* **1984**, *25*, 1490–1500.

pharmaceutics

MDPI

Article

Preparation, Characterization and Dermal Delivery of Methadone

Chin-Ping Kung [1,*], Bruno C. Sil [2], Jonathan Hadgraft [1], Majella E. Lane [1], Bhumik Patel [3] and Renée McCulloch [3]

1 Department of Pharmaceutics, UCL School of Pharmacy, 29-39 Brunswick Square, London WC1N 1AX, UK; jonathan.hadgraft@btinternet.com (J.H.); majella.lane@btinternet.com (M.E.L.)
2 School of Human Sciences, London Metropolitan University, 166-220 Holloway Road, London N7 8DB, UK; b.dasilvasildossantos@londonmet.ac.uk
3 Great Ormond Street Hospital for Children NHS Foundation Trust, Great Ormond Street, London, WC1N 3JH, UK; bhumik.patel@gosh.nhs.uk (B.P.); renee.mcculloch@gosh.nhs.uk (R.M.)
* Correspondence: c.kung@ucl.ac.uk

Received: 12 July 2019; Accepted: 24 September 2019; Published: 2 October 2019

Abstract: The use of methadone for the management of pain has received great interest in recent years. Currently, oral and intravenous formulations are available for clinical use. Dermal delivery represents an attractive alternative route of administration for this drug as it is associated with comparatively fewer side effects. The first stage of the work was the preparation of methadone free base as this form of the drug is expected to permeate the skin to a greater extent than the hydrochloride salt. Subsequently the molecule was characterized with Nuclear Magnetic Resonance (NMR) and thermal analysis, the distribution coefficient was determined and solubility studies were conducted in a range of solvents. In vitro permeation and mass balance studies were conducted under finite dose conditions (5 μL/cm^2) in porcine skin. The results confirmed the more favorable penetration of methadone free base compared with the salt. The highest cumulative amount of methadone (41 ± 5 μg/cm^2) permeated from d-limonene (LIM). Ethyl oleate (EO), Transcutol® P (TC) and octyl salicylate (OSAL) also appear to be promising candidate components of dermal formulations for methadone base. Future work will focus on further formulation optimization with the objective of progressing to evaluation of prototype dosage forms in clinical trials.

Keywords: dermal delivery; porcine skin; in vitro permeation; methadone; pain

1. Introduction

Neuropathic pain can be caused by injuries, surgery, chemotherapy and a number of disease conditions such as diabetes mellitus, cancer and human immunodeficiency virus infection [1]. It can also arise as a direct consequence of a lesion or disease affecting the peripheral nervous system or the central nervous system [2]. Patients' overall health-related quality of life is greatly impacted by neuropathic pain [3] and it is estimated to affect 7–10% of the general population in Europe [4]. The available current knowledge in terms of causes, diagnosis and treatment for peripheral neuropathic pain is more advanced than that for pain associated with the central nervous system [5]. However, to date, there are still very few effective treatments available for management of neuropathic pain.

Methadone has traditionally been used in the management of opioid dependence. However, there is increasing interest in the repurposing of methadone as a cost-efficient treatment for neuropathic pain [6,7]. Morley, et al. [8] reported the efficacy of oral methadone for the management of neuropathic pain in a double-blind randomized controlled crossover trial. 19 patients were enrolled in the trial and a statistically significant ($p < 0.05$) improvement in pain relief was reported. Methadone is not only a potent μ-opioid receptor agonist but also a non-competitive *N*-Methyl-D-aspartate (NMDA) receptor antagonist [9]. The combination of NMDA receptor antagonism and opioid receptor agonism induced by methadone is thought to result in enhanced analgesic efficacy. Animal studies have demonstrated that the antinociception effect of methadone is mediated by both opioid agonism and NMDA receptor antagonism in neuropathic pain [10]. The peripheral effect of morphine, a μ-opioid receptor agonist, was enhanced by combined administration of (+)-HA966, an NMDA receptor antagonist, in a rat model of neuropathic pain [11]. In addition, Stoetzer, et al. [12] also suggested that methadone is an unselective blocker of a number of voltage-gated sodium (Nav) channels including Nav1.2, Nav1.3, Nav1.7, and Nav1.8 with comparable potency to bupivacaine. These studies suggest that methadone is a promising candidate to be developed for the management of peripheral neuropathic pain.

Dermal delivery of drugs offers a number of advantages compared with other routes of administration. Constant drug levels in the plasma can be achieved with a decrease in dosing frequency. Moreover, the avoidance of first pass metabolism results in less intra- and inter-patient variability. Dermal delivery should also provide higher concentrations of methadone in skin tissues, thus targeting pain at its source. The peripheral actions of methadone also suggest a lower concentration of methadone can be delivered via the skin for pain relief compared with oral administration. To our knowledge, there are only three published papers that have examined the in vitro skin absorption of methadone. Fullerton, et al. [13] examined the permeation of methadone in human cadaver skin from simple ethanol solutions. Ghosh and Bagherian [14] also investigated the delivery of methadone free base from a transdermal patch in human skin. Recently, Muñoz, et al. [15] reported in vitro permeation studies using porcine skin to evaluate the efficiency of methadone hydrochloride patches. No studies have examined the in vivo delivery of this compound through the skin.

The aims of the present work were (i) to prepare and characterize methadone free base and (ii) to identify effective solvents for the dermal delivery of methadone. A concentration of 5% *w/v* methadone base solutions was selected based on available formulations for oral use. A range of solvents, spanning different physicochemical parameters such as polarity and solubilization properties, were selected as candidate vehicles. These solvents are generally recognized as safe (GRAS) and are already used in other topical and transdermal dosage forms.

2. Materials and Methods

2.1. Materials

Methadone hydrochloride, tripropylene glycol (TriPG), dipropylene glycol (DiPG), 1-octanol, 1,3-butanediol (1,3-BD), Brij™ O20, isopropyl myristate (IPM), octyl salicylate (OSAL), oleic acid (OA) and ethyl oleate (EO) were purchased from Sigma-Aldrich, Dorset, UK. Propylene glycol (PG), ethyl acetate, d-limonene (LIM), high performance liquid chromatography (HPLC) grade water, acetonitrile, orthophosphoric acid, 85+%, sodium dihydrogen phosphate, sodium hydrogen phosphate and sodium hydroxide were supplied by Fisher Scientific, Loughborough, UK. Chloroform-*d* ($CDCl_3$) was purchased from Cambridge Isotope Laboratories Tewksbury, MA, USA. Labrafac™ lipophile WL 1349 (medium-chain triglycerides of caprylic and capric acids, WL 1349), Transcutol® (TC), propylene glycol monocaprylate (PGMC) Type II and propylene glycol monolaurate (PGML) Type II were gifts from Gattefossé, St. Priest, France. Phosphate buffered saline (PBS) (pH 7.3 ± 0.2 at 25 °C) was prepared using Dulbecco A tablets supplied by Oxoid, Cheshire, UK. Full thickness porcine ear skin was obtained from a local abattoir.

2.2. Preparation of Methadone Base

Methadone hydrochloride (1.730 g, 0.005 mol) was placed in a dry 250 mL round-bottom flask with a Teflon coated magnetic stirrer. 20 mL of HPLC grade water was added and the mixture was stirred for 10 min. The pH was then adjusted to 11.0 with 1 M sodium hydroxide solution. The newly formed precipitate was stirred for 30 min. 100 mL of ethyl acetate was added to the suspension with stirring for 60 min at 25 °C. The organic layer was then collected, and the aqueous layer washed with 45 mL (3 × 15 mL) of ethyl acetate. All organic layers were collected together and dried with magnesium sulfate. Ethyl acetate was removed using a rotary evaporator (Heidolph, Schwabach, Germany) using a high vacuum line for 5 h. Structural characterization was conducted using proton nuclear magnetic resonance (^{1}H-NMR) spectroscopy. The spectrum was obtained in chloroform-*d* using a Bruker Avance 500 MHz NMR spectrometer (Bruker Corporation, Billerica, MA, USA) and processed using MestReNova 11.0.4 (Mestrelab Research, Santiago de Compostela, Spain). The Fourier transform infrared (FTIR) spectra were obtained with a Bruker Alpha Spectrometer with a Platinum ATR accessory (Bruker Optics, Coventry, UK) in transmittance mode. Spectral analysis and instrument control were performed with OPUS software v.7.0 (Bruker Optics). The spectrum of each sample was measured by taking the average of 64 scans at a resolution of 2 cm^{-1} at room temperature. The reference background spectrum was recorded before collecting IR spectra.

2.3. *Thermal Analysis*

The melting points of methadone hydrochloride and methadone free base were measured using thermogravimetric analysis (TGA) and differential scanning calorimetry (DSC). Discovery TGA (TA instruments, Waters, LLC, USA) was used for the degradation temperature identification. Approximately 3 mg of sample was placed in a tared aluminium pan. A heating ramp of 10 °C/min to 550 °C was used during the analysis. A nitrogen flow of 25 mL/min was supplied to create an inert atmosphere around the sample. A DSC Q2000 (TA instruments) system was used to measure the melting point. The sample was weighed in a hermetic aluminium pan which was subsequently sealed with a hermetic aluminium lid using a Tzero press. An empty hermetic aluminium pan sealed with a hermetic aluminium lid was used as a reference. Sample and reference pans were heated with a heating ramp of 10 °C/min with nitrogen as the purge gas (50 mL/min).

2.4. *HPLC Analysis*

The HPLC system used in this study consisted of an Agilent G1322A degasser, G1311A quaternary pump, G1313A auto sampler, G1316A thermostat column compartment and G1315B diode array detector (Agilent Technologies, Palo Alto, CA, USA.). The software used to acquire and analyze the data was ChemStation® for LC 3D, Rev. A. 09.03 (Agilent Technologies). Analysis was performed with a Luna® Omega 5 μm PS C_{18} 150 × 4.60 mm column (Phenomenex, Macclesfield, UK), equipped with a universal HPLC guard column packed with a SecurityGuard™ C_{18} cartridge. The mobile phase consisted of 20 mM sodium phosphate buffer at pH 3 ± 0.2 and acetonitrile (60:40, *v/v*) and the flow rate was 1 mL/min. The column temperature and injection volume were set to 30 °C and 10 μL, respectively. Ultraviolet (UV) detection at 213 nm was employed. The HPLC method was validated in terms of specificity, linearity, accuracy, precision, limit of detection (LOD) and limit of quantification (LOQ) according to the International Conference of Harmonization guidelines [16]. Calibration curves in the concentration range of 0.5–100 μg/mL were constructed ($r^2 \geq 0.99$) and the LOD and LOQ values were 0.23 and 0.69 μg/mL, respectively.

2.5. *Log D*

The method used for Log D measurement was the shake flask method, adapted from the Organization for Economic Co-operation and Development (OECD) guidelines [17]. 0.2 M sodium phosphate buffer solutions were prepared at pH 6.0, 6.5, 7.0, 7.4 and 11.0 and mutually saturated with 1-octanol by slow-stirring (at 130 rpm) for 48 h at 25 °C. The solutions were equilibrated in a separation funnel for 24 h before separation. Methadone solutions in octanol were prepared at 0.1 and 0.5 mmol/L. These solutions were then mixed with the aqueous phase (sodium phosphate buffers) at three different ratios (1:1, 2:1 and 1:2). To reach equilibrium, the mixtures were rotated approximately one hundred times through 180° at room temperature. Before sampling, the mixtures were centrifuged at 25 °C and at 13,000 rpm for 30 min. Samples were taken from each phase with suitable dilution using methanol and analyzed using the HPLC method described in Section 2.4.

2.6. Solubility and Stability

Stability studies of methadone free base in the Franz cell receptor medium (6% *w/v* Brij™ O20 in pH 7.4 PBS) and a range of neat solvents were conducted for 96 h. A known quantity of methadone free base was dissolved in the receptor medium or neat solvent. These solutions were placed in Eppendorf® tubes and sealed with Parafilm® before being placed in a shaker (VWR, Leicestershire, UK) at 32 ± 1 °C. Samples were taken at 0, 24, 48, 72 and 96 h. The samples were diluted when necessary and analyzed using the HPLC method described in Section 2.4.

The solubility parameter values (δ) of the solvents were calculated by the van Krevelen-Hoftyzer approach [18] using Molecular Modelling Pro® Version 6.3.3 software (ChemSW, Fairfield, CA, USA). In total, 13 different single solvents were selected for solubility studies in order to ensure that solvents with a wide range of solubility parameter values were investigated. Solubility studies were also conducted with PBS and PBS with 6% Brij™ O20 (*w/v*) solution to confirm that sink conditions would be maintained during the in vitro permeation studies.

For solubility determinations, an excess amount of methadone hydrochloride or free base was added to 0.5 mL of each solvent in Eppendorf® tubes ($n = 3$). The tubes were sealed with Parafilm® and placed on a rotator at 32 ± 2 °C for at least 48 h. These samples were then centrifuged at 12,000 rpm for 15 min at 32 ± 1 °C. The supernatant was suitably diluted to lie within the range of the calibration curve of the validated HPLC method, described in Section 2.4.

2.7. In Vitro Permeation and Mass Balance Studies

In vitro permeation studies were carried out as reported previously by Santos, et al. [19] using vertical glass Franz diffusion cells. Full thickness porcine ear skin was separated from the underlying tissue at room temperature and then stored at −20 °C before use. Skin integrity was assessed by measuring impedance at a frequency of 50 Hz before applying formulations [20]. The diffusion area was ~1 cm^2 and was accurately measured before application of finite doses (5 μL/cm^2) of 5% *w/v* methadone base solutions. The complete dissolution of methadone in all solvents was confirmed in the preparation of formulations. 6% *w/v* Brij™ O20 was added to the receptor phase, PBS pH 7.3 ± 0.2 to ensure the concentration of methadone never exceeded 10% of its solubility without affecting the integrity of the skin [21,22]. Sink conditions in this medium were therefore confirmed during experiments. Permeation studies were performed for 24 h at 32 ± 1 °C. 200 μL samples were withdrawn from the receptor compartment and replaced with 200 μL of fresh receptor medium at 0, 2, 4, 6, 8, 10, 12, 24 h.

Validated mass balance studies were performed after each permeation study. The skin surfaces were washed three times with 1 mL of methanol. The skin was then placed in Eppendorf® tubes with 1 mL of methanol. The samples for skin extraction were placed in a shaker overnight to extract methadone. All Eppendorf ® tubes were centrifuged at 13,000 rpm at 32 °C for 15 min before sampling. The supernatants were sampled and diluted where necessary and analyzed by HPLC.

2.8. Statistical Analysis

Microsoft Excel® 2016 was used for data processing and the calculation of mean and standard deviation (SD). IBM® SPSS Statistics® 24.0 (IBM SPSS Statistics, Feltham, UK) was used for statistical analysis. The Shapiro-Wilk test was used to assess the normality of the data. If the p value calculated from the test was higher than 0.05, the data were assumed to be normally distributed. For normally distributed data (parametric data), the independent-samples t test and one-way analysis of variance (ANOVA) with Tukey's HSD post hoc test were used to analyze two groups and ≥3 groups respectively. For non-normally distributed data (non-parametric data), the Mann-Whitney U test was used to test statistical significance between two groups and the Kruskal-Wallis one-way ANOVA test was performed to investigate statistical differences among different groups (≥3 groups). A probability of $p < 0.05$ was considered as a statistically significant difference.

3. Results and Discussion

3.1. Characterization of Methadone Free Base with NMR and IR Spectroscopy

The ^{1}H-NMR spectrum of methadone hydrochloride is shown in Figure 1. A singlet at 12.00 ppm suggests the protonation of the tertiary amine while the ^{1}H-NMR spectrum of methadone free base shows that there is no singlet around 12.00 ppm for the hydrochloride proton (Figure 2). In addition, all spectral peaks were assigned for both methadone hydrochloride and free base. A water singlet at 1.61 ppm in both spectra may reflect small amounts of water present in the samples [23]. These results confirm the successful conversion of methadone hydrochloride to the free base. Methadone free base was obtained as a white powder, with a yield of 92%. The IR spectra of methadone free base and methadone hydrochloride also support the conclusion that methadone hydrochloride was successfully converted to methadone free base (Figure S1). Characteristic peaks for methadone were obtained for both methadone hydrochloride and free base; a broad band at 2399 cm^{-1} was assigned to the NH$^+$ stretching of methadone hydrochloride.

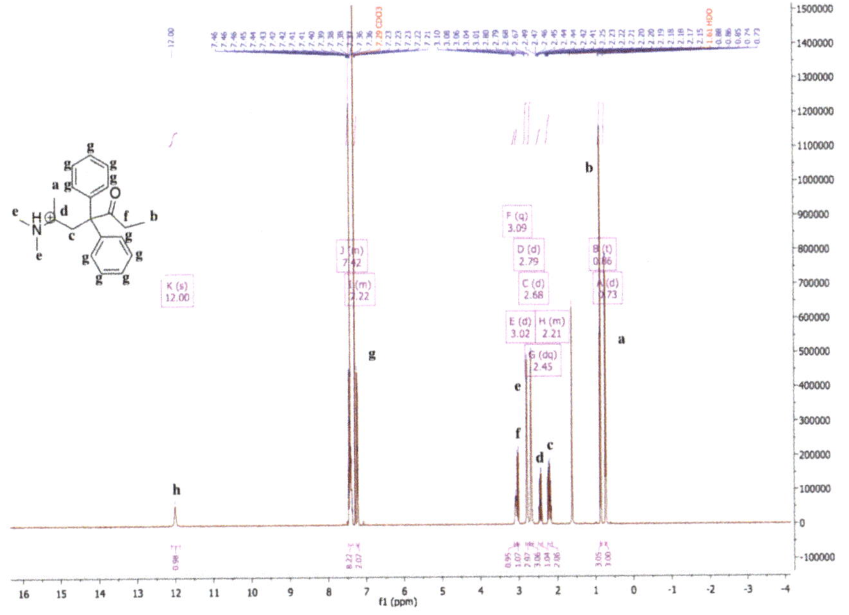

Figure 1. ^{1}H-NMR spectrum of methadone hydrochloride in chloroform-*d*. ^{1}H-NMR (500 MHz, Chloroform-*d*) δ 12.00 (s, 1H), 7.48–7.35 (m, 8H), 7.25–7.19 (m, 2H), 3.09 (q, 1H), 3.02 (d, 1H), 2.79 (d, 3H), 2.68 (d, 3H), 2.45 (dq, 1H), 2.26–2.14 (m, 2H), 0.86 (t, 3H), 0.73 (d, 3H). A singlet at 12.00 ppm suggests the protonation of the tertiary amine.

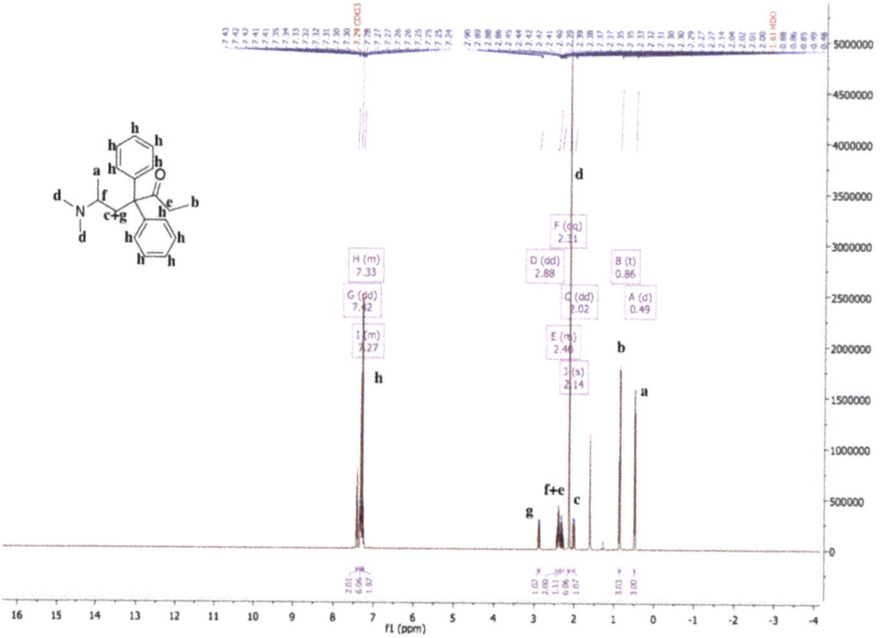

Figure 2. ^{1}H-NMR spectrum of methadone free base in chloroform-d. ^{1}H-NMR (500 MHz, Chloroform-*d*) δ 7.42 (dd, 1.6 Hz, 2H), 7.36–7.30 (m, 6H), 7.28–7.24 (m, 2H), 2.88 (dd, *J* = 13.9, 5.5 Hz, 1H), 2.46–2.36 (m, 2H), 2.31 (dq, 7.2 Hz, 1H), 2.14 (s, 6H), 2.02 (dd, *J* = 13.9, 5.6 Hz, 1H), 0.86 (t, 3H), 0.49 (d, 3H). The ^{1}H-NMR spectrum of methadone free base shows that there is no singlet around 12.00 ppm for the hydrochloride proton.

3.2. Thermal Analysis

The thermogravimetric analysis of methadone hydrochloride and methadone free base is shown in Figure S3. The decomposition of methadone hydrochloride is evident from 167 to 261 °C (onset: 230.12 °C) while that of methadone free base occurs from 134 to 230 °C (onset: 194.35 °C).

The DSC thermograms of methadone hydrochloride and the free base are shown in Figure 3. The melting points of methadone free base and methadone hydrochloride were obtained as the onset temperatures. The melting point of methadone hydrochloride (235.54 °C) is very close to the degradation temperature of the compound. Only one endothermic event which occurs between 73.5 °C and 79.8 °C was observed for methadone free base. The obtained melting point of methadone free base is 74.00 °C which is consistent with the literature (76 °C) [24].

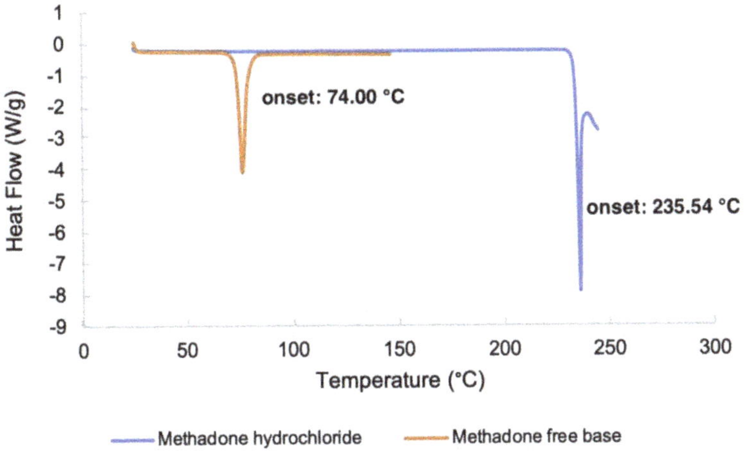

Figure 3. DSC thermograms of methadone hydrochloride and methadone free base.

3.3. *Log D Measurement*

The predicted values of the Log P for methadone base from ChemAxon and ACD/Labs were 5.0 and 4.2, respectively. These values are higher than the experimental Log P value of 3.93 reported previously [25]. The measurement of the partition coefficient of an ionizable species should be made in the non-ionized form according to the OECD guidelines [17]. An appropriate buffer with a pH of at least one unit above the dissociation constant (pK_a) of methadone (pK_a = 8.94) [26] should be used to ensure the compound is present as the free base. Hence, 20 mM pH 11 PBS was used in this study to measure the partition coefficient of methadone base. The value obtained in this measurement was 4.85 ± 0.03. The Log D values obtained at different pH values are listed in Table 1. The log D value at pH 7.4 is lower than the experimental value previously reported (Log $D_{7.4}$ = 2.1) [27], however no details of the buffer or ionic strength used were given for this earlier measurement.

Table 1. Distribution coefficient of methadone for different pH values at 25 ± 1 °C.

pH	Log D
6.0	0.31 ± 0.01
6.5	0.80 ± 0.01
7.0	1.35 ± 0.01
7.4	1.82 ± 0.01
11.0 (free base)	4.85 ± 0.03

3.4. *Stability and Solubility*

After 96 h stability studies at 32 ± 1 °C, the recovery values of methadone base in all solvents was >97%. The chemical stability of methadone free base over 96 h in the receptor medium for permeation studies and common solvents, including LIM, EO, IPM, WL 1349, OA, PGML, PGMC, TC, OSAL, TriPG, DiPG, PG, 1,3-BD and ethyl acetate, was confirmed (Figure S4).

The solubility values for methadone hydrochloride in water and ethanol have been reported previously as 120 and 80 mg/mL, respectively [28]. The solubility of methadone hydrochloride and free base at 32 ± 1 °C was measured in a range of solvents (Table 2). As expected, methadone hydrochloride is poorly soluble in solvents such as LIM, EO, IPM and OSAL and relatively high solubility was observed for hydrophilic solvents. The highest solubility of methadone hydrochloride was observed in PG. The solubility values for methadone free base and its hydrochloride salt in PBS are 0.49 ± 0.01 and 86.66 ± 0.95 mg/mL, respectively. The addition of 6% *w/v* Brij™ O20 in PBS increased the solubility of methadone free base and methadone hydrochloride to 2.61 ± 0.02 and 107.45 ± 1.35 mg/mL, respectively. Methadone free base has a calculated van Krevelen and Hoftyzer solubility parameter of 10.07 $(cal/cm^3)^{1/2}$ and its solubility in solvents with solubility parameters, ranging from 8 to 11 $(cal/cm^3)^{1/2}$ was >100 mg/mL (Figure 4). These results are consistent with the theory proposed by Hancock, et al. [29] i.e., when the solubility parameters of solute and solvent are similar, high solubility is expected compared with solvents that do not have similar solubility parameters. On the other hand, solubility parameters only provide an indication of solubility characteristics and cannot account for all circumstances. Molecules may take up different conformations in the various solvents and anomalies are possible. It is interesting to note that methadone base has relatively low solubility in hydrophilic solvents with solubility parameter value above 11 $(cal/cm^3)^{1/2}$ and it showed a lower solubility in TriPG compared with OSAL. The anomalous solubility behavior of caffeine was also reported previously [30–32].

Table 2. Summary of the solubility of methadone hydrochloride and free base in neat solvents at 32 ± 1 °C. The solubility parameter of methadone free base is 10.07 $(cal/cm^3)^{1/2}$.

Solvent	Solubility of Methadone base (mg/mL)	Solubility of Methadone Hydrochloride (mg/mL)
LIM	342.38 ± 2.99	0.08 ± 0.002
EO	205.46 ± 1.69	0.08 ± 0.01
IPM	179.80 ± 0.89	0.03 ± 0.001
WL 1349	217.66 ± 3.73	0.05 ± 0.001
OA	438.76 ± 2.56	2.53 ± 0.03
PGML	209.43 ± 0.54	19.68 ± 0.79
PGMC	250.74 ± 2.17	28.65 ± 0.46
TC	247.68 ± 0.95	21.96 ± 0.46
OSAL	277.20 ± 6.96	0.05 ± 0.001
TriPG	105.90 ± 0.25	18.03 ± 0.93
DiPG	85.94 ± 0.41	43.97 ± 1.28
PG	24.78± 0.49	201.33 ± 1.30
1,3-BD	26.24 ± 0.05	88.40 ± 0.79
PBS	0.49 ± 0.01	86.66 ± 0.95
PBS + 6% *w/v* Brij™ O20	2.61 ± 0.02	107.45 ± 1.35

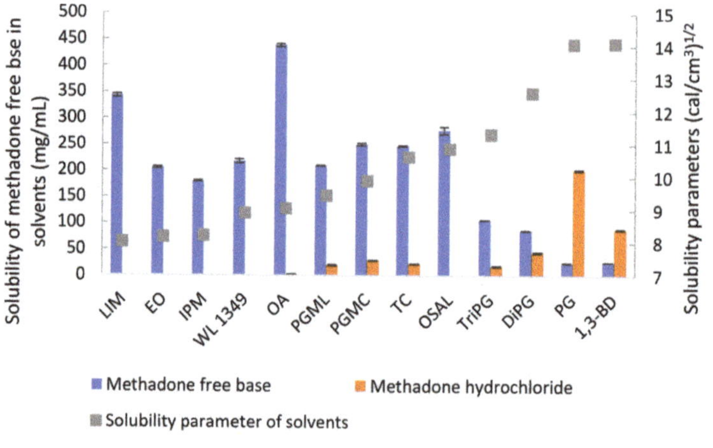

Figure 4. Solubility of methadone free base and methadone hydrochloride in solvents at 32 ± 1 °C and solubility parameters of solvents.

3.5. In Vitro Permeation and Mass Balance Studies of Methadone Base in Porcine Ear Skin

Eight solvents were selected for in vitro permeation studies of methadone free base in porcine skin under finite dose conditions (5 μL/cm^2). The permeation profiles are shown in Figure 5. The highest permeation of methadone was observed for LIM ($p < 0.01$). The cumulative amount of methadone that permeated after 24 h was 41.3 ± 4.7 μg/cm^2 (20.7 ± 2.3% of the applied dose). The results also suggest EO, TC and OSAL are promising vehicles for methadone. Although methadone hydrochloride permeation in PG was investigated also, the maximum cumulative amount that permeated through porcine skin after 24 h was only 2.5 ± 0.6 μg/cm^2.

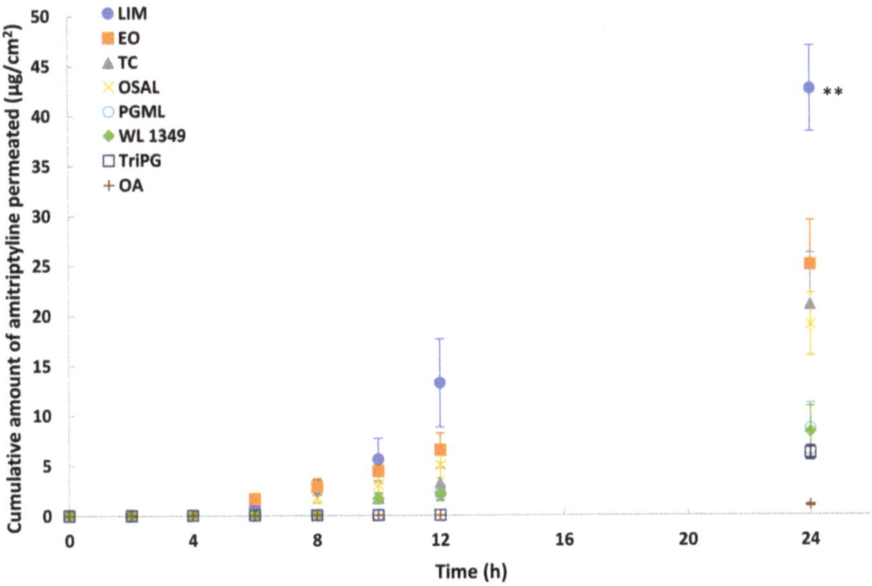

Figure 5. Cumulative permeation profiles of methadone in porcine skin after application of 5% (*w/v*) methadone free base in LIM (●), EO (■), TC (▲), OSAL (×), PGML (○), WL 1349 (♦), TriPG (□) and OA (+) for finite dose (5 μL/cm^2) at 32 ± 1 °C. Each data point represents the mean ± SD (mean ± SD; $4 \leq n \leq 5$). ** $p < 0.01$.

Mass balance studies confirm that high permeation of methadone generally was associated with high amounts of drug extracted from the skin (Figure 6). Except for LIM, the overall recoveries for other formulations were within the recovery range (90–110%) recommended in the OECD guidelines [33]. Although the stability of methadone free base in formulations and the receptor fluid was confirmed, the overall recovery of methadone for LIM was only 86.33 ± 2.15%. However, LIM still delivered significantly higher ($p < 0.05$) percentages of methadone into the skin and through the skin compared with the other solvents. The results confirm that the lowest percentage of methadone recovered from the skin surface was observed for LIM, followed by EO, OSAL and TC (Figure 6). Except for LIM, the percentages of applied methadone recovered from the skin surface were significantly higher compared with the percentages of methadone inside skin and permeated across skin.

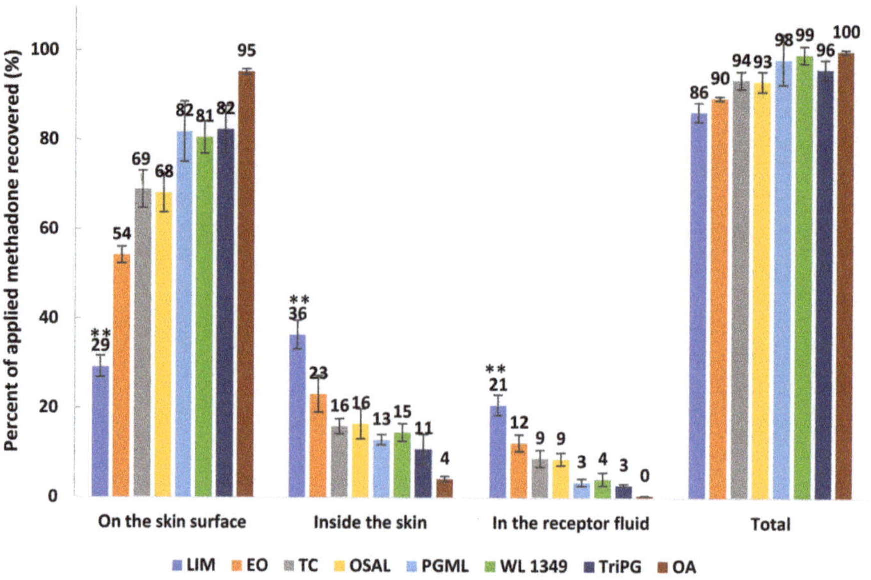

Figure 6. Mass balance results after 24 h finite dose (5 μL/cm^2) permeation studies in porcine skin for 5% (*w/v*) methadone free base in LIM, EO, TC, OSAL, PGML, WL 1349, TriPG and OA at 32 ± 1 °C (mean ± SD; $4 \leq n \leq 5$). ** $p < 0.01$.

A proposed mechanism of penetration enhancement for LIM is the disruption of the highly ordered structure of intercellular lipids which may result in an increase in drug diffusion [34]. The permeation of LIM through human skin and high affinity of LIM for the epidermis were reported by Cal, et al. [35]. This indicates another potential mechanism that may contribute to high permeation of methadone in the present study. With the exception of OA, the highest solubility of methadone base was observed for LIM. The uptake of LIM into skin may create a more favorable environment for methadone and thus increase the partition of methadone into the stratum corneum (SC). In addition, both skin uptake and evaporation of LIM can also contribute to an increase in the thermodynamic activity of methadone and the partition into skin. On the other hand, drug crystallization inside the skin or on the skin surface may occur as well when LIM permeates through skin. LIM is generally recognized as a safe ingredient in topical products [36]; the highest concentration used in FDA approved topical products is 10% *w/w* [37].

EO is derived from the esterification of OA with ethanol. Both EO and OA have a double bond in the *cis* configuration, forming a "kinked" shape [38]. This kink conformation may disrupt SC lipid packing by introducing a separate phase in the intercellular lipid domain and thus increase the diffusion of solute through skin [39,40]. The permeation of methadone for OA was significantly lower than that for EO and other solvents ($p < 0.05$). This may reflect electrostatic interaction between methadone free base and the carboxylic acid group of OA. The presence of ionized methadone might also be expected to reduce the partition of methadone from OA into SC lipids, thus reducing the permeation of methadone. FTIR was subsequently used to confirm an interaction between methadone free base and OA (Figure S2). The high solubility of methadone in OA reported above also supports the possibility of an interaction between OA and methadone free base.

The cumulative amount of methadone that permeated through skin for OSAL was significantly higher than for PGML and medium-chain triglycerides of caprylic and capric acids (WL 1349) ($p < 0.05$) while there is no significant difference between the amounts of methadone extracted from skin for these solvents ($p > 0.05$). This indicates that OSAL is more likely to enhance permeation by increasing the diffusion of methadone through skin rather than altering the partition of methadone into stratum corneum. Santos, et al. [41] reported that OSAL is taken up to a high extent by the skin but no effect on lipid fluidity was observed using DSC and FTIR. The authors proposed that OSAL may enhance drug diffusion by creating "pools" of solvent within the gel lipid phase.

The cumulative amount of methadone that permeated through porcine skin from TC after 24 h was 21.07 ± 5.12 μg/cm^2. Almost double the amount of methadone was recovered following skin extraction compared with the amount that permeated for this vehicle. TC is miscible with both polar and non-polar solvents and it has been widely used as a penetration enhancer. Haque, et al. [42] reported that 53.4% of TC permeated through human skin in Franz cell studies by 19 h. The rapid skin uptake of TC suggest that TC is likely to enhance permeation by increasing drug solubility in intracellular lipids. TC may therefore play a key role in driving the partition of methadone into skin and increasing permeation. Increasing thermodynamic activity of methadone resulting from TC evaporation and skin uptake may also contribute to the skin permeation of methadone. The highest concentrations of TC, OSAL and EO used in FDA approved topical products are 49.91% *w/w*, 8.5% *w/w* and 0.14 mg/mL, respectively [37].

Fullerton et al. [13] evaluated the transdermal delivery of methadone free base using human cadaver skin over 24 h. Solutions of methadone base were prepared in ethanol and propylene glycol and in ethanol and propylene glycol with either oleic acid or Azone®. The highest amount of methadone permeated from the ethanol: PG: Azone solution (~400 μg/cm^2), however the concentration of methadone (720 μg/μL) was more than 10-fold greater than that evaluated in the present work. Ghosh and Bagherian [14] also investigated a transdermal patch containing methadone free base in human skin. Patches with or without 5% *w/w* Azone® or 5% *w/w* *n*-decylmethyl sulfoxide were tested. The cumulative amounts of methadone permeation at 24 h in human skin ranged from 1 to 3 mg/cm^2. Again, comparisons with the present work are limited because of the comparatively larger doses of methadone in the patches compared with the formulations examined here. It is also important to note that the objectives of these two earlier studies were systemic delivery of methadone for management of substance abuse rather than local delivery.

4. Conclusions

Methadone free base was prepared from its hydrochloride salt, followed by a series of characterization studies. A range of solvents was evaluated using in vitro permeation and mass balance studies in porcine skin and a maximum skin flux of 2.54 ± 0.19 μg/cm^2/h was estimated. The results suggest that TC, LIM, OSAL and EO appear to be promising candidate vehicles for dermal delivery of methadone base. This is the first study to confirm skin permeation of methadone base under finite dose conditions. However, for most formulations the majority of the active remained on the skin surface after 24 h. Future work will focus on development of more complex vehicles with further optimization and evaluation of skin permeation in human skin. The most promising formulations will be progressed for investigation in the clinic.

Supplementary Materials: The following are available online at http://www.mdpi.com/1999-4923/11/10/509/s1, Figure S1: IR spectra of (A) methadone free base and (B) methadone hydrochloride, Figure S2: IR spectra of (A) oleic acid and (B) 10mg methadone free base dissolved in 0.1 mL oleic acid (OA), Figure S3: Thermogravimetric analysis of methadone hydrochloride and methadone free base, Figure S4: Recovery (%) of methadone free base in a series of neat after 24, 48, 72 and 96 h at 32 ± 1 °C (n = 3; mean ± SD).

Author Contributions: Conceptualization, R.M. and M.E.L.; methodology, C.-P.K., B.C.S.; software, C.-P.K.; validation, M.E.L., J.H. and C.-P.K.; formal analysis, C.-P.K., B.C.S.; investigation, C.-P.K., B.C.S.; resources, M.E.L., C.-P.K.; data curation, C.-P.K.; writing—original draft preparation, C.-P.K.; writing—review and editing, C.-P.K., M.E.L., J.H., B.C.S., R.M., B.P.; visualization, C.-P.K., M.E.L., J.H.; supervision, J.H., M.E.L.; project administration, M.E.L.; funding acquisition, C.-P.K.

Funding: This research received no external funding.

Acknowledgments: We thank our colleagues from the UCL Skin Research Group who provided insight and expertise that greatly assisted the research.

Conflicts of Interest: The authors declare no conflict of interest.

Abbreviations

1,3-BD	1,3-butanediol
^{1}H-NMR	Proton Nuclear Magnetic Resonance
ANOVA	One-way Analysis of Variance
CDCl3	Chloroform-d
DiPG	Dipropylene Glycol
DSC	Differential Scanning Calorimetry
EO	Ethyl Oleate
FTIR	Fourier Transform Infrared
GRAS	Generally Recognized as Safe
HPLC	High Performance Liquid Chromatography
IPM	Isopropyl Myristate
LIM	d-limonene
LOD	Limit of Detection
Log D	Logarithm to the Base 10 of Distribution Coefficient
Log P	Logarithm to the Base 10 of Partition Coefficient
LOQ	Limit of Quantification
Nav	Voltage-gated Sodium (Nav) Channels
NMDA	*N*-Methyl-D-aspartate
OA	Oleic Acid
OECD	Organisation for Economic Co-operation and Development
OSAL	Octyl Salicylate
PBS	Phosphate Buffered Saline
PG	Propylene Glycol
PGMC	Propylene Glycol Monocaprylate
PGML	Propylene Glycol Monolaurate
pK_a	Dissociation Constant
SD	Standard Deviation
TC	Transcutol®
TGA	Thermogravimetric Analysis
TriPG	Tripropylene Glycol
UV	Ultraviolet
WL 1349	Labrafac™ lipophile WL 1349

References

1. O'Connor, A.B.; Dworkin, R.H. Treatment of neuropathic pain: An overview of recent guidelines. *Am. J. Med.* **2009**, *122*, S22–S32. [CrossRef] [PubMed]
2. Treede, R.-D.; Jensen, T.S.; Campbell, J.; Cruccu, G.; Dostrovsky, J.; Griffin, J.; Hansson, P.; Hughes, R.; Nurmikko, T.; Serra, J. Neuropathic pain redefinition and a grading system for clinical and research purposes. *Neurology* **2008**, *70*, 1630–1635. [CrossRef] [PubMed]
3. Jensen, M.P.; Chodroff, M.J.; Dworkin, R.H. The impact of neuropathic pain on health-related quality of life Review and implications. *Neurology* **2007**, *68*, 1178–1182. [CrossRef] [PubMed]
4. Van Hecke, O.; Austin, S.K.; Khan, R.A.; Smith, B.; Torrance, N. Neuropathic pain in the general population: A systematic review of epidemiological studies. *Pain* **2014**, *155*, 654–662. [CrossRef]
5. Colloca, L.; Ludman, T.; Bouhassira, D.; Baron, R.; Dickenson, A.H.; Yarnitsky, D.; Freeman, R.; Truini, A.; Attal, N.; Finnerup, N.B.; et al. Neuropathic pain. *Nat. Rev. Dis. Primers* **2017**, *3*, 17002. [CrossRef]
6. Altier, N.; Dion, D.; Boulanger, A.; Choinière, M. Management of chronic neuropathic pain with methadone: A review of 13 cases. *Clin. J. Pain* **2005**, *21*, 364–369. [CrossRef]
7. Sandoval, J.A.; Furlan, A.D.; Mailis-Gagnon, A. Oral methadone for chronic noncancer pain: A systematic literature review of reasons for administration, prescription patterns, effectiveness, and side effects. *Clin. J. Pain* **2005**, *21*, 503–512. [CrossRef]

8. Morley, J.S.; Bridson, J.; Nash, T.P.; Miles, J.B.; White, S.; Makin, M.K. Low-dose methadone has an analgesic effect in neuropathic pain: A double-blind randomized controlled crossover trial. *Palliat. Med.* **2003**, *17*, 576–587. [CrossRef]
9. McLean, S.; Twomey, F. Methods of rotation from another strong opioid to methadone for the management of cancer pain: A systematic review of the available evidence. *J. Pain Symptom Manag.* **2015**, *50*, 248–259.e241. [CrossRef]
10. Sotgiu, M.L.; Valente, M.; Storchi, R.; Caramenti, G.; Biella, G.E.M. Cooperative N-methyl-d-aspartate (NMDA) receptor antagonism and μ-opioid receptor agonism mediate the methadone inhibition of the spinal neuron pain-related hyperactivity in a rat model of neuropathic pain. *Pharmacol. Res.* **2009**, *60*, 284–290. [CrossRef]
11. Martinez, V.; Christensen, D.; Kayser, V. The glycine/NMDA receptor antagonist (+)-HA966 enhances the peripheral effect of morphine in neuropathic rats. *Pain* **2002**, *99*, 537–545. [CrossRef]
12. Stoetzer, C.; Kistner, K.; Stüber, T.; Wirths, M.; Schulze, V.; Doll, T.; Foadi, N.; Wegner, F.; Ahrens, J.; Leffler, A. Methadone is a local anaesthetic-like inhibitor of neuronal Na+ channels and blocks excitability of mouse peripheral nerves. *Br. J. Anaesth.* **2015**, *114*, 110–120. [CrossRef] [PubMed]
13. Fullerton, A.; Christrup, L.; Bundgaard, H. Evaluation of the transdermal route for administration of narcotic analgesics: Human skin permeability studies of methadone and pethidine. *Acta Pharm. Nord.* **1991**, *3*, 181–182. [PubMed]
14. Ghosh, T.K.; Bagherian, A. Development of a transdermal patch of methadone: In vitro evaluation across hairless mouse and human cadaver skin. *Pharm. Dev. Technol.* **1996**, *1*, 285–291. [CrossRef] [PubMed]
15. Muñoz, M.; Castán, H.; Ruiz, M.; Morales, M. Design, development and characterization of transdermal patch of methadone. *J. Drug Deliv. Sci. Technol.* **2017**, *42*, 255–260. [CrossRef]
16. ICH. Q2 (R1). Validation of analytical procedures: Text and methodology. In Proceedings of the International Conference on Harmonization, Geneva, Switzerland, 10 November 2005.
17. OECD. *Test No. 107: Partition Coefficient (N-Octanol/Water): Shake Flask Method*; Organisation for Economic Cooperation and Development: Paris, France, 1995.
18. Van Krevelen, D.W. *Properties of Polymers: Their Correlation with Chemical Structure, Their Numerical Estimation and Prediction from Additive Group Contributions*, 3rd ed.; Elsevier Scientific Pub. Co.: Amsterdam, The Netherlands, 1990; pp. 200–225.
19. Santos, P.; Watkinson, A.; Hadgraft, J.; Lane, M. Oxybutynin permeation in skin: The influence of drug and solvent activity. *Int. J. Pharm.* **2010**, *384*, 67–72. [CrossRef] [PubMed]
20. Woo, E.; Hua, P.; Webster, J.; Tompkins, W.; Pallas-Areny, R. Skin impedance measurements using simple and compound electrodes. *Med. Biol. Eng. Comput.* **1992**, *30*, 97–102. [CrossRef]
21. Bronaugh, R.L.; Stewart, R.F. Methods for in vitro percutaneous absorption studies III: Hydrophobic compounds. *J. Pharm. Sci.* **1984**, *73*, 1255–1258. [CrossRef]
22. Brain, K.R.; Walters, K.A.; Watkinson, A.C. Methods for Studying Percutaneous Absorption. In *Dermatological and Transdermal Formulations*; Walters, K.A., Roberts, M.S., Eds.; Marcel Dekker, lnc: New York, NY, USA, 2002; pp. 197–270.
23. Gottlieb, H.E.; Kotlyar, V.; Nudelman, A. NMR chemical shifts of common laboratory solvents as trace impurities. *J. Org. Chem.* **1997**, *62*, 7512–7515. [CrossRef]
24. Lemberg, K.; Kontinen, V.K.; Viljakka, K.; Kylänlahti, I.; Yli-Kauhaluoma, J.; Kalso, E. Morphine, oxycodone, methadone and its enantiomers in different models of nociception in the rat. *Anesth. Analg.* **2006**, *102*, 1768–1774. [CrossRef]
25. Hansch, C.; Leo, A.; Hoekman, D.; Livingstone, D. *Exploring QSAR: Hydrophobic, Electronic, and Steric Constants*; American Chemical Society: Washington, DC, USA, 1995.
26. Perrin, D. *Dissociation Constants of Organic Acids and Bases*; Butterworths: London, UK, 1965.
27. Moffat, A.C.; Osselton, M.D.; Widdop, B.; Watts, J. *Clarke's Analysis of Drugs and Poisons*; Pharmaceutical press London: London, UK, 2011; Volume 3.
28. O'Neil, M.J. *The Merck Index: An Encyclopedia of Chemicals, Drugs, and Biologicals*; RSC Publishing: Cambridge, UK, 2013.
29. Hancock, B.C.; York, P.; Rowe, R.C. The use of solubility parameters in pharmaceutical dosage form design. *Int. J. Pharm.* **1997**, *148*, 1–21. [CrossRef]

30. Herrador, M.A.; González, A.G. Solubility prediction of caffeine in aqueous N,N-dimethylformamide mixtures using the extended Hildebrand solubility approach. *Int. J. Pharm.* **1997**, *156*, 239–244. [CrossRef]
31. Bustamante, P.; Navarro, J.; Romero, S.; Escalera, B. Thermodynamic origin of the solubility profile of drugs showing one or two maxima against the polarity of aqueous and nonaqueous mixtures: Niflumic acid and caffeine. *J. Pharm. Sci.* **2002**, *91*, 874–883. [CrossRef] [PubMed]
32. Dias, M.; Hadgraft, J.; Lane, M.E. Influence of membrane-solvent-solute interactions on solute permeation in model membranes. *Int. J. Pharm.* **2007**, *336*, 108–114. [CrossRef] [PubMed]
33. OECD. *Test No. 28: Guidance Document for the Conduct of Skin Absorption Studies*; Organisation for Economic Cooperation and Development: Paris, France, 2004.
34. Williams, A.C.; Barry, B.W. Terpenes and the lipid–protein–partitioning theory of skin penetration enhancement. *Pharm. Res.* **1991**, *8*, 17–24. [CrossRef]
35. Cal, K.; Janicki, S.; Sznitowska, M. In vitro studies on penetration of terpenes from matrix-type transdermal systems through human skin. *Int. J. Pharm.* **2001**, *224*, 81–88. [CrossRef]
36. Herman, A.; Herman, A.P. Essential oils and their constituents as skin penetration enhancer for transdermal drug delivery: A review. *J. Pharm. Pharmacol.* **2015**, *67*, 473–485. [CrossRef]
37. FDA. Inactive Ingredient Search for Approved Drug Products. Available online: https://www.accessdata.fda.gov/scripts/cder/iig/index.cfm (accessed on 10 October 2018).
38. Small, D.M. Lateral chain packing in lipids and membranes. *J. Lipid Res.* **1984**, *25*, 1490–1500.
39. Ongpipattanakul, B.; Burnette, R.R.; Potts, R.O.; Francoeur, M.L. Evidence that oleic acid exists in a separate phase within stratum corneum lipids. *Pharm. Res.* **1991**, *8*, 350–354. [CrossRef]
40. Walker, M.; Hadgraft, J. Oleic acid—A membrane "fluidiser" or fluid within the membrane? *Int. J. Pharm.* **1991**, *71*, R1–R4. [CrossRef]
41. Santos, P.; Watkinson, A.; Hadgraft, J.; Lane, M. Influence of penetration enhancer on drug permeation from volatile formulations. *Int. J. Pharm.* **2012**, *439*, 260–268. [CrossRef] [PubMed]
42. Haque, T.; Rahman, K.M.; Thurston, D.E.; Hadgraft, J.; Lane, M.E. Topical delivery of anthramycin I. Influence of neat solvents. *Eur. J. Pharm. Sci.* **2017**, *104*, 188–195. [CrossRef] [PubMed]

pharmaceutics

MDPI

Article

In Situ Hydrogel-Forming/Nitric Oxide-Releasing Wound Dressing for Enhanced Antibacterial Activity and Healing in Mice with Infected Wounds

Juho Lee [1], Shwe Phyu Hlaing [1], Jiafu Cao [1], Nurhasni Hasan [1], Hye-Jin Ahn [2], Ki-Won Song [2] and Jin-Wook Yoo [1,*]

[1] College of Pharmacy, Pusan National University, Busan 46241, Korea; jhlee2350@gmail.com (J.L.); shwephyuhlaing@gmail.com (S.P.H.); caojiafu1985@163.com (J.C.); hasni1986.nh@gmail.com (N.H.)

[2] Department of Organic Material Science and Engineering, Pusan National University, Busan 46241, Korea; hyejin-asu@hanmail.net (H.-J.A.); kwsong@pusan.ac.kr (K.-W.S.)

* Correspondence: jinwook@pusan.ac.kr; Tel.: +82-51-510-2807

Received: 6 September 2019; Accepted: 25 September 2019; Published: 27 September 2019

Abstract: The eradication of bacteria from wound sites and promotion of healing are essential for treating infected wounds. Nitric oxide (NO) is desirable for these purposes due to its ability to accelerate wound healing and its broad-spectrum antibacterial effects. We developed an in situ hydrogel-forming/NO-releasing powder dressing (NO/GP), which is a powder during storage and forms a hydrogel when applied to wounds, as a novel NO-releasing formulation to treat infected wounds. An NO/GP fine powder (51.5 μm) was fabricated by blending and micronizing S-nitrosoglutathione (GSNO), alginate, pectin, and polyethylene glycol (PEG). NO/GP remained stable for more than four months when stored at 4 or 37 °C. When applied to wounds, NO/GP absorbed wound fluid and immediately converted to a hydrogel. Additionally, wound fluid triggered a NO release from NO/GP for more than 18 h. The rheological properties of hydrogel-transformed NO/GP indicated that NO/GP possesses similar adhesive properties to marketed products (Vaseline). NO/GP resulted in a 6-log reduction in colony forming units (CFUs) of methicillin resistant *Staphylococcus aureus* (MRSA) and *Pseudomonas aeruginosa,* which are representative drug-resistant gram-positive and -negative bacteria, respectively. The promotion of wound healing by NO/GP was demonstrated in mice with full-thickness wounds challenged with MRSA and *P. aeruginosa*. Thus, NO/GP is a promising formulation for the treatment of infected wounds.

Keywords: in situ hydrogel-forming powder; nitric oxide-releasing formulation; S-nitrosoglutathione (GSNO); antibacterial; wound dressing; wound healing

1. Introduction

Cutaneous wound infections are a global problem whose cost of treatment runs into millions of dollars per year, and these infections can lead to severe complications including sepsis, for which mortality remains around 30% in the United States [1,2]. Wound healing proceeds spontaneously through three sequential phases; inflammation, proliferation, and remodeling [3–6]. However, when wounds are infected, the healing process is delayed during the inflammation phase, since bacteria induce continuous inflammation at the infected site [7,8]. Thus, eradicating bacteria from the injured site is essential for the treatment of infected wounds.

In recent years, nitric oxide (NO) has gained attention as a novel agent for the treatment of infected wounds because it facilitates wound healing processes such as skin cell proliferation and tissue remodeling, and it also exerts broad-spectrum antibacterial effects [9–12]. NO enhances re-epithelialization and collagen synthesis during wound healing [5,13]. In addition, NO possesses broad-spectrum antibacterial properties through the formation of reactive nitrogen species such as peroxynitrile, nitrogen dioxide, and dinitrogen trioxide, which can interact with various bacterial proteins, DNA, and enzymes to result in bacterial cell death [14]. Since NO exerts bactericidal effects via multiple biochemical pathways, it exhibits antibacterial effects against drug-resistant bacteria, including methicillin resistant *Staphylococcus aureus* (MRSA) [15]. Moreover, NO does not develop drug resistance due to its diverse antibacterial mechanisms, which require multiple mutations for resistance to develop [16]. However, despite these beneficial effects of NO, its clinical application remains challenging because of its short half-life and gaseous nature. Therefore, the development of an NO-releasing formulation with a sustained NO-release and good storage stability is required.

We hypothesized that a powder dressing that forms a hydrogel in situ maintains a powder state during storage and converts to hydrogel immediately when applied to wounds could be an ideal NO-releasing formulation for the treatment of infected wounds. An in situ hydrogel-forming/NO-releasing powder dressing possesses the benefits of both powders and hydrogels. Since a water-free powder ensures high storage stability, the stability of easily hydrolyzable pharmaceutical ingredients can be markedly improved. When applied to the wound site, an in situ hydrogel-forming powder dressing can fit the irregular surface of the wound without wrinkles or fluting [17–19]. In addition, in situ hydrogel-forming powders are easy to apply to bendable areas of the human body, such as elbows, finger joints, ankles, or wide wound beds resulting from burn and pressure ulcers. Once applied to the wound, they can absorb the wound fluid and form an adhesive hydrogel, which can protect the wound site from the external environment and maintain a humid environment to aid wound healing [20,21]. At the same time, a NO release triggered by the absorbed wound fluid may assist wound healing via the elimination of bacteria and stimulation of wound-healing processes [22].

In this study, a novel in situ hydrogel-forming/NO-releasing powder dressing (NO/GP) possessing the benefits of both powders and hydrogels was developed using S-nitrosoglutathione (GSNO), alginate, pectin, and polyethylene glycol (PEG) for the treatment of infected wounds. GSNO is a widely used endogenous NO donor that can generate NO over several hours under physiological conditions, which may be beneficial properties for NO releasing wound dressings [23]. Sodium alginate was selected to form a bioadhesive hydrogel. In addition, it can absorb wound exudate up to approximately 20-times its weight [24]. Pectin was used to form a hydrogel structure and accelerate the powder-to-hydrogel transition [19]. PEG was added to modulate the ability of the formulation to uptake fluid to prevent potential wound drying caused by the excessive absorption of exudate. Following the characterization of NO/GP, the storage stability, in situ hydrogel-forming ability, rheological properties, and NO-release profiles were evaluated in a series of in vitro and in vivo experiments. The antibacterial effects of NO/GP were examined against MRSA and *Pseudomonas aeruginosa*, which are drug-resistant gram-positive and -negative bacteria, respectively. The in vivo therapeutic effects of NO/GP were evaluated using a bacteria-challenged full-thickness wound mouse model.

2. Materials and Methods

2.1. Materials

Glutathione (reduced form) was purchased from Wako Pure Chemical (Osaka, Japan). Pectin and agar were purchased from Yakuri Co., Ltd. (Osaka, Japan). Sodium alginate, PEG (average molecular weight: 8000), sodium nitrite, crystal violet, Lugol's solution, 2,2,2 tribromoethanol, *tert*-amyl alcohol, Mayer's hematoxylin, and eosin-Y disodium were purchased from Sigma-Aldrich (St. Louis, MO, USA). Bacto™ tryptic soy broth (TSB) and Difco™ cetrimide-agar media were purchased from BD Biosciences (San Jose, CA, USA). A Twort's Gram stain set was purchased from Newcomer Supply (Middleton, WI, USA). Masson's trichrome stain kit was purchased from Abcam (Cambridge, MA, USA). The LIVE/DEAD® *Bac*Light™ bacterial viability kit was purchased from Thermo Fisher

Scientific (Waltham, MA, USA). All other reagents and solvents were of the highest analytical grade commercially available.

2.2. GSNO Synthesis

GSNO was synthesized following a previously reported method with some modifications [25]. Briefly, sodium nitrite and reduced glutathione were added to a cold HCl solution with stirring for 40 min in an ice bath (the final concentration of $NaNO_2$, glutathione, and HCl was 0.625 M). To precipitate GSNO, acetone was added and stirred for 20 min. The precipitate was collected by filtration and washed once with 80% acetone, twice with 100% acetone, and three times with diethyl ether. After drying, GSNO was stored in a −20 °C refrigerator for subsequent experiments.

2.3. Preparation and Characterization of the NO-Releasing In Situ Hydrogel-Forming Powder

To prepare the in situ hydrogel-forming agent, sodium alginate, pectin, and PEG were micronized, sieved (90 μm), and blended. The ratio of alginate, pectin, and PEG used for the in situ hydrogel-forming powder (GP) was optimized with sodium alginate:pectin:PEG at a 2:1:6 ratio in several pilot studies. To prepare the NO-releasing in situ hydrogel-forming powder (NO/GP), GSNO was added to the GP (final content of GSNO was 4 wt %). GSNO was sieved before blending with GP to eliminate the GSNO aggregates, which could induce undesirable effects in the content uniformity. NO/GP was stored in a −20 °C refrigerator.

NO/GP was characterized by determining particle size, GSNO content, content homogeneity, and powder flowability. Briefly, the particle sizes of NO/GP and the non-micronized mixture were analyzed by ImageJ software (National Institutes of Health, Bethesda, MA, USA) using microscopic images. More than 100 particles were used to assess particle size. GSNO contents were determined using 10 samples of each NO/GP and non-micronized mixture, which were dissolved in distilled water (DW), and then the absorbance was detected using a UV/Vis spectrophotometer (U-5100, Hitachi, Tokyo, Japan) at 335 nm. From the absorbance values, GSNO content and relative standard deviation (RSD) were calculated to investigate GSNO content and content homogeneity, respectively. Powder flowability was evaluated as previously reported, with some modifications [26]. Briefly, 40 mg of NP/GP was loaded in a 1 mL syringe and tapped until no change in volume was detected. The bulk and tapped density were calculated from the tapped and untapped volume of NO/GP, and the Hausner ratio was calculated based on the tap density/bulk density ratio.

2.4. Rheological Properties of NO/GP in Hydrogel Form

The rheological properties of the hydrogel-form of NO/GP were evaluated as previously reported, with some modification [27–29]. The steady shear and dynamic viscoelastic properties of the hydrogel-form of NO/GP were measured using a strain-controlled rheometer (Advanced Rheometric Expansion System [ARES], Rheometric Scientific, Piscataway, NJ, USA) equipped with a parallel-plate fixture with a radius of 12.5 mm and a gap size of 1.0 mm. All rheological measurements were performed at a fixed temperature of 37 °C over a wide range of shear rates and strain amplitudes. In this study, simulated wound fluid (SWF) [30,31] was used to induce NO/GP swelling. The SWF consisted of 0.64% NaCl, 0.22% KCl, 2.5% $NaHCO_3$, and 0.35% NaH_2PO_4 in double distilled water with pH 7.4. Three different conditions of NO/GP in hydrogel form (NO/GP that absorbed 200%, 350%, and 500% of SWF absorbed per weight) were examined with SWF. Before initiating the experiments, 2, 3.5, or 5 mL of SWF were added to 1 g of NO/GP and mixed well to obtain the homogeneous hydrogel. In all experiments, a fresh sample was used and rested for 15 min after loading to allow for material relaxation and temperature equilibration. To evaluate the steady shear flow behaviors of the hydrogel-form of NO/GP, steady rate-sweep tests were performed over a range of shear rates from 1 to 1000 s^{-1} with a logarithmically increasing scale. Next, strain-sweep tests were conducted to investigate both the linear viscoelastic region and nonlinear viscoelastic behavior over a strain amplitude range of 0.0625%–500% at a fixed angular frequency of 10 rad/s.

2.5. *Storage Stability*

The storage stability of NO/GP was evaluated by determining GSNO degradation under two temperature conditions: 4 and 37 °C. Two milligrams of NO/GP were placed in each tube, which were then stored in either a 4 °C refrigerator or a 37 °C incubator. At previously set time points, three tubes from each group were sampled, and the absorbance at 335 nm was measured to determine the GSNO content following dilution with DW.

2.6. *Behavior of NO/GP After Exposure to Wound Fluid*

2.6.1. Morphological Changes of NO/GP at the Wound Site

All animal experiments in this study have been reviewed and approved by the Pusan National University Institutional Animal Care and Use Committee (PNU-IACUC) on 01 February 2018 (Approval Number: PNU-2018-1800). To investigate the ability of NO/GP to form hydrogel in situ, macroscopic images of wounds treated with NO/GP were taken at each time point. Briefly, imprinting control region (ICR) mice (7 weeks old, male, Samtako Bio Korea) were purchased and acclimated for 7 days. To induce anesthesia, 0.5–0.6 mg/g of avertin (tribromoethanol) were administered intraperitoneally. Then, hair was removed from the dorsal side of the mouse by electric trimmers and hair removal cream (Veet for sensitive skin, Reckitt Benckiser, France). After hair removal, a full-thickness wound was created on the dorsal area of the mouse via an 8 mm diameter disposable biopsy punch (Kai medical, Japan). Macroscopic images were taken at each time point following treatment of the wound with 28.5 mg NO/GP.

2.6.2. Fluid Uptake Ability

The ability of NO/GP to uptake fluid was measured as previously described, with some modifications [26,32]. A three-station Franz diffusion cell apparatus (PermeGear, Inc., Hellertown, PA, USA) was used to measure the water uptake ability. A regenerated cellulose membrane (pore size = 0.45 μm) was placed between the donor and receiver compartments. In the receiver compartment, SWF was filled and thermostated at 37 °C. After SWF was loaded into the receiver compartment, 40 mg of NO/GP were placed on the regenerated cellulose membrane (donor compartment). The amount of SWF was maintained at 8 mL. At each time point, the weight of the donor compartment was measured to calculate the amount of absorbed fluid.

2.6.3. NO Release from NO/GP

The NO release from NO/GP was calculated by measuring the GSNO decomposition. The amount of GSNO remaining was determined using a UV/Vis spectrophotometer at a wavelength of 335 nm. Fifty milligrams of NO/GP powder were placed in a 2 mL microtube, and different amounts of SWF were added to mimic swelling (NO/GP that absorbed 200%, 350%, and 500% of SWF per weight). All microtubes were placed in a 37 °C incubator. At the set time points, the remaining GSNO was measured by determining the absorbance of the supernatant at 335 nm after dilution and centrifugation. The NO released from NO/GP at each time point ($[NO]_t$) was calculated using an Equation (1) ($[GSNO]_0$: Initial GSNO concentration; $[GSNO]_t$: GSNO concentration at each time point) [25,33].

$$[NO]_t = [GSNO]_0 - [GSNO]_t \quad (1)$$

2.7. Antibacterial Assay

The bactericidal effect of NO/GP was evaluated against *P. aeruginosa* PAO1 (wild-type prototroph) [34] and MRSA (USA 300) [35]. Each pathogen was incubated overnight in TSB at 37 °C, and the bacterial suspension was adjusted with TSB media to approximately 10^8 colony forming unit (CFU)/mL until the optical density at 600 nm reached 0.15–0.2 (0.5 of the McFarland scale) [36]. The adjusted bacterial suspension (100 µL) was inoculated into each tube. Then, 28.5 mg of NO/GP and GP were added to each well and incubated for 24 h at 37 °C. To calculate the number of living bacterial cells, tubes were diluted with an additional 1.9 mL of the TSB medium. After serial dilution, 100 µL of each aliquot were plated on the TSB agar and incubated for 24 h at 37 °C. CFUs were determined by counting the colonies on the agar plates after incubation. To visualize the antibacterial activity of NO/GP, bacteria treated with or without GP and NO/GP were stained with SYTO9 (Thermo Fisher Scientific, Waltham, MA, USA) (final concentration was 66.8 µM) for 15 min. After incubation, bacteria were collected by centrifugation at 3000 *g* for 10 min. Each sample was washed three times and resuspended in 5 mL of normal saline. Green fluorescence from stained bacteria was imaged by an in vivo imaging system (FOBI, Neoscience, Suwon, Korea). For confocal laser scanning microscopy, bacteria were washed three times with normal saline after 24 h incubation with or without GP and NO/GP. Then, the bacteria were stained with SYTO 9 dye and propidium iodide (LIVE/DEAD® *Bac*Light™ bacterial viability kit) according to the manufacturer's protocol. Images were obtained at 20× magnification using the LSM 800 (Carl Zeiss, Oberkochen, Germany).

2.8. In Vivo Wound Healing Study in a Bacteria-Challenged Full Thickness Wound Model

2.8.1. Evaluation of Wound Size Reduction

In this study, mouse models of *P. aeruginosa*- and MRSA-challenged full thickness wounds were used to evaluate the ability of NO/GP to heal infected wounds. For *P. aeruginosa*-challenged wound healing study, 8 mm-sized wounds were created using above-mentioned method. Then, 10^9 CFU of *P. aeruginosa* suspension was inoculated at the wound site. Each wound was covered with Tegaderm film and fastened by surgical tape (Durapore™, 3M) for protection. Mice were then incubated for 2 days with no treatment for wound infection. Two days after wounding, mice were treated with 28.5 mg of NO/GP and GSNO-free NO/GP every 2 days. Untreated mice were used as a control group (changing Tegaderm film and surgical tape only). Photographs were obtained every 2 days, and the size of the wound was analyzed by ImageJ software. For the MRSA-challenged wound healing study, a 2×10^6 CFU of MRSA suspension was used instead of *P. aeruginosa*, and the procedure described above was followed.

2.8.2. Quantification of *P. aeruginosa* at the Wound Site

In the *P. aeruginosa*-challenged wound study, bacteria were quantified at the wound as previously reported, with some modifications [37]. Briefly, wound samples were harvested from representative mice on predetermined days with an 8 mm diameter biopsy punch. Each sample was placed in 1 mL of PBS, chopped, and sonicated to detach bacteria from the tissue samples. Then, 100 µL of each tissue-bacteria suspension was plated on an agar plate after serial dilution (1:10). To quantify the amount of *P. aeruginosa* at the wound site, a cetrimide-agar plate was used as a pseudomonas-selective media [38]. CFUs were determined by counting the colonies on the agar plates after 24 h of incubation.

2.8.3. Histological Examination

In the *P. aeruginosa*-challenged wound healing study, mice were euthanized 14 days after the initiation of drug treatment, and each wound site was sampled with an 8 mm diameter biopsy punch. Each sample was immediately immersed in 10% buffered formalin for fixation. Fixed wound samples were placed in paraffin blocks, sectioned to obtain 5 µm wound samples, and prepared for hematoxylin and eosin (H&E) staining, Twort's Gram staining, and Masson's trichrome staining. Each staining procedure was performed according to the manufacturer's protocol with some modifications. After staining, each slide was photographed using a light microscope at 20× magnification for H&E and Masson's trichrome staining, as well as 100× for Twort's gram staining.

2.9. Statistical Analysis

The statistical analysis was performed using a one-way analysis of variance (ANOVA) with a Bonferroni posttest in GraphPad Prism 5.0 (GraphPad Software, Inc., La Jolla, CA, USA). *p*-values less than 0.05 were considered statistically significant.

3. Results and Discussion

3.1. Powder Characterization

NO/GP was successfully prepared by micronizing, sieving, and blending GSNO, sodium alginate, pectin, and PEG. To examine the homogeneous fabrication of NO/GP, particle size distribution was analyzed using more than 100 particles, and GSNO contents were measured from 10 different samples. As shown in Figure 1A, pink GSNO particles were homogeneously dispersed in NO/GP. After micronizing, the average particle size and standard deviation decreased (from 85.2 ± 47.3 to 51.5 ± 22 μm, respectively) (Table 1, Figure 1A,B). In addition, the RSD of GSNO contents was reduced (16.06–4.77) due to the removal of large GSNO particles which interfere with content homogeneity (Table 1, Figure 1C). Flowability was measured to investigate the movement of NO/GP at the wound site before conversion to hydrogel. The flowability of in situ hydrogel-forming powders should be low because highly flowable powders can be easily cleared from the wound site prior to hydrogel formation. In this experiment, the flowability of NO/GP was expressed by the Hausner ratio. After the blending and micronizing process, the Hausner ratio of NO/GP increased from 1.34 to 1.97 (Table 1). Due to the decreased particle size, flowability decreased after micronization. In general, powders with a Hausner ratio exceeding 1.6 possess extremely poor flowability [39]. Low flowability can prevent the removal of the powder and is essential for the in situ hydrogel-forming powder system; the powder should remain on the wound site until it is converted to a hydrogel. For this reason, the Hausner ratios of previously developed powder dressings are around 1.7 [18,19,26], as this ratio allows the powders to resist the flow. Therefore, NO/GPs with a Hausner ratio of 1.97 could also resist flow away from the wound site before hydrogel formation.

Table 1. Content homogeneity and flowability of in situ hydrogel-forming/nitric oxide (NO)-releasing powder dressing (NO/GP).

	Particle Size (μm)	GSNO Contents (%)	RSD of GSNO Contents (%)	Hausner Ratio
Non-micronized mixture	85.2 ± 47.3	4 ± 0.64	16.06	1.34 ± 0.04
NO/GP	51.5 ± 22	4 ± 0.19	4.77	1.97 ± 0.06

Particle size was analyzed by ImageJ software from microscopic images ($n > 100$). S-nitrosoglutathione (GSNO) contents and relative standard deviation (RSD) were calculated from 10 samples of NO/GP. The Hausner ratio was calculated from the tap/bulk density ratio ($n = 3$).

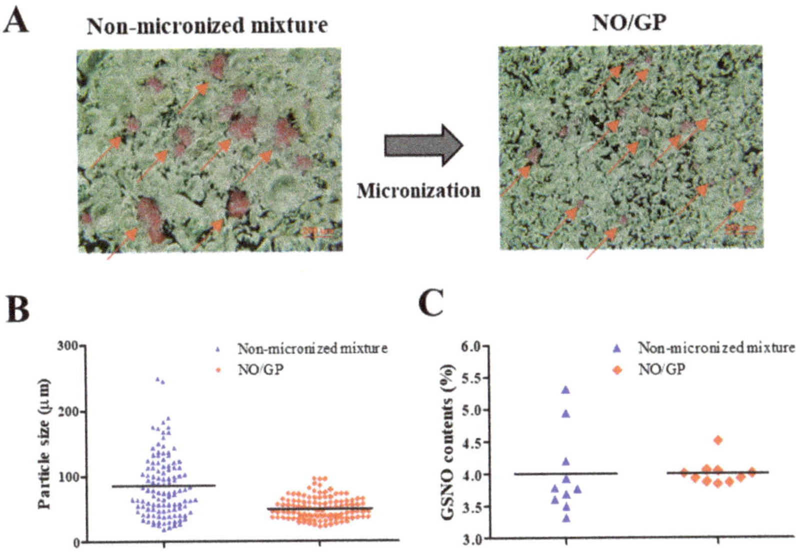

Figure 1. Characterization of NO/GP in powder form. Microscopic images (**A**), particle size distribution ($n > 100$) (**B**), and S-nitrosoglutathione (GSNO) contents of non-micronized mixture and NO/GP ($n = 10$) (**C**). Red arrows indicate GSNO particles (pink particles).

3.2. Rheological Properties of NO/GP in Hydrogel Form

Rheological properties, including viscosity, storage modulus, and loss modulus, were evaluated to investigate the adhesiveness of NO/GP in hydrogel form against various steady shear strains or oscillatory shear strains. Adhesiveness is an important factor of hydrogel dressings because hydrogels should adhere to the damaged site to protect the wound and maintain humid conditions, which is an essential role of hydrogel dressings. Figure 2A,B show the dependence of shear stress and steady shear viscosity on shear rate for NO/GP following the absorption of 200%, 350%, and 500% SWF per weight. In all steady rate-sweep tests, the shear stress tended to level off and approach a limiting constant value (usually referred to as "yield stress") as the shear rate approached zero. Yield stress plays an important role in predicting the adhesiveness of semi-solid formulations because stress is related to the level of internal structures that can exhibit resistance to flow. Steady shear viscosity decreased sharply as the shear rate increased, indicating that NO/GP exhibited a marked non-Newtonian shear-thinning flow behavior. In a previous study, petroleum jelly, which is a widely used and marketed product, demonstrated similar behavior in the 350% swollen condition, and the values of shear stress and steady shear viscosity were also similar to those of the swollen condition [40]. These results indicate that the NO/GP hydrogel could maintain a gel-like structure and resist small shear stress such as gravitational force or brushing against clothes. Figure 2C,D,E indicate the storage modulus, G', and loss modulus, G'', as a function of strain amplitude under three different swelling conditions of NO/GP hydrogels with a fixed angular frequency of 10 rad/s. The storage modulus was found to be larger than the loss modulus within a relatively smaller strain amplitude, indicating that the rheological behavior in this region is dominated by an elastic (solid-like) rather than a viscous (liquid-like) property. However, as the strain amplitude gradually increased, viscous behavior became superior to elastic behavior because the storage modulus demonstrated a sharper decrease with increasing strain amplitude compared with the loss modulus. These results indicate that adhesiveness to a relatively large imposed deformation (such as scrubbing motion) is weakened; therefore, the NO/GP hydrogels could easily flow and be removed from the wound site.

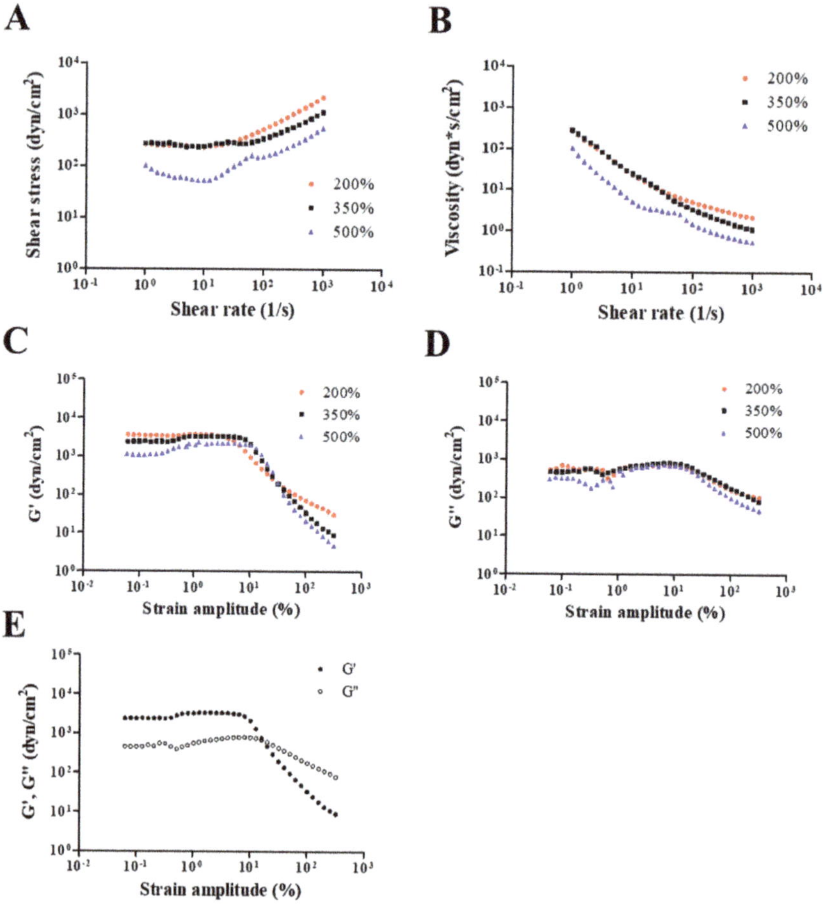

Figure 2. Rheological properties of NO/GP in hydrogel form. Shear stress and viscosity (**A** and **B**, respectively) of NO/GP following absorption of 200%, 350%, and 500% of simulated wound fluid (SWF) per weight as a function of shear rate. Storage modulus (*G*′) and loss modulus (*G*″) of each swollen condition as a function of strain amplitude (**C** and **D**, respectively). *G*′ and *G*″ of 350% swollen NO/GP hydrogel as a function of strain amplitude (**E**). Strain-sweep tests were performed at a fixed angular frequency of 10 rad/s.

3.3. Storage Stability

The storage stability of NO/GP was evaluated by detecting GSNO decomposition under two temperature conditions (4 and 37 °C). Since GSNO can be easily degraded by hydrolysis, storage stability is an important factor in the development of GSNO-containing formulations. Though several GSNO-containing hydrogel dressings have been developed to accelerate wound healing [41–44], those formulations did not present long-term stability because GSNO hydrolysis is inevitable in water-containing formulations. Conversely, no significant GSNO decomposition was noted in NO/GP up to 140 days under both the 4 and 37 °C conditions (Figure 3). Since GSNO in the NO/GP remained in a powder state, which was a water-free condition during storage, the hydrolysis of GSNO was prevented. Thus, NO/GP could remain stable whilst in storage without any concerns relating to GSNO degradation. In addition, there were no significant changes in particle size, Hausner ration and rheological properties during the storage period (data not shown).

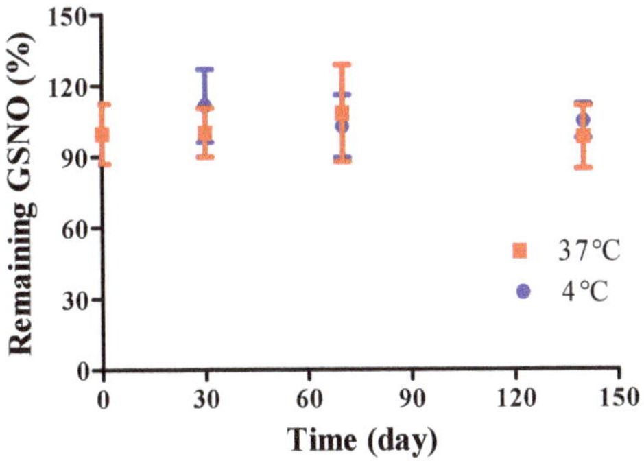

Figure 3. Storage stability of NO/GP at 4 (blue) and 37 °C (red). Remaining GSNO percentage compared with that of initial NO/GP was calculated to evaluate storage stability. Each point represents the mean ± standard deviation (n = 3).

3.4. Behavior of NO/GP After Exposure to Wound Fluid

3.4.1. Morphological Changes in NO/GP at the Wound Site

To investigate the ability of NO/GP to form hydrogel in situ, morphological changes in NO/GP were observed following application of 28.5 mg of NO/GP to the full-thickness wounds in mice. The amount of NO/GP was sufficient to cover 1 cm^3 of a full-thickness wound. As shown in Figure 4A, following its application to the wound, the NO/GP powder was immediately converted to a glittering hydrogel, and more than 50% of the NO/GP powders converted to a hydrogel within 1 min. All of the NO/GP applied was converted to hydrogel within 10 min. After 10 min, no morphological changes in NO/GP were observed due to the completion of the hydrogel structure.

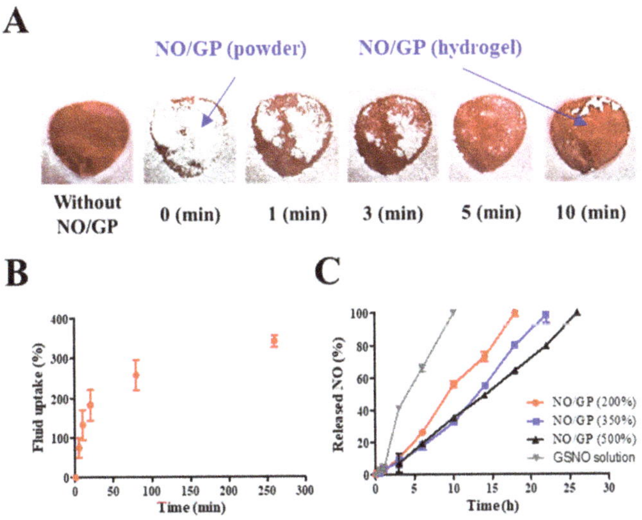

Figure 4. Behavior of NO/GP following exposure to wound fluid. Morphological changes in NO/GP applied to the mouse full-thickness wound model (**A**). Fluid uptake profile of NO/GP (amount of absorbed SWF is presented as the percent per initial NO/GP powder weight) (**B**). NO release profiles of NO/GP under different swelling conditions and the GSNO solution at the equivalent concentration to 350% swollen NO/GP (**C**). Each point represents the mean ± standard deviation (n = 3).

3.4.2. Fluid Uptake Ability

Since hydrogel formation is initiated by the absorption of wound fluid, an investigation of fluid uptake ability is essential for evaluation of powder dressings that form hydrogels in situ. To evaluate the fluid uptake ability of NO/GP, the dressings were exposed to SWF at 37 °C, and the amount of absorbed fluid was calculated by measuring the change in weight of NO/GP. The amount of absorbed fluid was presented as a percentage of weight gained by fluid uptake per initial NO/GP. As shown in Figure 4B, NO/GP absorbed SWF rapidly, and around 200% of SWF was absorbed within 20 min. After the initial rapid absorption of the SWF, the rate of fluid uptake by NO/GP was decreased, and NO/GP absorbed up to 375% of SWF in 270 min. After that, no further significant fluid absorption was observed during the experiment. In the initial state, the swellable polymers in NO/GP (pectin and alginate) absorbed SWF and rapidly formed a hydrogel structure. Following hydrogel formation, SWF was slowly captured in the intermolecular space of the hydrogel structure, because hydrophilic polymers in NO/GP are able to trap SWF by hydrogen bonding between polymers and water molecules. Finally, since the intermolecular space was filled with SWF, no more fluid could be absorbed. Since NO/GP could efficiently absorb fluid, hydrogel formation and subsequent NO release was initiated rapidly.

3.4.3. NO Release from NO/GP

Since NO released from GSNO in NO/GP exerts therapeutic effects, the NO release profiles of NO/GP were investigated by exposing NO/GP to SWF at 37 °C. The NO release from NO/GP was investigated under three swollen conditions (200%, 350%, and 500% of SWF per initial NO/GP weight) that represented an amount of low, medium and high wound exudate, respectively. As GSNO generates NO via hydrolytic cleavage of the S–N bond, the NO release from NO/GP is initiated by wound fluid. Thus, the amount of NO released from NO/GP was calculated by measuring GSNO degradation (released NO = initial GSNO − remaining GSNO). Regardless of swelling, NO/GP exhibited a linear NO release without a burst release (Figure 4C). In addition, lower levels of NO/GP swelling resulted in a slightly faster NO release rate compared with higher levels of swelling, and NO was released up to 18, 22, and 26 h in the 200%, 350%, and 500% conditions, respectively. Due to the presence of polymeric compounds (alginate, pectin, and PEG) in the NO/GP hydrogel structure, GSNO molecules or NO radicals were surrounded by polymeric molecules which restrict the diffusion of radicals in what is termed the "cage effect" [45,46]. Compared with the GSNO solution, NO/GP presented a prolonged NO-release profile, which was due to the restricted diffusion of radicals over the cage (NO was released 100% within 12 h at the GSNO concentration equivalent to 350% swollen NO/GP). The release profiles different under different levels of swelling because the rate of NO release from GSNO was affected by its initial concentration; thus, the higher initial concentration resulted in faster NO release due to the increased amount of radicals contributing to the degradation of GSNO molecules [47]. Therefore, 200% SWF added to the NO/GP group (high GSNO concentration) resulted in a faster NO release compared with the 350% and 500% groups. In addition, since NO/GP exhibited a linear NO release under all levels of swelling, this indicates that dressings can be changed any time without concerns of toxicity caused by burst-released NO.

3.5. *In Vitro Antibacterial Assay*

Antibacterial efficacy is the most important characteristic of a dressing for the treatment of infected wounds. To investigate the antibacterial activity of NO/GP, an in vitro antibacterial assay was performed using the CFU method against MRSA and *P. aeruginosa*, which are representative drug-resistant gram-positive and -negative bacteria. Following incubation for 24 h with or without NO/GP in TSB media, a 6-log reduction in bacterial CFUs was observed in the NO/GP-treated group compared to the GP-treated group against both MRSA and *P. aeruginosa* (Figure 5A). After CFU examination, the antibacterial activity of NO/GP was visualized by staining with SYTO 9, which is a green fluorescence dye that can stain bacterial DNA. Since only living bacteria were collected by centrifugation, green fluorescence indicated the presence of live bacteria. As shown in Figure 5B, distinct green fluorescence was detected in the untreated and GP-treated groups for both MRSA and *P. aeruginosa*. Furthermore, signals from the NO/GP-treated group were significantly reduced, owing to the high number of bacteria killed by NO in both the MRSA and *P. aeruginosa* groups. The antibacterial effect of NO/GP was also examined via confocal microscopy using the LIVE/DEAD® *Bac*Light™ bacterial viability kit. Since propidium iodide can only penetrate damaged bacterial membranes, living bacteria were stained with SYTO 9 (green fluorescence) and damaged bacteria were stained with propidium iodide (red fluorescence). As shown in Figure 5C, confocal images of the GP-treated and untreated groups exhibited distinct green fluorescence, while those of the NO/GP-treated group exhibited strong red fluorescence. This indicates that most of the bacteria survived in the GP-treated and untreated groups, while few bacteria survived in the NO/GP-treated group. Since NO possesses broad-spectrum antibacterial effects and NO/GP can release NO in a sustained manner, these results indicate that NO/GP exhibited significant bactericidal activity against both gram-negative *P. aeruginosa* and gram-positive MRSA without bacterial re-growth for 24 h. Broad-spectrum antibacterial and potent bactericidal effects against drug-resistant bacteria are essential for the treatment of infected wounds, since the infection of cutaneous wounds by drug-resistant bacteria is increasing and it is hard to immediately distinguish bacterial species. Moreover, the multiple antibacterial mechanisms of NO may prevent the emergence of NO-resistant bacteria [16]. Thus, these findings indicate that NO/GP possesses desirable antibacterial properties and may be beneficial for the treatment of infected wounds.

3.6. *In Vivo Wound Healing Study*

3.6.1. Evaluation of Wound Size Reduction Effect

The therapeutic effects of NO/GP were evaluated in mice using the bacteria-challenged full-thickness wound model. The acceleration of infected wound recovery with NO/GP was evaluated by observing morphological changes in the wound and measuring wound size change every 2 days. In both *P. aeruginosa*- and MRSA-challenged full-thickness wound models, the NO/GP treatment resulted in a significant reduction in wound size compared with GP treatment and no treatment after 4 days (Figure 6). In NO/GP-treated groups, wound size was reduced to less than 20% of the initial size 14 and 8 days after treatment initiation in the *P. aeruginosa*- and MRSA-challenged models, respectively. Conversely, in the GP treated groups, no significant acceleration of wound healing was observed in either the *P. aeruginosa*- or MRSA-challenged models compared to the untreated groups. Accelerated wound healing in the NO/GP groups can be attributed to the action of NO released from GSNO in NO/GP [22]. In particular, broad and potent antibacterial effects could effectively eradicate infection with gram-positive or -negative bacteria [48,49]. Moreover, NO facilitates wound healing by promoting fibroblast proliferation, collagen formation, and tissue remodeling [13,50]. Therefore, NO/GP may facilitate wound healing in *P. aeruginosa*- and MRSA-challenged full-thickness wounds in mice.

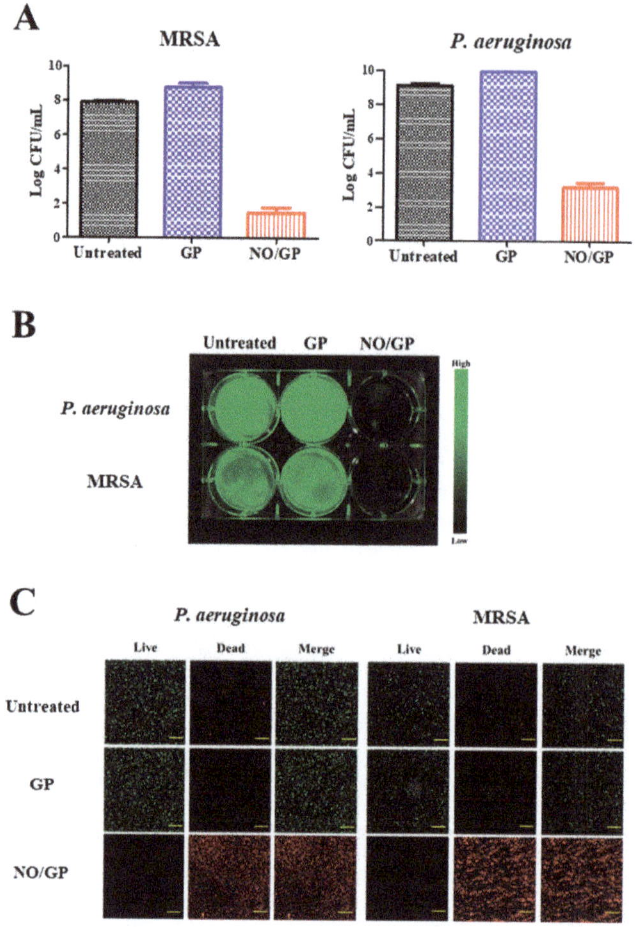

Figure 5. Antibacterial effects of NO/GP. Antibacterial effects of NO/GP against *Pseudomonas aeruginosa* and methicillin-resistant *Staphylococcus aureus* (MRSA) by the colony forming unit (CFU) method. The results are presented as the mean ± standard deviation (n = 3) (**A**). Visualization of bacteria by SYTO9 staining. Green fluorescence indicates the presence of live bacteria (**B**). Confocal laser scanning microscopic images of cells treated and untreated with GP and NO/GP. Green fluorescence indicates live bacteria and red fluorescence indicates dead bacteria. Images were taken at 20× magnification. Scale bar represents 50 μm (**C**).

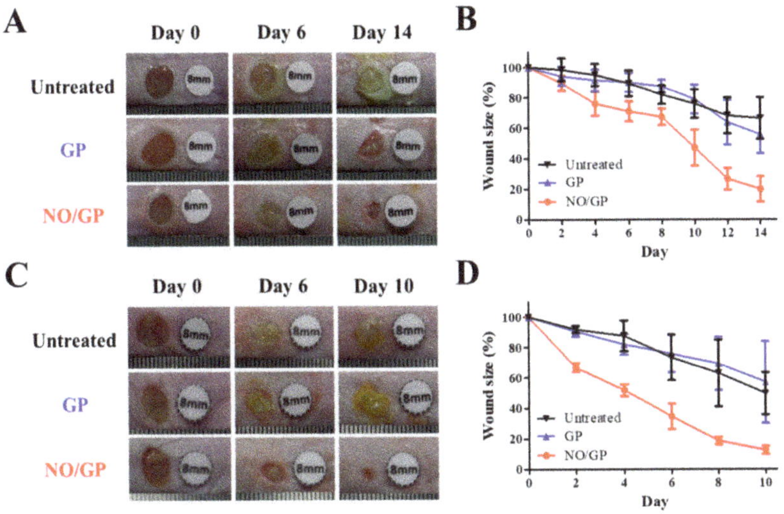

Figure 6. Representative macroscopic images of *P. aeruginosa*-challenged full-thickness wounds in mice 0, 6, and 14 days after treatment initiation (**A**). Changes in wound size in mice with *P. aeruginosa*-challenged full-thickness wounds (**B**). Representative macroscopic images of MRSA-challenged full-thickness wounds in mice 0, 6, and 14 days after treatment initiation (**C**). Changes in wound size in mice with MRSA-challenged full-thickness wounds (**D**). Values are presented as the mean ± standard deviation (n = 4).

3.6.2. Quantification of P. aeruginosa at the Wound Site

To investigate the in vivo antibacterial effects of NO/GP, wound samples were harvested 2, 8, and 14 days after treatment initiation, and CFUs were assessed with *Pseudomonas*-selective agar plates, which exclude other bacterial species. As shown in Figure 7A, there was no decrease in the number of *P. aeruginosa* 2 days after treatment initiation; however, on day 8, significant bactericidal effects were observed in the NO/GP-treated group (around 3-log CFU reduction). Only 4.1 and 4.8 CFU/cm^2 *P. aeruginosa* were observed in the NO/GP-treated group, while 6.7 and 7.6 CFU/cm^2 and 6.4 and 6.5 CFU/cm^2 *P. aeruginosa* were observed in untreated and GP-treated groups 8 and 14 days after treatment initiation, respectively. To visualize the antibacterial effects in vivo, Twort's Gram-staining was performed. Because *P. aeruginosa* is a rod-shaped gram-negative bacteria 1–2 μm in size, it can be detected by Twort's gram staining in tissue samples containing more than 10^5 CFU (low levels of bacteria are hard to detect by Gram staining) [51,52]. Fourteen days after treatment initiation, rod-shaped, brown-colored bacteria (*P. aeruginosa*) were observed in GP-treated and -untreated groups in the damaged epidermal region, indicating that at least 10^5 CFU *P. aeruginosa* was present in the samples (Figure 7B). Conversely, no bacteria were observed in the NO/GP-treated group or in the healthy control. Since NO released from NO/GP was able to efficiently eradicate *P. aeruginosa* from infected wound sites, wound healing may have occurred subsequent to inflammation. Furthermore, high numbers of *P. aeruginosa* in GP-treated and untreated groups resulted in consistent inflammation and, consequently, in impaired re-epithelization.

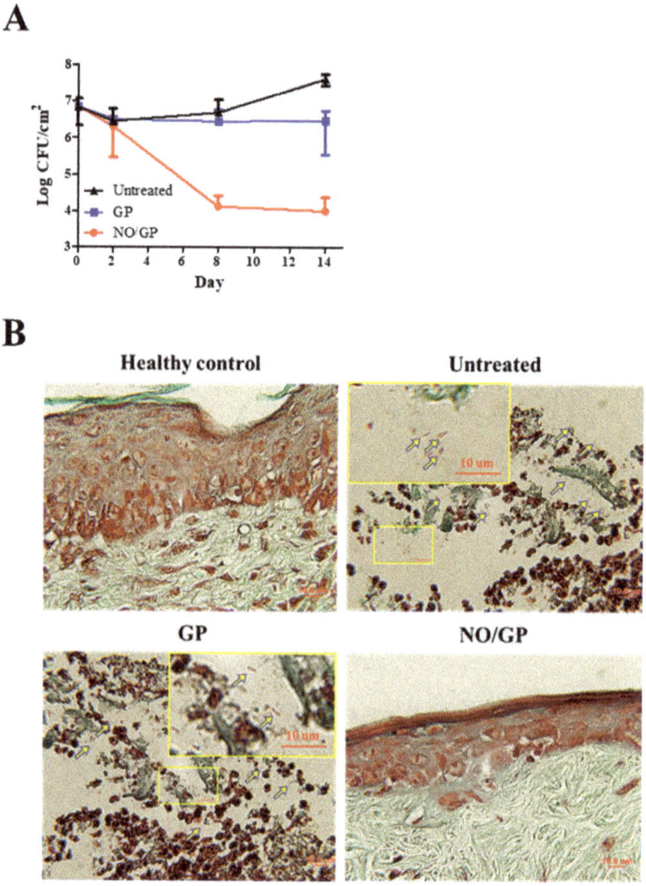

Figure 7. Bacterial quantification at the wound site (n = 3) (**A**). Twort's gram staining of wound samples from mice treated with or without GP or NO/GP. The epidermal region of the tissue samples was imaged with a microscope at a magnification of 100×. Arrows indicate *P. aeruginosa* (1–2 µm sized, rod-shaped, and brown). Scale bar represents 10 µm (**B**).

3.6.3. Histological Examination

Tissue regeneration and collagen synthesis in full thickness wounds challenged with *P. aeruginosa* were evaluated by H&E and Masson's trichrome staining. Fourteen days after the initiation of drug treatment, more organized skin morphology and higher collagen abundance were observed in the NO/GP-treated group compared with the GP-treated and untreated groups (Figure 8). Well-differentiated epidermis was observed in the NO/GP-treated group, whilst damaged epidermis was observed in the GP-treated and untreated groups following H&E staining. In addition, skin cells, such as keratinocytes and fibroblasts, were abundant in the NO/GP-treated group. Conversely, granulation and large numbers of immune cells were observed in GP-treated and untreated groups. The amount of collagen in wound samples was visualized by Masson's trichrome staining (blue color indicates collagen). As shown in Figure 8, samples from the NO/GP-treated group exhibited a prominent blue color similar to that of healthy skin tissue. However, GP-treated and untreated groups exhibited less collagen in the dermis region. Since inflammation was ongoing in these groups, the collagen synthesis and tissue remodeling processes were inhibited, resulting in delayed wound healing.

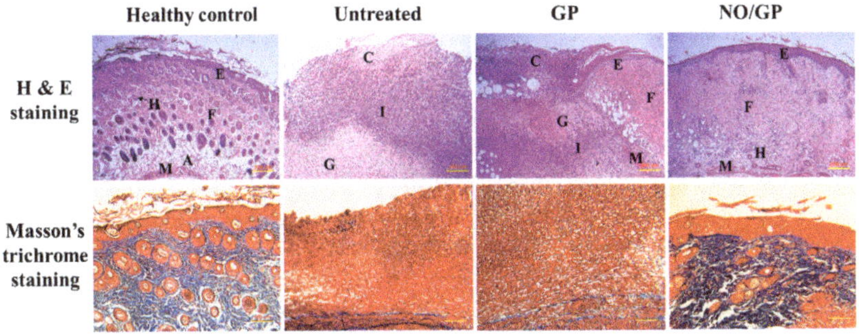

Figure 8. H&E (hematoxylin and eosin) and Masson's trichrome straining of wound tissues from *P. aeruginosa*-challenged full-thickness wound mice threated with or without GP or NO/GP for 14 days. A: Adipose tissue; C: Cell debris; E: Epidermis; F: Fibrous tissue; G: Granulation tissue; H: Hair follicle; I: Immune cells; M: Muscle. Scale bar represents 200 and 100 μm for the H&E and Masson's trichrome images, respectively.

4. Conclusions

In this study, we successfully developed an in situ hydrogel-forming/NO-releasing wound dressing (NO/GP) composed of alginate, pectin, PEG, and GSNO, with a controlled NO release property and good storage stability for the effective treatment of infected wounds (Figure 9). Since NO/GP maintained a water-free powder form until use on the wound, the degradation of GSNO in NO/GP was prevented for more than 3 months when stored at 4 and 37 °C. When applied to wounds, NO/GP absorbed up to 350% of wound fluid and was quickly transformed from a dry powder to an adhesive hydrogel. Simultaneously, a NO release was triggered by absorbed wound exudates, followed by a sustained NO release over 24 h without an initial burst release. Rheological studies indicated that the hydrogel structure of NO/GP exhibited sufficient adhesiveness to remain stable on the wound surface. The results of an in vitro antibacterial study demonstrated that NO/GP leads to a 6-log reduction in MRSA and *P. aeruginosa* over 24 h. Finally, in vivo antibacterial effects and accelerated wound healing were observed in mice with infected wounds treated with NO/GP. These results suggest that the in situ hydrogel-forming/NO releasing formulation presented in this study can be fabricated by a simple and cost-effective manufacturing process and thus would be a promising alternative to dressings for the treatment of infected wounds.

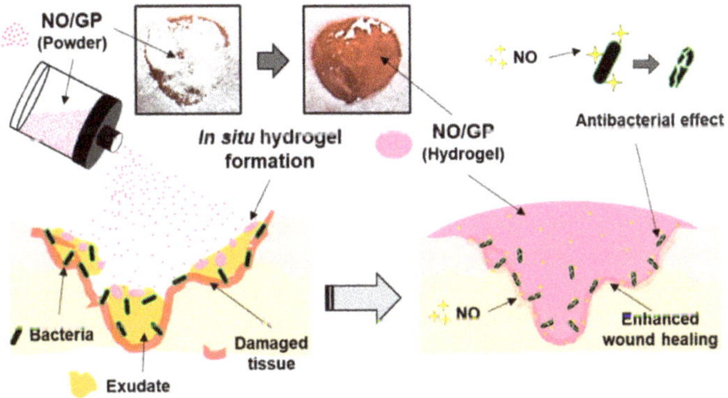

Figure 9. Schematic illustration of NO/GP for the treatment of infected wounds.

Author Contributions: Conceptualization, J.L. and J.-W.Y.; methodology, J.L., N.H., S.P.H., H.-J.A. and J.C.; formal analysis, J.L. and H.-J.A.; investigation, J.L.; writing—original draft preparation, J.L.; writing—review and editing, J.L., K.-W.S. and J.-W.Y.; supervision, J.-W.Y.; project administration, J.-W.Y.

Funding: This research was supported by a grant from the Korean Healthcare Technology R&D Project, Ministry for Health and Welfare Affairs, Republic of Korea (HI15C2558) and by a Basic Science Research Program through the National Research Foundation of Korea (NRF) funded by the Ministry of Education (2019R1I1A3A01057849).

Conflicts of Interest: The authors declare no conflict of interest.

References

1. Daeschlein, G. Antimicrobial and antiseptic strategies in wound management. *Int. Wound J.* **2013**, *10*, 9–14. [CrossRef] [PubMed]
2. Fleischmann, C.; Scherag, A.; Adhikari, N.K.; Hartog, C.S.; Tsaganos, T.; Schlattmann, P.; Angus, D.C.; Reinhart, K. Assessment of global incidence and mortality of hospital-treated sepsis. Current estimates and limitations. *Am. J. Respir. Crit. Care Med.* **2016**, *193*, 259–272. [CrossRef] [PubMed]
3. Bello, Y.M.; Phillips, T.J. Recent advances in wound healing. *JAMA* **2000**, *283*, 716–718. [CrossRef] [PubMed]
4. Muzzarelli, R.A. Chitins and chitosans for the repair of wounded skin, nerve, cartilage and bone. *Carbohydr. Polym.* **2009**, *76*, 167–182. [CrossRef]
5. Janis, J.; Attinger, C. The basic science of wound healing. *Plast. Reconstr. Surg.* **2006**, *117*, 12S–34S. [CrossRef]
6. Witte, M.B.; Barbul, A. General principles of wound healing. *Surg. Clin. North Am.* **1997**, *77*, 509–528. [CrossRef]
7. Yurt, R.W.; McManus, A.T.; Mason, A.D.; Pruitt, B.A. Increased susceptibility to infection related to extent of burn injury. *Arch. Surg.* **1984**, *119*, 183–188. [CrossRef]
8. Percival, S.L.; Hill, K.E.; Williams, D.W.; Hooper, S.J.; Thomas, D.W.; Costerton, J.W. A review of the scientific evidence for biofilms in wounds. *Wound Repair Regen.* **2012**, *20*, 647–657. [CrossRef]
9. Kevil, C.G.; Kolluru, G.K.; Pattillo, C.B.; Giordano, T. Inorganic nitrite therapy: Historical perspective and future directions. *Free Radic. Biol. Med.* **2011**, *51*, 576–593. [CrossRef]
10. Schäffer, M.R.; Tantry, U.; Gross, S.S.; Wasserkrug, H.L.; Barbul, A. Nitric oxide regulates wound healing. *J. Surg. Res.* **1996**, *63*, 237–240. [CrossRef]
11. Fatima, A.D.; Modolo, L.V.; Conegero Sanches, A.C.; Porto, R.R. Wound healing agents: The role of natural and non-natural products in drug development. *Mini Rev. Med. Chem.* **2008**, *8*, 879–888. [CrossRef] [PubMed]
12. Rizk, M.; Witte, M.B.; Barbul, A. Nitric oxide and wound healing. *World J. Surg.* **2004**, *28*, 301–306. [CrossRef] [PubMed]
13. Witte, M.B.; Barbul, A. Role of nitric oxide in wound repair. *Am. J. Surg.* **2002**, *183*, 406–412. [CrossRef]
14. Jones, M.L.; Ganopolsky, J.G.; Labbé, A.; Wahl, C.; Prakash, S. Antimicrobial properties of nitric oxide and its application in antimicrobial formulations and medical devices. *Appl. Microbiol. Biotechnol.* **2010**, *88*, 401–407. [CrossRef] [PubMed]
15. Schairer, D.O.; Chouake, J.S.; Nosanchuk, J.D.; Friedman, A.J. The potential of nitric oxide releasing therapies as antimicrobial agents. *Virulence* **2012**, *3*, 271–279. [CrossRef] [PubMed]
16. Privett, B.J.; Broadnax, A.D.; Bauman, S.J.; Riccio, D.A.; Schoenfisch, M.H. Examination of bacterial resistance to exogenous nitric oxide. *Nitric Oxide* **2012**, *26*, 169–173. [CrossRef] [PubMed]
17. Balakrishnan, B.; Mohanty, M.; Umashankar, P.; Jayakrishnan, A. Evaluation of an in situ forming hydrogel wound dressing based on oxidized alginate and gelatin. *Biomaterials* **2005**, *26*, 6335–6342. [CrossRef] [PubMed]
18. De Cicco, F.; Reverchon, E.; Adami, R.; Auriemma, G.; Russo, P.; Calabrese, E.C.; Porta, A.; Aquino, R.P.; Del Gaudio, P. In situ forming antibacterial dextran blend hydrogel for wound dressing: SAA technology vs. spray drying. *Carbohydr. Polym.* **2014**, *101*, 1216–1224. [CrossRef]
19. De Cicco, F.; Porta, A.; Sansone, F.; Aquino, R.P.; Del Gaudio, P. Nanospray technology for an in situ gelling nanoparticulate powder as a wound dressing. *Int. J. Pharm.* **2014**, *473*, 30–37. [CrossRef]
20. Dabiri, G.; Damstetter, E.; Phillips, T. Choosing a wound dressing based on common wound characteristics. *Adv. Wound Care* **2016**, *5*, 32–41. [CrossRef]

21. Del Gaudio, P.; Amante, C.; Civale, R.; Bizzarro, V.; Petrella, A.; Pepe, G.; Campiglia, P.; Russo, P.; Aquino, R.P. In situ gelling alginate-pectin blend particles loaded with Ac2-26: A new weapon to improve wound care armamentarium. *Carbohydr. Polym.* **2019**, *227*, 115305. [CrossRef]
22. Carpenter, A.W.; Schoenfisch, M.H. Nitric oxide release: Part II. Therapeutic applications. *Chem. Soc. Rev.* **2012**, *41*, 3742–3752. [CrossRef] [PubMed]
23. Broniowska, K.A.; Diers, A.R.; Hogg, N. S-nitrosoglutathione. *Biochim. Biophys. Acta* **2013**, *1830*, 3173–3181. [CrossRef] [PubMed]
24. Kannon, G.A.; Garrett, A.B. Moist wound healing with occlusive dressings: A clinical review. *Dermatol. Surg.* **1995**, *21*, 583–590. [CrossRef] [PubMed]
25. Yoo, J.W.; Acharya, G.; Lee, C.H. In vivo evaluation of vaginal films for mucosal delivery of nitric oxide. *Biomaterials* **2009**, *30*, 3978–3985. [CrossRef] [PubMed]
26. Romic, M.D.; Klaric, M.S.; Lovric, J.; Pepic, I.; Cetina-Cizmek, B.; Filipovic-Grcic, J.; Hafner, A. Melatonin-loaded chitosan/Pluronic(R) F127 microspheres as in situ forming hydrogel: An innovative antimicrobial wound dressing. *Eur. J. Pharm. Biopharm.* **2016**. [CrossRef]
27. Balakrishnan, P.; Park, E.K.; Song, C.K.; Ko, H.J.; Hahn, T.W.; Song, K.W.; Cho, H.J. Carbopol-incorporated thermoreversible gel for intranasal drug delivery. *Molecules* **2015**, *20*, 4124–4135. [CrossRef]
28. Cho, H.J.; Balakrishnan, P.; Park, E.K.; Song, K.W.; Hong, S.S.; Jang, T.Y.; Kim, K.S.; Chung, S.J.; Shim, C.K.; Kim, D.D. Poloxamer/cyclodextrin/chitosan-based thermoreversible gel for intranasal delivery of fexofenadine hydrochloride. *J. Pharm. Sci.* **2011**, *100*, 681–691. [CrossRef] [PubMed]
29. Kwak, M.S.; Ahn, H.J.; Song, K.W. Rheological investigation of body cream and body lotion in actual application conditions. *Korea-Aust. Rheol. J.* **2015**, *27*, 241–251. [CrossRef]
30. Lin, S.Y.; Chen, K.S.; Run-Chu, L. Design and evaluation of drug-loaded wound dressing having thermoresponsive, adhesive, absorptive and easy peeling properties. *Biomaterials* **2001**, *22*, 2999–3004. [CrossRef]
31. Homsy, C.A. Bio-Compatibility in selection of materials for implantation. *J. Biomed. Mater. Res.* **1970**, *4*, 341–356. [CrossRef] [PubMed]
32. Phaechamud, T.; Lertsuphotvanit, N.; Issarayungyuen, P.; Chantadee, T. Design, fabrication and characterization of xanthan gum/liquid-loaded porous natural rubber film. *J. Pharm. Investig.* **2019**, *49*, 149–160. [CrossRef]
33. Levin, R.J. The mechanisms of human female sexual arousal. *Annu. Rev. Sex Res.* **1992**, *3*, 1–48. [CrossRef]
34. Pearson, J.P.; Pesci, E.C.; Iglewski, B.H. Roles of Pseudomonas aeruginosa las and rhl quorum-sensing systems in control of elastase and rhamnolipid biosynthesis genes. *J. Bacteriol.* **1997**, *179*, 5756–5767. [CrossRef] [PubMed]
35. McDougal, L.K.; Steward, C.D.; Killgore, G.E.; Chaitram, J.M.; McAllister, S.K.; Tenover, F.C. Pulsed-field gel electrophoresis typing of oxacillin-resistant Staphylococcus aureus isolates from the United States: Establishing a national database. *J. Clin. Microbiol.* **2003**, *41*, 5113–5120. [CrossRef] [PubMed]
36. Castro, J.; Rivera, D.; Franco, L.A. Topical anti-inflammatory activity in TPA-induced mouse ear edema model and in vitro antibacterial properties of Cordia alba flowers. *J. Pharm. Investig.* **2019**, *49*, 331–336. [CrossRef]
37. Rojas, I.G.; Padgett, D.A.; Sheridan, J.F.; Marucha, P.T. Stress-induced susceptibility to bacterial infection during cutaneous wound healing. *Brain Behav. Immun.* **2002**, *16*, 74–84. [CrossRef] [PubMed]
38. Kominos, S.D.; Copeland, C.E.; Grosiak, B.; Postic, B. Introduction of Pseudomonas aeruginosa into a hospital via vegetables. *Appl. Microbiol.* **1972**, *24*, 567–570. [CrossRef] [PubMed]
39. Lebrun, P.; Krier, F.; Mantanus, J.; Grohganz, H.; Yang, M.; Rozet, E.; Boulanger, B.; Evrard, B.; Rantanen, J.; Hubert, P. Design space approach in the optimization of the spray-drying process. *Eur. J. Pharm. Biopharm.* **2012**, *80*, 226–234. [CrossRef]
40. Park, E.K.; Song, K.W. Rheological evaluation of petroleum jelly as a base material in ointment and cream formulations: Steady shear flow behavior. *Arch. Pharmacal Res.* **2010**, *33*, 141–150. [CrossRef]
41. Amadeu, T.P.; Seabra, A.B.; De Oliveira, M.G.; Costa, A.M. S-nitrosoglutathione-containing hydrogel accelerates rat cutaneous wound repair. *J. Eur. Acad. Dermatol. Venereol.* **2007**, *21*, 629–637. [CrossRef] [PubMed]

42. Schanuel, F.S.; Santos, K.S.R.; Monte-Alto-Costa, A.; de Oliveira, M.G. Combined nitric oxide-releasing poly (vinyl alcohol) film/F127 hydrogel for accelerating wound healing. *Colloids Surf. B Biointerfaces* **2015**, *130*, 182–191. [CrossRef] [PubMed]
43. Georgii, J.; Amadeu, T.; Seabra, A.; de Oliveira, M.; Monte-Alto-Costa, A. Topical S-nitrosoglutathione-releasing hydrogel improves healing of rat ischaemic wounds. *J. Tissue Eng. Regen. Med.* **2011**, *5*, 612–619. [CrossRef] [PubMed]
44. Champeau, M.; Póvoa, V.; Militão, L.; Cabrini, F.M.; Picheth, G.F.; Meneau, F.; Jara, C.P.; de Araujo, E.P.; de Oliveira, M.G. Supramolecular poly(acrylic acid)/F127 hydrogel with hydration-controlled nitric oxide release for enhancing wound healing. *Acta Biomater.* **2018**, *74*, 312–325. [CrossRef] [PubMed]
45. Herk, L.; Feld, M.; Szwarc, M. Studies of "cage" reactions. *J. Am. Chem. Soc.* **1961**, *83*, 2998–3005. [CrossRef]
46. Shishido, S.M.; Oliveira, M.G. Polyethylene glycol matrix reduces the rates of photochemical and thermal release of nitric oxide from S-nitroso-N-acetylcysteine. *Photochem. Photobiol.* **2000**, *71*, 273–280. [CrossRef]
47. De Oliveira, M.G.; Shishido, S.M.; Seabra, A.B.; Morgon, N.H. Thermal stability of primary S-nitrosothiols: Roles of autocatalysis and structural effects on the rate of nitric oxide release. *J. Phys. Chem. A* **2002**, *106*, 8963–8970. [CrossRef]
48. Hetrick, E.M.; Shin, J.H.; Paul, H.S.; Schoenfisch, M.H. Anti-biofilm efficacy of nitric oxide-releasing silica nanoparticles. *Biomaterials* **2009**, *30*, 2782–2789. [CrossRef]
49. Raulli, R.; McElhaney-Feser, G.; Hrabie, J.; Cihlar, R. Antimicrobial properties of nitric oxide using diazeniumdiolates as the nitric oxide donor. *Rec. Res. Dev. Microbiol.* **2002**, *6*, 177–183.
50. CHEN, A.F. Nitric oxide: A newly discovered function on wound healing. *Acta Pharmacol. Sin.* **2005**, *26*, 259–264.
51. Heggers, J.P.; Robson, M.C.; Doran, E.T. Quantitative assessment of bacterial contamination of open wounds by a slide technique. *Trans. R. Soc. Trop. Med. Hyg.* **1969**, *63*, 532–534. [CrossRef]
52. Robson, M.C. Wound infection: A failure of wound healing caused by an imbalance of bacteria. *Surg. Clin. N. Am.* **1997**, *77*, 637–650. [CrossRef]

pharmaceutics

Article

Dermal Delivery of the High-Molecular-Weight Drug Tacrolimus by Means of Polyglycerol-Based Nanogels

Fiorenza Rancan [1,*], Hildburg Volkmann [1], Michael Giulbudagian [2], Fabian Schumacher [3,4], Jessica Isolde Stanko [1], Burkhard Kleuser [3], Ulrike Blume-Peytavi [1], Marcelo Calderón [2,5,6] and Annika Vogt [1]

1 Clinical Research Center for Hair and Skin Science, Department of Dermatology and Allergy, Charité—Universitätsmedizin Berlin, Corporate Member of Freie Universität Berlin, Humboldt-Universität zu Berlin, and Berlin Institute of Health, 10117 Berlin, Germany
2 Institut für Chemie und Biochemie, Freie Universität Berlin, 14195 Berlin, Germany
3 Institute of Nutritional Science, Department of Nutritional Toxicology, University of Potsdam, 14558 Nuthetal, Germany
4 Department of Molecular Biology, University of Duisburg-Essen, 45147 Essen, Germany
5 POLYMAT and Applied Chemistry Department, Faculty of Chemistry, University of the Basque Country UPV/EHU, Paseo Manuel de Lardizabal 3, 20018 Donostia-San Sebastián, Spain
6 IKERBASQUE, Basque Foundation for Science, 48013 Bilbao, Spain
* Correspondence: fiorenza.rancan@charite.de; Tel.: +49-30-450-518-347

Received: 30 June 2019; Accepted: 31 July 2019; Published: 5 August 2019

Abstract: Polyglycerol-based thermoresponsive nanogels (tNGs) have been shown to have excellent skin hydration properties and to be valuable delivery systems for sustained release of drugs into skin. In this study, we compared the skin penetration of tacrolimus formulated in tNGs with a commercial 0.1% tacrolimus ointment. The penetration of the drug was investigated in ex vivo abdominal and breast skin, while different methods for skin barrier disruption were investigated to improve skin permeability or simulate inflammatory conditions with compromised skin barrier. The amount of penetrated tacrolimus was measured in skin extracts by liquid chromatography tandem-mass spectrometry (LC-MS/MS), whereas the inflammatory markers IL-6 and IL-8 were detected by enzyme-linked immunosorbent assay (ELISA). Higher amounts of tacrolimus penetrated in breast as compared to abdominal skin or in barrier-disrupted as compared to intact skin, confirming that the stratum corneum is the main barrier for tacrolimus skin penetration. The anti-proliferative effect of the penetrated drug was measured in skin tissue/Jurkat cells co-cultures. Interestingly, tNGs exhibited similar anti-proliferative effects as the 0.1% tacrolimus ointment. We conclude that polyglycerol-based nanogels represent an interesting alternative to paraffin-based formulations for the treatment of inflammatory skin conditions.

Keywords: tacrolimus formulation; nanogels; skin penetration; drug delivery; human excised skin; Jurkat cells

1. Introduction

Tacrolimus, also known as FK 506, is an immunosuppressive drug acting predominantly via inhibition of T cell proliferation. This macrolide molecule builds a complex with the FK binding protein, which in turn binds to calcineurin and inhibits the dephosphorylation of the nuclear factor of activated T cells (NFATs) and its translocation to the nucleus [1–3]. As a consequence, the expression of IL-2, which is required for T cell proliferation, is inhibited. Tacrolimus also binds to isoforms of the FK binding protein, which have a cell type-specific expression pattern. This results in inhibitory or toxic effects towards other types of cells, e.g., mast and Langerhans cells [4–6]. In addition, induction of T cell apoptosis was found by Hashimoto and co-workers [7] and confirmed by Chung et al., who showed that tacrolimus induced apoptosis in Jurkat cells via activation of caspases 3 and 12 [8]. Furthermore, interference with the activation of the mitogen-activated protein kinase (MAPK) signaling pathways in primary human T lymphocytes was described by Matsuda et al. [9].

While the compound is widely used as topical agent to treat certain inflammatory skin diseases, its limited penetration across the skin barrier is a major limitation for a wider clinical use. Because of the poor solubility, the marketed formulation (Protopic®) consists of a paraffin-based ointment containing 0.03% or 0.1% tacrolimus in hard, liquid and white soft paraffin. In addition to insufficient drug penetration rates, mis-sensations such as skin stinging, burning and pruritus at the application site frequently lead to treatment discontinuation [10]. These side effects probably result from drug-induced chemical irritation and release of pro-inflammatory cytokines such as IL-6, as demonstrated for UVB-activated keratinocytes [11] and fibroblasts [12].

The hydrophobic paraffins in the ointment can reduce skin water loss and have therefore moisturizing properties. However, besides the fact that greasy excipients may be unpleasant for daily skin care, increasing concerns have been expressed because of symptom exacerbation in eczema sufferers. Furthermore, paraffin is a flammable excipient and consumers are often not aware of this fact [13]. Thus, several aspects indicate that new alternative formulations could result in significant improvements of current therapeutic strategies. Consequently, new formulations for the delivery of tacrolimus into the skin have been investigated in the last years, including lipid-based nanocarriers [14], liposomes [15], micelles [16–18], or transferosomes [19]. In all these works, the investigated nanocarrier formulation improved skin penetration of tacrolimus with respect to the marketed formulation.

Almost all studies used lipid-based carriers or delivery systems formulated with surfactants or permeabilizing components like ethanol that may cause side effects when applied on inflamed skin. In contrast, in this study, we investigated an alternative formulations based on thermoresponsive nanogels (tNGs) made of dendritic polyglycerol, which is cross-linked with thermoresponsive polymers, namely poly(glycidyl methyl ether-co-ethyl glycidyl ether) (tPG) and poly(*N*-isopropylacrylamide) (pNIPAM). During inflammatory skin diseases, skin temperature is slightly enhanced compared to unaffected skin. The concept of thermoresponsive nanogels implies sensing of such temperature differences with preferential release of drug in diseased skin. In fact, the progressive temperature increment after topical application has been shown to influence nanogel softness and the release of the drug [20]. More specifically, nanogels are soft when applied on skin surface and can penetrate deep in the stratum corneum (SC), where local temperature increase induces a change of conformation that results in the release of the incorporated active compound. The investigated nanogels were shown to enhance SC hydration [21–23] and exhibited promising drug delivery properties [24] along with low cytotoxicity [25,26].

In most previous studies, tacrolimus penetration was investigated using animal skin [18,27], which is anatomically and immunologically different from human skin, with little consideration of skin barrier impairment or skin inflammatory status. In this study, we used excised human skin from two distinct anatomical regions, breast as well as abdomen, and different methods to induce barrier disruption and inflammatory reactions. In this way, we could monitor the effects of barrier-disruption on tacrolimus skin penetration and release of inflammatory markers like IL-6 and IL-8. The additional use of a trans-well set up to co-culture ex vivo human skin and Jurkat cells enabled the assessment of tacrolimus anti-proliferative effects.

2. Materials and Methods

2.1. Nanogel Preparation and Characterization

Commercially available chemicals from standardized sources were used as delivered. Solvents were purchased as reagent grade and distilled if necessary. Anhydrous solvents were either purchased as ultra-dry solvent (Acros Organics®, Geel, Belgium) or received from solvent purification system.

For the tPG polymerization reactions, dry toluene was obtained from MBRAUN SPS 800 solvent purification system (Garching, Germany). Water was purified by Millipore water purification system. Dendritic polyglycerol with average molecular weight of 10 kDa (PDI = 1.27) was purchased from Nanopartica GmbH (Berlin, Germany). Glycidyl methyl ether (85%) and ethyl glycidyl ether (98%; both TCI Europe, Eschborn, Germany) were dried over CaH_2, distilled, and stored over molecular sieves (5 Å). The crosslinking reagent (1R,8S,9s)-bicyclo[6.1.0]non-4-yn-9-ylmethyl (4-nitrophenyl) carbonate was purchased from Synaffix (Oss, the Netherlands). The cyanine dye indodicarbocyanine (IDCC) was purchased from Lumiprobe GmbH (Hannover, Germany).

The tNGs were synthesized according to previously reported methods. For detailed synthesis and characterization description, refer to the following publications [22,26,28]. Briefly, for the synthesis of poly(*N*-isopropylacrylamide) (pNIPAM)-based nanogels (NG-pNIPAM), NIPAM (66 mg), acrylated dendritic polyglycerol (dPG-$Ac_{10\%}$) (33 mg), sodium dodecyl sulfate (SDS) (1.8 mg), and ammonium persulfate (APS) (2.8 mg) were dissolved in 5 mL of distilled water. Argon was bubbled into the reaction mixture for 15 min, which was followed by stirring under argon atmosphere for another 15 min. The reaction mixture was transferred into a hot bath at 68 °C and polymerization was activated after 5 min with the addition of a catalytic amount of *N,N,N′,N′*-tetramethylethane-1,2-diamine (TEMED; 120 µL). The mixture was stirred at 500 rpm for at least 4 h, prior to purification by dialysis. For the synthesis of fluorescently labeled nanogels, a mixture of unlabeled dPG-$Ac_{10\%}$ (30 mg) and indodicarbocyanine (IDCC)-labelled dPG-$Ac_{10\%}$ (3 mg) was used.

For the synthesis of tPG-based nanogels (NG-tPG), dPG functionalized with (1R,8S,9s)-bicyclo[6.1.0]non-4-yn-9-ylmethyl carbonate (dPG-$BCN_{8\%}$) (10 mg) and di-azide functionalized tPG (tPG-$(N_3)_2$) (20 mg) were mixed in 1 mL of dimethylformamide (DMF), cooled in an ice bath and injected with a syringe into 20 mL of water at 45 °C. The mixture was stirred for 3 h and the unreacted alkynes were quenched with azidopropanol or alternatively with IDCC-N_3.

For loading tacrolimus, highly concentrated tNGs (10 mg) were added to a suspension of tacrolimus (5 mg) in 2 mL of MilliQ water. The nanogels were let to swell, followed by sonication in an ice water bath for 30 min. The suspension was stirred overnight at 25 °C and the encapsulated fraction was separated from the free drug by filtration with a 0.45 µm regenerated cellulose syringe filter. Following, 100 µL of the encapsulated fraction were lyophilized for determination of the total concentration, while the encapsulation capacity was determined by LC-MS/MS measurements. The nanogels with the encapsulated drugs were stored at 4 °C. The characterization of the investigated nanogels is reported in Table 1.

Table 1. Properties and drug loading of the investigated nanogels.

Nanogel	Size (PDI) [a]	Cloud Point Temperature [b]	Tacrolimus Loading [c]	ζ Potential [mV] [d]
NG-pNIPAM	110.5 nm (0.194)	34.6 °C	0.9 wt.%	−1.07
NG-tPG	132.9 nm (0.073)	28.9 °C	2.5 wt.%	0.332

[a] Size and polydispersity index (PDI) by dynamic light scattering (DLS) in water at 25 °C. Measurements were performed in triplicates; intensity average mean value presented; [b] Cloud point temperature determined as the temperature at 50% transmittance by UV-Vis (λ = 500 nm); [c] Refer to Gerecke, et al., *Nanotoxicology* **2017**, *11*, 267–277 [26] for detailed information; [d] ζ potential determined by Zeta-sizer in phosphate buffer. Measurements were performed in triplicates; intensity average mean value presented. NG-pNIPAM: poly(*N*-isopropylacrylamide-based nanogels; NG-tPG: poly(glycidyl methyl ether-co-ethyl glycidyl ether)-based nanogels.

2.2. *Skin Samples*

Breast and abdominal skin were obtained after informed consent from healthy donors undergoing plastic surgery. The study was conducted after approval by the Ethics Committee of the Charité–Universitätsmedizin Berlin (approval EA1/135/06, renewed on January 2018) and in accordance with the Declaration of Helsinki guidelines. The excised skin was used between 3 and 6 h after surgery and was examined to exclude injured parts, including macroscopic skin surface damages but also deeper structural defects like stretch marks. Subcutaneous fat tissue was partially removed (approximately 0.5 cm was kept) and skin was stretched and fixed on a Styrofoam block using needles. Skin areas of 2 cm^2 were marked. In order to induce skin barrier disruption, three methods were used: tape stripping 50 times (50 × TS), laser poration (LP), and sodium lauryl sulfate (SLS). TS was performed with adhesive, polyethylene tape (19-mm diameter, TESA film no. 5529, Beiersdorf, Hamburg, Germany). For LP, a P.L.E.A.S.E® Professional system (Pantec Biosolutions, Ruggell, Lichtenstein) was used with the following setting: delivered energy 73.1 J/cm^2, pulse length 125 µs, repetition rate 300 Hz, 10 pulses per pore, treated surface 10 × 10 mm, pore density 8%. For SLS treatment, 20 µL/cm^2 of 5 % SLS (*w*/*v*) in deionized distilled water were applied on a filter paper disc (12 mm^2 diameter for Finn Chambers®, SmartPractice, Hillerød, Denmark) and incubated for 4 h at 37 °C. Thereafter, skin was carefully cleaned with a paper towel.

A total amount of 5 µg tacrolimus per square centimeter was applied either incorporated in an aqueous suspension of nanogels or as 0.1% marketed formulation (Protopic®, manufactured by LEO Laboratories Ltd., Dublin, Ireland). Safety margins of at least 0.5 cm were left. Controls consisted of skin treated with 20 µL/cm^2 of sterile 0.9% NaCl solution. Samples and controls were placed in humid chambers (plastic boxes with lid filled with humidified towels) and incubated for 24 h at 37 °C, 5% CO_2 and 100% humidity. After incubation, non-penetrated material was removed with a paper towel, the untreated safety margins were cut and the treated tissue blocks were plunge frozen in liquid nitrogen and stored at −80°C for further processing.

2.3. Preparation of Skin Extracts

In order to separate epidermis from dermis and prepare extracts for tacrolimus and cytokine analyses, skin samples were cut horizontally (thickness 50 µm) with a microtome (Frigocut 2800 N, Leica, Bensheim, Germany): the first 100 µm corresponding roughly to epidermis and the remaining 900 µm to dermis. The sections were put in 500 µL of extraction buffer (100 mM Tris-HCl; 150 mM NaCl; 1 mM EDTA; 1 g Triton-X-100; 10% EtOH), homogenized (GLH OMNI homogenizer, Kennesaw, GA, USA) for 10 s, and incubated on ice for 45 min. Then, samples were sonicated at 4 °C for 10 min, vortexed and centrifuged for 5 min at 450× *g*. The pellets were then added of 500 µL of extraction buffer and the above described procedure was repeated once more. The supernatants were pooled and stored at −80°C.

2.4. Determination of Tacrolimus in Skin Extracts by Isotope-Dilution Liquid Chromatography Tandem-Mass Spectrometry (LC-MS/MS)

Skin extracts were thawed at room temperature, spiked with stable-isotope labeled internal standard [$^{13}C_1$,D_4]tacrolimus (Alsachim, Illkirch-Graffenstaden, France), vortexed, and centrifuged at 9300× *g* for 3 min (4 °C). Analyses were conducted with an Agilent 1260 Infinity LC system coupled to an Agilent 6490 triple quadrupole-mass spectrometer (both from Waldbronn, Germany) interfaced with an electrospray ion source operating in the positive ion mode (ESI+). Chromatographic separation was carried out using an Agilent Zorbax SB-C18 column (1.8 µm, 2.1 × 50 mm). Aqueous ammonium formate (20 mM, pH 3.5) and methanol (VWR, Darmstadt, Germany) were used as eluents A and B, respectively. Samples (5 µL) were injected into a mobile phase consisting of 90% eluent A. Tacrolimus and its internal standard [$^{13}C_1$,D_4]tacrolimus were eluted from the column, which was tempered at 30 °C, with a 4-min linear gradient to and a subsequent isocratic stage for 5 min at 2:98 (*v*:*v*) eluent A/B at a flow rate of 0.35 mL/min. Tacrolimus and [$^{13}C_1$,D_4]tacrolimus co-eluted from the separation column at 5.3 min. The total run time for one analysis was 13 min, including re-equilibration of the LC system. The following ion source parameters were taken from Koster et al. [29], who used a comparable mass spectrometric configuration for detection of four immunosuppressants including tacrolimus: drying gas temperature = 200 °C, drying gas flow = 13 L/min of nitrogen, sheath gas temperature = 200 °C, sheath gas flow = 12 L/min of nitrogen, nebulizer pressure = 18 psi, capillary voltage = 4500 V, and nozzle voltage = 0 V. The ion funnel parameters were: high pressure RF voltage = 150 V and low pressure RF voltage = 60 V. Quantification of tacrolimus in relation to the internal standard [$^{13}C_1$,D_4]tacrolimus was carried out using the multiple reaction monitoring (MRM) approach.

Ammonium adducts $[M+NH_4]^+$ were selected as precursor ions by the first quadrupole. The following mass transitions were recorded (optimized collision energies in parentheses): tacrolimus: *m/z* 821.5 → 786.5 (16 eV), *m/z* 821.5 → 768.5 (20 eV), *m/z* 821.5 → 576.2 (24 eV); $[^{13}C_1,D_4]$tacrolimus: *m/z* 826.5 → 791.5 (16 eV), *m/z* 826.5 → 773.6 (20 eV), *m/z* 826.5 → 581.4 (24 eV). Thereby, the loss of two hydroxyl groups and ammonium from the precursor ion, represented by *m/z* 821.5 → 768.5 for tacrolimus and *m/z* 826.5 → 773.6 for $[^{13}C_1,D_4]$tacrolimus, was used for quantification. The dwell time for each of the six mass transitions recorded was 150 ms.

2.5. Enzyme-linked Immunosorbent Assay (ELISA)

Human IL-6 and IL-8 were investigated using ELISA kits (Human IL-6 and IL-8 CytoSetTM (CHC1263, CHC1303) Invitrogen Corporation, Carlsbad, CA, USA) following the manufacturer instructions. The amounts of cytokines were normalized to total protein content measured with Pierce 660 nm Protein Assay (Thermo Fisher Scientific Inc., Rockford, IL, USA). Absorbance was measured with EnSpire® Multimode plate reader (Perkin Elmer, Akron, OH, USA).

2.6. Preparation of Cryosections and Fluorescence Microscopy

Skin samples treated with fluorescent nanogels were placed in tissue freezing medium (Leica Microsystems, Wetzlar, Germany) and plunge-frozen in liquid nitrogen. Cryosections of 5 µm thickness were prepared and observed by means of a fluorescence microscope (Olympus BX60F3, Olympus, Hamburg, Germany). The following filter combinations were used: bright pass = 545–580 nm, long pass > 610 nm for IDCC (red) and bright pass = 470–490 nm, long pass > 550 nm for FL. Pictures (magnification of 200×) of at least 20 randomly chosen skin sections per donor and skin sample were taken, and the mean fluorescence intensity of areas in the SC, viable epidermis, and dermis was calculated using the ImageJ software (Version 1.47).

2.7. Isolation of Cells, Flow Cytometry, and Confocal Fluorescence Microscopy

After incubation with nanogels, skin samples were cut in small pieces (0.2 × 0.2 cm) and incubated overnight at 4 °C in 2.4 U/mL dispase (Roche Applied Science, Penzberg, Germany) in order to detach epidermis from dermis. The epidermis sheets were incubated for 10 min at 37 °C in 5 mL of trypsin solution (0.025% trypsin and 1.5 mM $CaCl_2$ in PBS). Dermis tissue was digested by incubation for 2 h at 37 °C with an enzyme cocktail made of 0.6 g/mL collagenase II (Biochrom, Berlin, Germany), 0.3 g/mL hyaluronidase (Sigma-Aldrich, Hamburg, Germany), and 1 µg/mL DNase (Roche Diagnostics, Berlin, Germany). Enzymes were stopped with RPMI-1640 cell culture medium (PAA, Heidelberg, Germany) containing 10% fetal calf serum (PAA, Heidelberg, Germany) and cells were harvested by repeated pipetting, filtering through a 70 µm cell strainer (FalconTM, Becton Dickinson, Heidelberg, Germany) and washing twice with PBS (PAA, Heidelberg, Germany). After centrifugation at 300× *g* for 10 min, cells were fixed with 4% paraformaldehyde (Sigma-Aldrich, Taufkirchen, Germany) and stored at 4 °C until analysis by flow cytometry (FACS Calibur, BD, Heidelberg, Germany). At least 20,000 events were collected in the selected gate. The software FCS Express (De Novo Software, Version 3.1, Glendale, CA, USA) was used for data analysis. Pictures of isolated cells were taken by means of a confocal laser microscope (LSM Exciter, Zeiss, Jena, Germany).

2.8. Isolation and Culture of T cells

T cells were isolated from dermis after digestion as described above. Dermis cell suspension was cultured overnight in RPMI 1640 medium (Gibco, Darmstadt, Germany) supplemented with 10% fetal calf serum, 100 µg/mL streptomycin, and 100 I.E./mL penicillin. Non-adherent cells were collected and red blood cells were lysed with 1% Triton X-100 in PBS for 10 min on ice. Cells were then washed with PBS and incubated with carboxyfluorescein succinimide ester (CFSE, CellTraceTM, Life Technologies, Darmstadt, Germany) for 20 min at room temperature. Cells were washed with 1% bovine serum albumin and re-suspended in supplemented RPMI 1640 medium. Cells were left untreated, incubated with IL-2 (2.5 μg/mL) only, or incubated with IL-2 and tacrolimus in 10% ethanol or tacrolimus-loaded NG-tPG nanogels (final tacrolimus concentration of 5 μg/mL). Cell proliferation was measured after 5 days by flow cytometry. T cells were gated in forward vs. side scatter dot plots and at least 10,000 events were collected.

2.9. *Co-culture of Full-Thickness Human Skin and Jurkat Cells*

After topical application of tacrolimus formulations, skin samples were transferred on 8 μm-pore inserts (Cell Culture Inserts, BD Falcon™, Corning, New York, NY, USA). These were placed in a 6-well plate with 2 mL supplemented RPMI 1640 medium and 10^6 Jurkat cells (clone E6.1) per well. Jurkat cells had previously been stained with CFSE as described above. Skin was maintained at the air-liquid interface and co-cultured with Jurkat cells for 2 or 5 days (37 °C, 5% CO_2). 500 μL of fresh medium were replaced every 2 days. Jurkat cells were collected and analyzed by flow cytometry.

3. Results and Discussion

3.1. *Tacrolimus Penetration and Inflammatory Reaction in Ex Vivo Human Skin with Intact or Disrupted Barrier*

In order to compare the new nanogel-based tacrolimus formulations to the commercially available 0.1% tacrolimus ointment, we measured the amounts of penetrated drug and released inflammatory markers (IL-6 and IL-8) in ex vivo human skin. Different methods (TS, LP, and SLS) were applied to simulate a barrier dysfunction and improve drug penetration. Laser poration (at the used energy) induces a local removal of stratum corneum (micropores), whereas tape stripping reduces the thickness of the stratum corneum. Both methods result in a partial removal of both lipids and corneocytes [30,31]. On the other hand, the surfactant SLS acts predominantly on the lipid layers disrupting their structure [32]. Skin from eight donors and two different areas was used: abdomen (see Appendix A, Figure A1(D1–D3)) and breast (Figure 1(D4–D6), and Figure 2(D7,D8). After incubation, skin samples were processed as described in Material and Methods and the amounts of drug as well as cytokines were quantified by means of LC-MS/MS and ELISA, respectively. In general, the ointment formulation resulted in higher concentrations of penetrated tacrolimus. This better performance might be due to the permeabilizing effects of some of the excipients in the ointment formulation. However, it has to be considered that the detection of tacrolimus in epidermis extracts does not provide any spatially resolved information, i.e., the distribution of the drug between the SC and the viable epidermis remains unknown.

Low penetration of tacrolimus was measured in intact abdominal skin. Pretreatment with TS had no significant effects on drug penetration, independently on the tested formulation (Figure A1). Little effect was measured also with regard of the inflammatory markers IL-6 and IL-8. On the contrary, higher tacrolimus concentrations were detected in intact breast skin as compared to intact abdominal skin (Figure 1). In addition, slightly increased drug penetration and cytokine production were found after barrier disruption by LP.

These results suggest that breast skin is more permeable than abdominal skin, probably due to a thinner SC and a higher density of hair follicles, which have been shown to contribute to the skin permeation of topically applied substances [33–35]. The fact that skin from breast areas expressed also much more IL-6 and IL-8 than skin from abdominal region might be due to a higher number of immune active cells.

With regard to tacrolimus penetration in breast skin, TS pretreatment resulted in a marked increase of tacrolimus penetration for both ointment and nanogel formulations (Figure 2(D7,D8)), while application of 5% SLS, a standard procedure for chemical barrier disruption, had no effects. The results obtained after different time points (Figure 2(D8)) show that the penetration of tacrolimus in barrier disrupted skin treated with the ointment increased exponentially with time. On the contrary, the amount of drug penetrated in nanogel-treated samples after 100 min of incubation were similar to that measured after 24 h of incubation (Figure 2(D7)), suggesting a slower but constant delivery of drug by the nanogel formulations. Thus, the lower amounts of penetrated drug observed for the nanogel formulations after 24 h of incubation may also be a result of the slower drug delivery rate of the nanogel formulations.

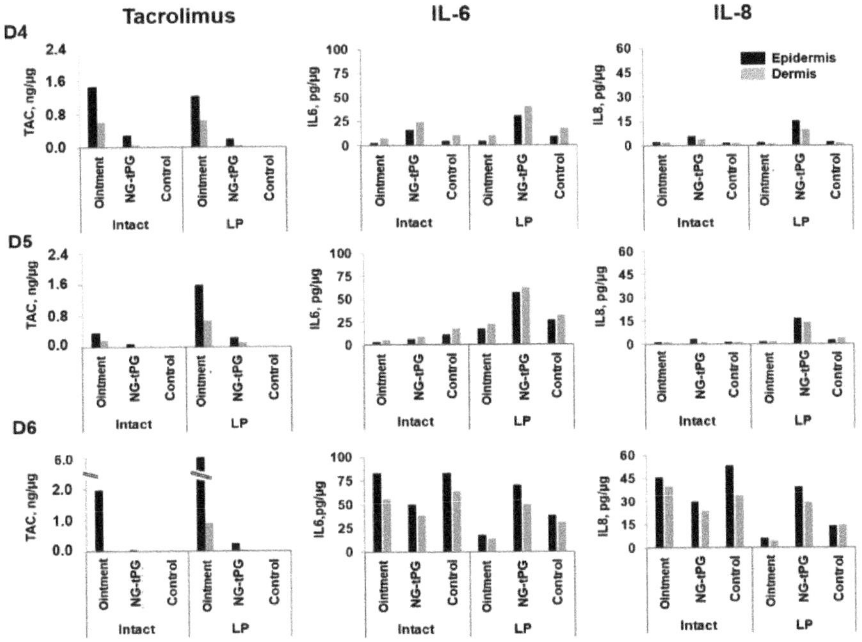

Figure 1. Tacrolimus skin penetration and expression of the inflammatory cytokines IL-6 and IL-8 after topical application of tacrolimus ointment or nanogel formulation (tacrolimus final dosage 5 µg/cm^2) on breast skin from three different donors (D4–6). Skin barrier was left intact or treated with LP prior to the application of the test formulations. Control skin was treated with 0.9% NaCl solution. TAC: tacrolimus; LP: laser poration; NG-tPG: nanogels based on thermoresponsive polyglycerol.

When considering cytokine release, a clear increase of both inflammatory markers was observed in control skin after LP or TS especially in the experiments performed on breast skin (Figures 1 and 2). An additional increase of IL-8 and IL-6 was registered in tacrolimus-treated barrier disrupted skin. This reaction might be attributed to activating or irritating effects of the nanogels themselves or of tacrolimus. While in previous experiments no toxicity was detected for the investigated nanogels [25,26], it is known that tacrolimus may have irritating effects [12]. Our findings point towards the fact that enhanced penetration, while beneficial for therapeutic effects, may pose new challenges with regard to tolerability, especially when the applied substances are capable of reaching cells of the viable epidermis that might be in an activated state as observed in inflammatory skin [36,37].

Overall, these results indicate that breast skin is more permeable to tacrolimus than abdominal skin, regardless of whether skin barrier was disrupted or not. After 24 h of incubation, higher amounts of tacrolimus were measured in ointment-treated samples. Nevertheless, biological effects, like the release of IL-6 and IL-8, were detected also in response to tacrolimus-loaded nanogel formulations.

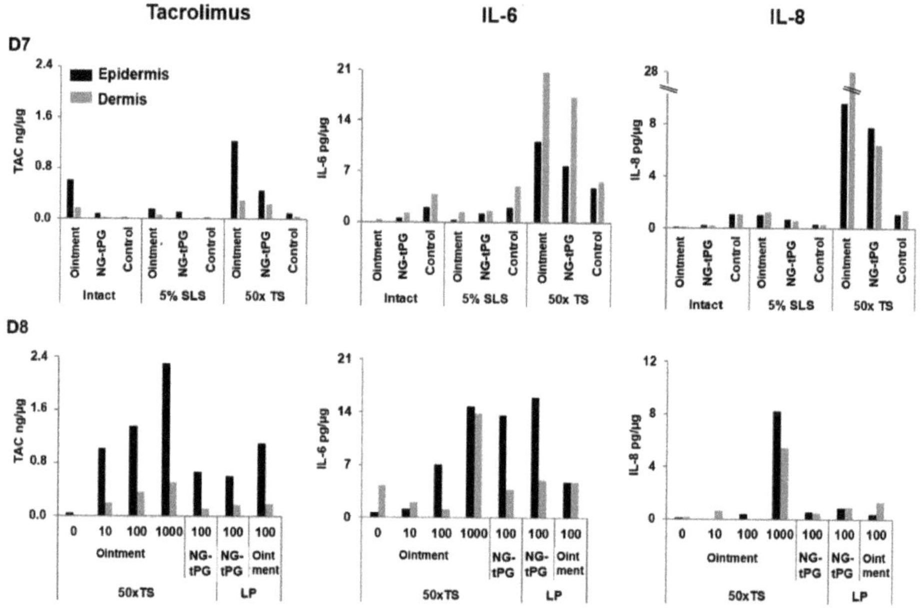

Figure 2. Effects of tape stripping (TS) on tacrolimus penetration and release of IL-6 and IL-8 in breast skin. The amounts of tacrolimus, IL-6, and IL-8 were measured in the epidermis and dermis of breast skin pre-treated to disrupt the skin barrier and incubated with the investigated tacrolimus formulations. (D7) Breast skin was treated with 50 × TS or with 5% SLS previous topical application of 0.1% tacrolimus ointment and tacrolimus-loaded NG-tPG (tacrolimus end concentration 5 µg/cm^2) after 24 h. (D8) Tacrolimus penetration and cytokine release in breast skin pre-treated with 50 × TS after 10, 100, and 1000 min of incubation with tacrolimus ointment and comparison with skin pre-treated with 50 × TS or LP and incubation for 100 min with NG-tPG or ointment formulations. Control skin was treated with 0.9% NaCl solution. 50 × TS: tape stripping 50 times; TAC: tacrolimus; LP: laser poration; 5% SLS: 5% sodium lauryl sulfate; NG-tPG: nanogels based on thermoresponsive polyglycerol.

3.2. Nanogel Skin Penetration and Cellular Uptake after Different Degrees of Barrier Disruption by TS

The SC is a key barrier which hinders the penetration of topically applied compounds. Especially size is one of the major determinants of penetration. With regard to nanoparticulate drug delivery systems, deformability and elasticity further contribute to their penetration properties. Large amounts of carrier material typically remain on the skin surface or in superficial SC compartments. However, the question as to how deep single nanogel particles are capable to penetrate is important with regard to the likelihood of exposure of viable cells to nanogels. Thus, possible translocation of small amounts of nanogel particles to the viable skin layers after skin barrier disruption by TS was investigated using IDCC-tagged nanogels loaded with fluorescein (FL) (Figure 3).

The degree of skin barrier disruption was assessed by measuring the SC thickness in images of skin sections from different regions of the sample. In Figure 3a,d, representative images and the average of at least 15 measurements from three different donors (D9–11) are shown. After 50 TS, a mild skin barrier disruption was achieved for one donor (Figure 3a(D9)), whereas a more severe skin barrier disruption with a stronger reduction of SC thickness was obtained in skin from two other donors (Figure 3d, D10 and D11). Such a different extent of barrier disruption reflects the individual variability of SC thickness and strength. The spatially resolved skin penetration of nanogels (IDCC, red fluorescence) and delivered model dye (fluorescein, FL, green fluorescence) served to clarify the drug delivery mechanism of nanogels. In the representative fluorescence images (Figure 3b,e), it is to recognize that the two fluorophores co-localized in the SC, which resulted in yellow fluorescence, whereas the released FL penetrated deeper in the viable epidermis, especially in the skin with severe barrier disruption. To quantify the extent of FL penetration, the mean fluorescence intensity (MFI) in the green channel was calculated for different skin areas of at least 20 skin sections per sample. For D9 (Figure 3b), a higher fluorescence signal was detected in the SC for the tNG sample as compared to free FL, confirming the ability of NG-tPG to create a depot in the outermost layer of the epidermis [22]. In skin from donors 10 and 11, where TS procedure had induced a severe skin barrier disruption, a better skin penetration of the released dye was observed not only in the SC but also in the viable epidermis and dermis (Figure 3e). The analysis of NG-tPG penetration (IDCC signal) by fluorescence microscopy showed penetration only in the SC for donor 9 and also in the viable epidermis for donors 10 and 11 (Figure 3c,f). To detect possible cellular association with penetrated nanogels, part of the treated skin was processed to isolate cells and analyze them by flow cytometry and confocal fluorescence microscopy. While after mild skin disruption (D9) only a small percent of cells had high fluorescent signal, over 50% of epidermis cells and 10% of dermis cells were associated with nanogels after severe barrier perturbation (D10 and D11). Especially in the two donors with severe skin barrier disruption, NG-tPG were found to be associated also with Langerhans cells.

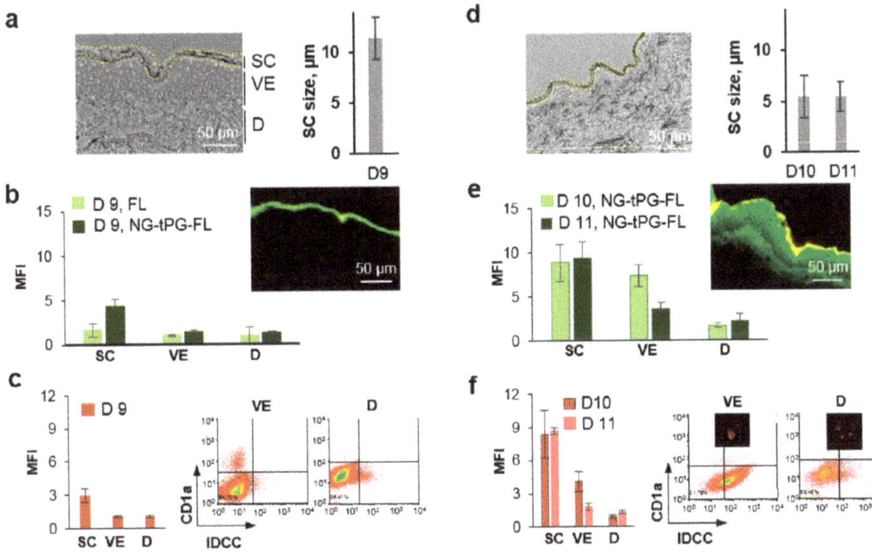

Figure 3. Skin penetration of topically applied nanogels and released dye depends on the degree of barrier disruption. Mild (**a**–**c**) and severe (**d**–**f**) skin barrier disruption was induced in breast skin by TS previous application of free fluorescein (green) or NG-tPG tagged with IDCC (red) and loaded with FL. After 16 h of incubation, skin was processed to prepare cryosections and isolate cells. (**a**,**d**) Representative transmission light microscopy images of skin sections showing the different degrees of barrier disruption and diagrams showing the average SC thickness; (**b**,**e**) analysis of FL penetration in SC, viable epidermis and dermis of skin sections by measurement of mean fluorescence intensity; (**c**,**f**) analysis of IDCC fluorescence on skin sections (diagrams) and in cells (flow cytometry, dot plots, and images of single cells) isolated from NG-tPG-treated skin and stained with anti-CD1a antibody (Langerhans cells). FL: fluorescein; SC: stratum corneum; VE: viable epidermis; D: dermis; MFI: mean fluorescence intensity; NG-tPG: nanogels based on thermoresponsive polyglycerol; IDCC: indodicarbocyanine.

These results clearly show that, when skin barrier is compromised, nanogels can penetrate to viable skin layers, be taken-up by epidermal and dermal cells and that uptake in dendritic cells is favored in pro-inflammatory environment. This observation may be of special advantage for the treatment of inflammatory skin diseases where, besides T cells, dendritic cells are key targets of therapeutics like tacrolimus. [5,6].

3.3. Effects of Tacrolimus Nanogels and Ointment on T Cells and Skin/Jurkat Cell Co-Cultures.

As outlined in the previous sections, assessment of a potential benefit of enhanced tacrolimus penetration on the cellular level is limited by its irritative effects on keratinocytes and fibroblasts. Given that immune cells are main therapeutic targets, we created an experimental set-up of skin tissue/T cell co-cultures to measure the effects of penetrated tacrolimus on T cell proliferation [3,10]. First, tacrolimus anti-proliferative effects was measured in vitro on T cells isolated from human excised skin and stimulated with recombinant human IL-2 (Figure 4a–c).

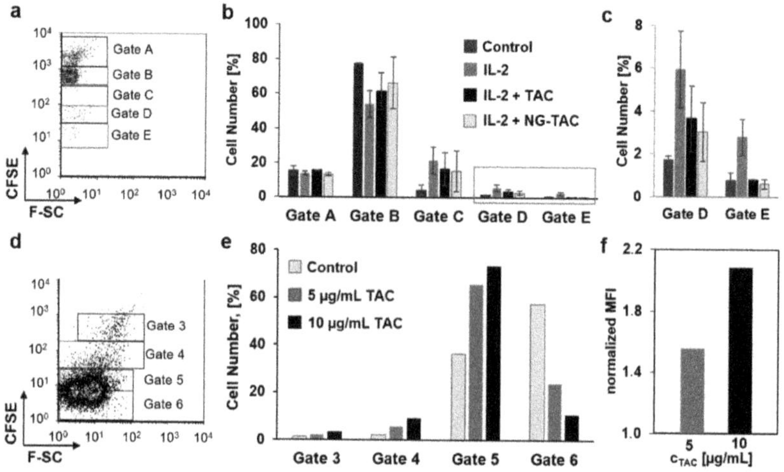

Figure 4. Effects of tacrolimus in solution or formulated in nanogels on Jurkat and T-cell proliferation in vitro. (**a–c**) Preliminary experiments on isolated dermal T-cells stimulated with IL-2 showed the inhibitory effects of tacrolimus (5 µg/mL) both in solution and in nanogels. Different cell populations were detected by flow cytometry (**a**) and the percentage of cells in each gate at day 5 of culture are plotted (**b**). Values in gates D and E are reported in (**c**) using a different axis scale. (**d–f**) Effects of tacrolimus were also detected in Jurkat cells after incubation with 5 and 10 µg/mL tacrolimus solution for 4 days. Cells were gated according to fluorescence intensity (**d**). The percentages of cells in each gate (e) as well as the normalized mean fluorescence intensity of all cells (**f**) showed a decrease of proliferation after treatment with tacrolimus. MFI: mean fluorescence intensity.

Approximately 20% of cells were stimulated to proliferate after addition of IL-2. Both tacrolimus in solution and loaded on NG-tPG reproducibly reduced the percentage of proliferating cells (Figure 4b,c). Tacrolimus was also reported to exert anti-proliferative effects on T cells and Jurkat cells via induction of apoptosis [7,8]. Accordingly, when Jurkat cells were incubated with tacrolimus, a concentration dependent anti-proliferative effect could be measured (Figure 4d–f). These results show the ability of nanogels to deliver tacrolimus to T cells in vitro and induce anti-proliferative effects in a degree similar to that of the free drug. In addition, it was shown that the pro-apoptotic effects of tacrolimus on Jurkat cells were measurable by CFSE assay (Figure 4e,f).

As next step, we cultured ex vivo skin at the air/liquid interface with Jurkat cells using a trans-well set-up (Figure 5a).

We hypothesized that, when tacrolimus is applied topically on skin, the penetrated drug would reach the medium compartment and affect the proliferation of Jurkat cells. In fact, all treated samples had higher MFI than the controls, as shown in the representative histogram in Figure 5b, confirming the anti-proliferative effects of the penetrated drug. A concentration-dependent effect was visible when Jurkat cells were co-cultured for 4 days with skin topically treated with 10 and 20 mg/cm^2 of 0.1% tacrolimus ointment, corresponding to 10 and 20 µg/cm^2 of tacrolimus, respectively (Figure 5c). When the ointment was compared to the NG-tPG tacrolimus formulation using a final tacrolimus concentration of 5 µg/cm^2 (Figure 5d,e), a clear reduction of proliferation was visible at day 5 (Figure 5e). Interestingly, at day 5, ointment and nanogels had similar effects for donors D14 and D15, while for donor D13 nanogels had even a higher anti-proliferative activity than the ointment. Thus, even if in the 24 h penetration experiments, low tacrolimus amounts were measured in the skin treated with nanogels, after longer incubation time in the skin/cell co-culture set up, nanogel formulations could exert anti-proliferative effects comparable to that of tacrolimus ointment.

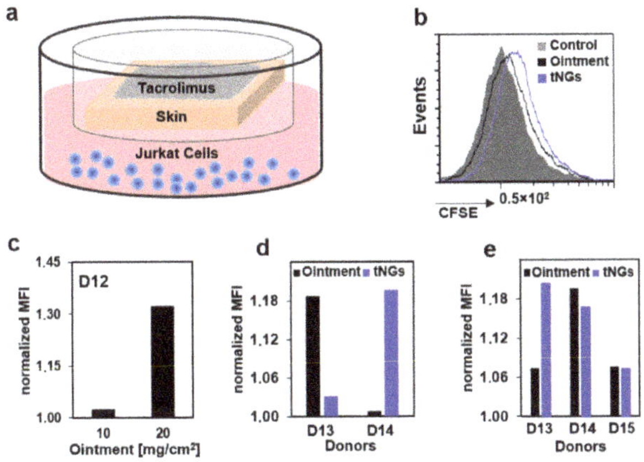

Figure 5. Penetration of tacrolimus across full thickness skin and inhibition of Jurkat cell proliferation. (**a**) Typical experimental procedure. Tacrolimus ointment or nanogels were applied topically on ex vivo skin with disrupted barrier (tape stripping 50 times) that was co-cultured with CFSE-labelled Jurkat cells in a trans-well set up. (**b**) Flow cytometry histogram of cells after treatment with tacrolimus ointment. (**c**) Normalized mean fluorescence intensity of cells cocultured with skin treated with 10 and 20 mg/cm^2 of ointment. (**d**,**e**) Normalized mean fluorescence intensity of Jurkat cells co-cultured for 2 (**d**) or 5 days (**e**) with skin treated with 5 µg/cm^2 of tacrolimus formulated as ointment or nanogel. Both ointment and tacrolimus-loaded NG showed inhibitory effects on Jurkat cell proliferation after topical application on co-cultured ex vivo skin. TAC: tacrolimus; CFSE: carboxyfluorescein succinimide ester; MFI: mean fluorescence intensity; tNGs: thermoresponsive nanogels.

4. Conclusions

This In this work, we show that tacrolimus formulated as ointment or nanogel suspension penetrates skin with different efficiency in dependence on SC thickness and integrity. Irritation effects of tacrolimus ointment and nanogel formulations, reflected by the released inflammatory cytokines IL-6 and IL-8, were more pronounced in barrier-disrupted and immuno-activated skin. Extensive barrier disruption by mechanical removal of SC resulted also in enhanced penetration of topically applied materials, including deformable macromolecules like nanogels, with consequent interaction and uptake by skin immune active cells. These results support the key role of the SC as barrier for drug and nanocarrier penetration. Our results further demonstrate the critical balance of penetration enhancement and potential increase of side effects. Slow release systems as observed herein already addresses this aspect. The slow drug release and delivery combined with SC hydration and special interaction with skin cells in inflamed skin may explain the good performance of nanogels with respect to tacrolimus ointment. Thus, we conclude that tNGs represent an attractive alternative water-based formulation for the topical delivery of high molecular weight, poorly water-soluble drugs like tacrolimus.

Author Contributions: Conceptualization, F.R., M.C., and A.V.; methodology, F.R., H.V.; formal analysis, F.R., M.G., and H.V.; investigation, H.V., M.G., F.S., and J.I.S.; resources, B.K., M.C., U.B.-P., and A.V.; writing—original draft preparation, F.R.; writing—review and editing M.G., F.S., M.C., and A.V.; visualization, F.R.; project administration, A.V., M.C., and B.K., funding acquisition, B.K., U.B.-P., M.C., and A.V.

Funding: This research was funded by the German Research Foundation (DFG), grant SFB1112, projects C04, A04, and Z0. We also acknowledge support from the German Research Foundation (DFG) and the Open Access Publication Fund of Charité—Universitätsmedizin Berlin for publication costs.

Conflicts of Interest: The authors declare no conflict of interest.

Appendix A

Tacrolimus penetration and inflammatory reaction in abdominal skin with or without barrier disruption. Tape stripping had no significant effects on drug penetration in abdominal skin. Only in skin from one donor and only for the ointment a high amount of tacrolimus, approximately 6 ng per μg of total extracted proteins, was detected after tape stripping (Figure A1, Donor 3). Little effect was measured also with regard of the inflammatory markers IL-6 and IL-8, with values around 0.2 pg per μg of total proteins and maximal of 4 pg/μg for NG-tPG in donor 3. While a moderate increase of IL-6 could be observed in tape-stripped skin controls, almost no IL-8 increase was measured in controls after barrier disruption, indicating that IL-6 might be a more sensitive marker for measuring the effect of mechanical damage to the SC. A moderate increase of IL-6 with respect to controls was observed only in the samples treated with the nanogel formulations, whereas a slight decrease of IL-6 with respect to control was measured in skin treated with 0.1% tacrolimus ointment.

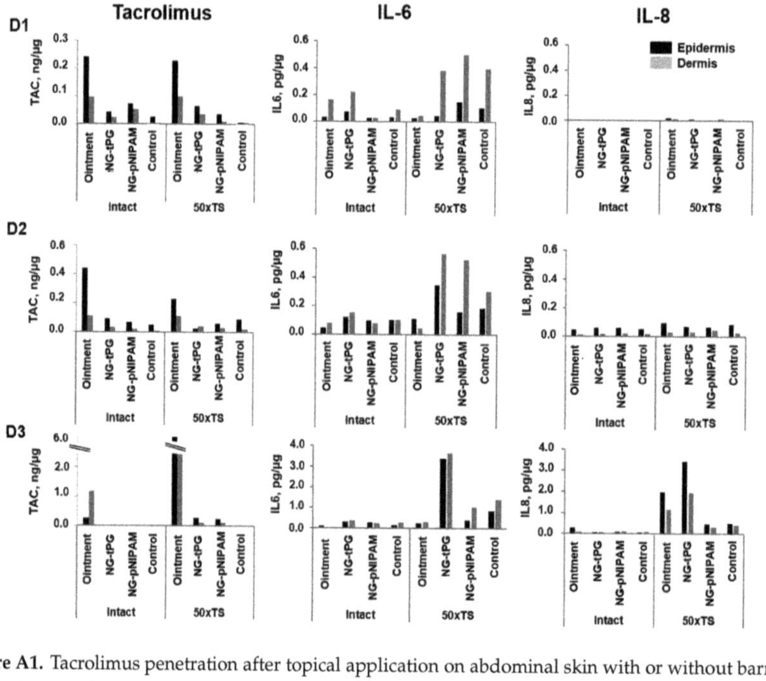

Figure A1. Tacrolimus penetration after topical application on abdominal skin with or without barrier disruption. Abdominal skin from three different donors (D1-3) was left intact or treated with tape stripping times (50 × TS). NG-pNIPAM (0.9 wt.% tacrolimus), NG-tPG (2.5 wt.% tacrolimus), and 0.1% tacrolimus ointment were applied for 24 h at a final tacrolimus concentration of 5 μg/cm^2. Tacrolimus as well as the inflammatory markers IL-6 and IL-8 were detected in skin extracts. TAC: tacrolimus.

References

1. Liu, J.; Farmer, J.D., Jr.; Lane, W.S.; Friedman, J.; Weissman, I.; Schreiber, S.L. Calcineurin is a common target of cyclophilin-cyclosporin A and FKBP-FK506 complexes. *Cell* **1991**, *66*, 807–815. [CrossRef]
2. McCaffrey, P.G.; Perrino, B.A.; Soderling, T.R.; Rao, A. NF-ATp, a T lymphocyte DNA-binding protein that is a target for calcineurin and immunosuppressive drugs. *J. Biol. Chem.* **1993**, *26*, 3747–3752.
3. Brazelton, T.R. Molecular mechanisms of action of new xenobiotic immunosuppressive drugs: Tacrolimus (FK506), sirolimus (rapamycin), mycophenolate mofetil and leflunomide. *Curr. Opin. Immunol.* **1996**, *8*, 710–720. [CrossRef]
4. De Paulis, A.; Stellato, C.; Cirillo, R.; Ciccarelli, A.; Oriente, A.; Marone, G. Anti-inflammatory effect of FK-506 on human skin mast cells. *J. Investig. Dermatol.* **1992**, *99*, 723–728. [CrossRef]
5. Panhans-Groß, A.; Novak, N.; Kraft, S.; Bieber, T. Human epidermal Langerhans' cells are targets for the immunosuppressive macrolide tacrolimus (FK506). *J. Aller. Clin. Immunol.* **2001**, *107*, 345–352.
6. Wollenberg, A.; Sharma, S.; von Bubnoff, D.; Geiger, E.; Haberstok, J.; Bieber, T. Topical tacrolimus (FK506) leads to profound phenotypic and functional alterations of epidermal antigen-presenting dendritic cells in atopic dermatitis. *J. Aller. Clin. Immunol.* **2001**, *107*, 519–525. [CrossRef]
7. Hashimoto, Y.; Matsuoka, N.; Kawakami, A.; Tsuboi, M.; Nakashima, T.; Eguchi, K.; Tomioka, T.; Kanematsu, T. Novel immunosuppressive effect of FK506 by augmentation of T cell apoptosis. *Clin. Exper. Immunol.* **2001**, *125*, 19–24. [CrossRef]
8. Chung, Y.; Chung, M.; Choi, S.; Choi, S.; Choi, S.; Chung, S. Tacrolimus-Induced Apoptosis is Mediated by Endoplasmic Reticulum–derived Calcium-dependent Caspases-3,-12 in Jurkat Cells. *Transplant. Proc.* **2018**, *50*, 1172–1177. [CrossRef]
9. Matsuda, S.; Shibasaki, F.; Takehana, K.; Mori, H.; Nishida, E.; Koyasu, S. Two distinct action mechanisms of immunophilin–ligand complexes for the blockade of T-cell activation. *EMBO Rep.* **2000**, *1*, 428–434. [CrossRef]
10. Soter, N.A.; Fleischer, A.B., Jr.; Webster, G.F.; Monroe, E.; Lawrence, I.; Group, T.O.S. Tacrolimus ointment for the treatment of atopic dermatitis in adult patients: Part II, safety. *J. Am. Acad. Dermatol.* **2001**, *44*, S39–S46. [CrossRef]
11. Lan, C.-C.E.; Yu, H.-S.; Huang, S.-M.; Wu, C.-S.; Chen, G.-S. FK506 induces interleukin-6 secretion from UVB irradiated cultured human keratinocytes via p38 mitogen-activated protein kinase pathway: Implication on mechanisms of tacrolimus-induced skin irritation. *J. Dermatol. Sci.* **2007**, *48*, 225–228. [CrossRef]
12. Muraoka, K.; Fujimoto, K.; Sun, X.; Yoshioka, K.; Shimizu, K.; Yagi, M.; Bose, H.; Miyazaki, I.; Yamamoto, K. Immunosuppressant FK506 induces interleukin-6 production through the activation of transcription factor nuclear factor (NF)-kappa (B). Implications for FK506 nephropathy. *J. Clin. Investig.* **1996**, *97*, 2433–2439. [CrossRef]
13. Shokrollahi, K. *Paraffin-Based Ointments and Fire Hazard: Understanding the Problem, Navigating the Media and Currently Available Downloadable Patient Information*; SAGE Publications Sage UK: London, UK, 2017.
14. Pople, P.V.; Singh, K.K. Development and evaluation of colloidal modified nanolipid carrier: Application to topical delivery of tacrolimus, Part II–In vivo assessment, drug targeting, efficacy, and safety in treatment for atopic dermatitis. *Eur. J. Pharm. Biopharm.* **2013**, *84*, 72–83. [CrossRef]
15. Erdogan, M.; Wright, J.; McAlister, V. Liposomal tacrolimus lotion as a novel topical agent for treatment of immune-mediated skin disorders: Experimental studies in a murine model. *Br. J. Dermatol.* **2002**, *146*, 964–967. [CrossRef]
16. Lapteva, M.; Mondon, K.; Möller, M.; Gurny, R.; Kalia, Y.N. Polymeric micelle nanocarriers for the cutaneous delivery of tacrolimus: A targeted approach for the treatment of psoriasis. *Mol. Pharm.* **2014**, *11*, 2989–3001. [CrossRef]
17. Li, G.; Fan, Y.; Fan, C.; Li, X.; Wang, X.; Li, M.; Liu, Y. Tacrolimus-loaded ethosomes: Physicochemical characterization and in vivo evaluation. *Eur. J. Pharm. Biopharm.* **2012**, *82*, 49–57. [CrossRef]
18. Yamamoto, K.; Klossek, A.; Fuchs, K.; Watts, B.; Raabe, J.; Flesch, R.; Rancan, F.; Pischon, H.; Radbruch, M.; Gruber, A. Soft X-ray microscopy for probing of topical tacrolimus delivery via micelles. *Eur. J. Pharm. Biopharm.* **2019**, *139*, 68–75. [CrossRef]
19. Lei, W.; Yu, C.; Lin, H.; Zhou, X. Development of tacrolimus-loaded transfersomes for deeper skin penetration enhancement and therapeutic effect improvement in vivo. *Asian J. Pharm. Sci.* **2013**, *8*, 336–345. [CrossRef]

20. Cuggino, J.C.; Blanco, E.R.O.; Gugliotta, L.M.; Igarzabal, C.I.A.; Calderón, M. Crossing biological barriers with nanogels to improve drug delivery performance. *J. Control. Release* **2019**, *307*, 221–246. [CrossRef]
21. Rancan, F.; Asadian-Birjand, M.; Dogan, S.; Graf, C.; Cuellar, L.; Lommatzsch, S.; Blume-Peytavi, U.; Calderón, M.; Vogt, A. Effects of thermoresponsivity and softness on skin penetration and cellular uptake of polyglycerol-based nanogels. *J. Control. Release* **2016**, *228*, 159–169. [CrossRef]
22. Giulbudagian, M.; Rancan, F.; Klossek, A.; Yamamoto, K.; Jurisch, J.; Neto, V.C.; Schrade, P.; Bachmann, S.; Rühl, E.; Blume-Peytavi, U. Correlation between the chemical composition of thermoresponsive nanogels and their interaction with the skin barrier. *J. Control. Release* **2016**, *243*, 323–332. [CrossRef]
23. Rancan, F.; Giulbudagian, M.; Jurisch, J.; Blume-Peytavi, U.; Calderon, M.; Vogt, A. Drug delivery across intact and disrupted skin barrier: Identification of cell populations interacting with penetrated thermoresponsive nanogels. *Eur. J. Pharm. Biopharm.* **2017**, *116*, 4–11. [CrossRef]
24. Giulbudagian, M.; Yealland, G.; Hönzke, S.; Edlich, A.; Geisendörfer, B.; Kleuser, B.; Hedtrich, S.; Calderón, M. Breaking the Barrier-Potent Anti-Inflammatory Activity following Efficient Topical Delivery of Etanercept using Thermoresponsive Nanogels. *Theranostics* **2018**, *8*, 450. [CrossRef]
25. Edlich, A.; Gerecke, C.; Giulbudagian, M.; Neumann, F.; Hedtrich, S.; Schäfer-Korting, M.; Ma, N.; Calderon, M.; Kleuser, B. Specific uptake mechanisms of well-tolerated thermoresponsive polyglycerol-based nanogels in antigen-presenting cells of the skin. *Eur. J. Pharm. Biopharm.* **2017**, *116*, 155–163. [CrossRef]
26. Gerecke, C.; Edlich, A.; Giulbudagian, M.; Schumacher, F.; Zhang, N.; Said, A.; Yealland, G.; Lohan, S.B.; Neumann, F.; Meinke, M.C. Biocompatibility and characterization of polyglycerol-based thermoresponsive nanogels designed as novel drug-delivery systems and their intracellular localization in keratinocytes. *Nanotoxicology* **2017**, *11*, 267–277. [CrossRef]
27. Dzhonova, D.; Olariu, R.; Leckenby, J.; Dhayani, A.; Vemula, P.K.; Prost, J.-C.; Banz, Y.; Taddeo, A.; Rieben, R. Local release of tacrolimus from hydrogel-based drug delivery system is controlled by inflammatory enzymes in vivo and can be monitored non-invasively using in vivo imaging. *PLoS ONE* **2018**, *13*, e0203409. [CrossRef]
28. Giulbudagian, M.; Asadian-Birjand, M.; Steinhilber, D.; Achazi, K.; Molina, M.; Calderón, M. Fabrication of thermoresponsive nanogels by thermo-nanoprecipitation and in situ encapsulation of bioactives. *Polym. Chem.* **2014**, *5*, 6909–6913. [CrossRef]
29. Koster, R.A.; Alffenaar, J.-W.C.; Greijdanus, B.; Uges, D.R. Fast LC-MS/MS analysis of tacrolimus, sirolimus, everolimus and cyclosporin A in dried blood spots and the influence of the hematocrit and immunosuppressant concentration on recovery. *Talanta* **2013**, *115*, 47–54. [CrossRef]
30. Döge, N.; Avetisyan, A.; Hadam, S.; Pfannes, E.K.B.; Rancan, F.; Blume-Peytavi, U.; Vogt, A. Assessment of skin barrier function and biochemical changes of ex vivo human skin in response to physical and chemical barrier disruption. *Eur. J. Pharm. Biopharm.* **2017**, *116*, 138–148. [CrossRef]
31. Bachhav, Y.; Summer, S.; Heinrich, A.; Bragagna, T.; Böhler, C.; Kalia, Y. Effect of controlled laser microporation on drug transport kinetics into and across the skin. *J. Control. Release* **2010**, *146*, 31–36. [CrossRef]
32. Yanase, K.; Hatta, I. Disruption of human stratum corneum lipid structure by sodium dodecyl sulphate. *Inter. J. Cosmet. Sci.* **2018**, *40*, 44–49. [CrossRef]
33. Otberg, N.; Patzelt, A.; Rasulev, U.; Hagemeister, T.; Linscheid, M.; Sinkgraven, R.; Sterry, W.; Lademann, J. The role of hair follicles in the percutaneous absorption of caffeine. *Br. J. Clin. Pharm.* **2008**, *65*, 488–492. [CrossRef]
34. Mohd, F.; Todo, H.; Yoshimoto, M.; Yusuf, E.; Sugibayashi, K. Contribution of the hair follicular pathway to Total skin permeation of topically applied and exposed chemicals. *Pharmaceutics* **2016**, *8*, 32. [CrossRef]
35. Tampucci, S.; Burgalassi, S.; Chetoni, P.; Lenzi, C.; Pirone, A.; Mailland, F.; Caserini, M.; Monti, D. Topical formulations containing finasteride. Part II: Determination of finasteride penetration into hair follicles using the differential stripping technique. *J. Pharm. Sci.* **2014**, *103*, 2323–2329. [CrossRef]
36. Rancan, F.; Amselgruber, S.; Hadam, S.; Munier, S.; Pavot, V.; Verrier, B.; Hackbarth, S.; Combadiere, B.; Blume-Peytavi, U.; Vogt, A. Particle-based transcutaneous administration of HIV-1 p24 protein to human skin explants and targeting of epidermal antigen presenting cells. *J. Control. Release* **2014**, *176*, 115–122. [CrossRef]
37. De Benedetto, A.; Kubo, A.; Beck, L.A. Skin barrier disruption: A requirement for allergen sensitization? *J. Investig. Dermatol.* **2012**, *132*, 949–963. [CrossRef]

pharmaceutics

MDPI

Article

Optimization of Rheological Behaviour and Skin Penetration of Thermogelling Emulsions with Enhanced Substantivity for Potential Application in Treatment of Chronic Skin Diseases

Markus Schmidberger [1], Ines Nikolic [2], Ivana Pantelic [2] and Dominique Lunter [1,*]

1 Department of Pharmaceutical Technology, Eberhard Karls University, Auf der Morgenstelle 8, 72076 Tuebingen, Germany
2 Department of Pharmaceutical Technology and Cosmetology, Faculty of Pharmacy, University of Belgrade, 450 Vojvode Stepe Street, 11221 Belgrade, Serbia
* Correspondence: dominique.lunter@uni-tuebingen.de; Tel.: +49-70712974558; Fax: +49-7071295531

Received: 28 June 2019; Accepted: 22 July 2019; Published: 24 July 2019

Abstract: Topical formulations are an important pillar in the therapy of skin diseases. Nevertheless, after application the formulation will be exposed to environmental effects. Contact with other surfaces will reduce the available amount of formulation and drug substance. The resulting consequences for therapy range from reduced effects to therapeutic failure. The removed active ingredient also contaminates patients' environment. The aim of this work was to develop preparations that remain at the application site. These will enhance safety and efficiency and thus improve of skin disease therapies. Therefore, we developed polymer-stabilised emulsions that show thermogelling properties. Emulsions with different methyl cellulose concentrations and macrogols of different molecular weights were investigated. The dispersed phase consisted of nonivamide as the active pharmaceutical ingredient, dissolved in medium-chain triglycerides. Rheological properties, droplet size, substantivity and ex vivo penetration experiments were performed to characterise the developed formulations. Droplet size and rheological parameters were affected by the composition of the preparations. The tested formulations showed benefits in their substantivity compared to a conventional semi-solid cream. We found a residual amount of up to 100% at the application site. The drug levels in viable epidermis were in a therapeutic range. The developed emulsions are a promising vehicle to improve therapy for chronic skin diseases.

Keywords: nonivamide; methyl cellulose; skin penetration; substantivity; thermogel

1. Introduction

The vehicle of a topical formulation plays an important role with respect to disease control and therapeutic outcome. It controls the penetration profile of the preparation [1–5] and has an effect on the skin barrier function [6,7]. This can improve or worsen the healing process of diseased skin. However, the applied formulation is partly removed, e.g., by touching skin surfaces or clothing. As a result, the drug and vehicle can be removed from the application site and thus cannot achieve the desired outcome. Higher drug concentration or repeated application will conceal this problem but will not solve it. Additionally, active pharmaceutical ingredients (API) can pollute the patients' environment. Consequently, other people can come into contact with the drug substance, resulting in irritations or undesired effects. Topical formulations that are more resistant to contact with the environment and remain at the application site are a promising approach to improve patients' compliance and reduce the consumption of such formulations. Safety aspects are another benefit. If the preparation stays at the application site, unintentional contact will be minimised. Furthermore, formulations that remain on the skin surface are possible drug reservoirs for topical preparations that exhibit sustained release.

The ability of a topical formulation to remain on the skin surface is called substantivity [8]. It has been shown that different types of formulations show notable differences in their substantivity. A substantial amount of semi-solid formulations and liquid preparations are removed from the skin surface by contact with other surfaces, whereas film-forming formulations are not affected [9,10]. These preparations differ in their rheological properties. Thus, it is a promising approach to tune the rheological behaviour of a topical formulation to increase its substantivity. We hypothesise that formulations that change their rheological behaviour to a more elastic character upon application to the skin, e.g., by thermogelation, will show enhanced substantivity. We thus developed emulsions that are stabilised with methyl cellulose (MC). Cellulose derivates, such as hydroxypropyl methylcellulose or methyl cellulose, are known to be suitable for preparing oil-in-water emulsions and show thermogelation [11–15].

In this work, we focus on nonivamide as a drug substance for chronic skin diseases. The compound is an agonist on the transient receptor vanilloid type 1 ion channel (TRPV1) [16]. This non-specific ion channel is present in human skin, especially in sensory nerve fibres [17]. The short-term activation of TRPV1 results in different symptoms. Most pronounced are warming and burning, in addition to stinging and itching [18,19]. With long-term use, the intracellular amount of calcium increases due to calcium influx and after a certain time the cellular processes modify. As a result, neurons are defunctionalised and the stimulus of itch is not conducted. Therefore, nonivamide and other capsaicinoids have a certain analgesic and antipruritic potential. They are thus agents used to treat neuralgic pain or chronic pruritus [20,21], which presents in many skin diseases. Their use in clinical practise is limited due to the necessity of multiple dosing and thus impaired patient compliance. Formulations with enhanced substantivity might therefore offer a beneficial approach to promote the use of capsaicinoids.

The substantivity of dermal preparations is less investigated and little is known about the influencing factors. A further aim of this work was thus to understand the rheological factors that influence substantivity and to employ this knowledge in the development of a topical formulation that remains at the application site due to optimised rheological properties.

2. Material and Methods

2.1. Materials

Methyl cellulose (Metolose SM-25) was kindly donated by Shin-Etsu Chemical Co., Tokyo, Japan. Avobenzone was provided by Symrise AG, Holzminden, Germany. All other materials were obtained from the named supplier: sodium citrate (Carl Roth GmbH + Co. KG, Karlsruhe, Germany), nonivamide (Sigma Aldrich Chemie GmbH, Steinheim, Germany), white soft paraffin (Hansen and Rosenthal KG, Hamburg, Germany), medium-chain triglycerides (Myritol® 312), propylene glycole and macrogol 200 and 4000 (BASF SE, Ludwigshafen, Germany) and cetyl alcohol (Ceasar and Loretz, Hilden, Germany). PEG-20-glyceryl stearate (Tagat S2®) and glycerol stearate (Fagron GmbH and Co. KG, Barsbüttel, Germany). Solvents methanol and acetonitril were HPLC gradient grade. Sodium chloride, disodium phosphate, potassium dihydrogen phosphate, magnesium sulphate and phosphoric acid were of European Pharmacopeia grade.

2.2. Preparation of Oil-in-Water Emulsions

The formulation was prepared by a syringe-to-syringe technique. Methyl cellulose, long-chain macrogol and sodium citrate were weighed into a syringe. Water was heated up to boiling and then weighed into a second syringe of the same size. The water had a temperature of 85–90 °C. Water-miscible liquids such as ethanol or liquid (short-chain) macrogol were added to the hot water. The two syringes were connected by an adapter and then mixed until no solid particles were visible. A white dispersion was the result. To avoid the incorporation of air in the formulation, the syringes were disconnected and the air in the headspace was removed. Subsequently, the syringes were connected again and the dispersion was mixed 100 times by transferring the mixture from one syringe to the other. The formulation was stored at 5 °C for 24 h. The preparation of such aqueous methyl cellulose preparations has already been described by Takeuchi et al. [22]. As a final step, nonivamide was dissolved in medium-chain triglycerides. The oily solution was weighed into a syringe and connected to the prepared aqueous phase. For a preparation with 0.9% API, the concentration of the oily solution was 3.6% nonivamide in medium-chain triglycerides. For an emulsion with 0.3% nonivamide, the concentration of API in the lipophilic phase was 1.2%. The two phases were mixed 100 times. As a result, a white oil-in-water emulsion was formed. The percentage composition of the emulsions is given in Table 1. The liquid formulation was filled into a glass vial and tightly sealed. Due to the preparation in a closed system, it was not necessary to add evaporated water.

Table 1. Percentage composition of thermogelling emulsions. The amount of nonivamide varied between 0.3 and 0.9% with regard to the final mass of the formulation.

	A	B	C
Substance		Amount (% m/m)	
Methyl cellulose	0.5	1.0	4.8
Sodium citrate	2.1	2.1	2.1
Macrogol 200 or 4000	6.0	6.0	6.0
Ethanol	9.0	9.0	9.0
Medium-chain triglycerides with nonivamide	25.0	25.0	25.0
Purified water	to 100	to 100	to 100

The composition and preparation of Hydrophilic Nonivamide Cream (HNC) is described in "Neues Rezeptur-Formularium". The cream was prepared as described in the monograph [23]. Capsaicin was replaced by nonivamide.

Formulations used in the in vivo substantivity measurements contained avobenzone instead of nonivamide. Formulations were prepared as described above.

2.3. Rheoloigcal Measurements

A rotational viscometer (Physica MCR 501, Anton Paar, Graz, Austria) with a plate/plate measuring arrangement (d = 25 mm) was used to characterise the rheological behaviour of the formulations. Oscillatory tests were performed at 5 °C and 32 °C. A temperature of 5 °C ensured that the measurement was below the gelling point. The rheological behaviour on skin surface was determined at 32 °C. The frequency was 1 Hz and the deformation was increased from 0.01 to 1000%. The gap size was set to 0.2 mm. Storage modulus G′ and loss modulus G″ were determined in the linear viscoelastic region. The dissipation factor was calculated as shown in Equation (1). All formulations contained 0.9% nonivamide. Experiments were performed in triplicate.

$$Dissipation\ factor = \frac{G''}{G'} \quad (1)$$

2.4. Preparation of Dermatomed Pig Ear Skin

For ex vivo substantivity tests and penetration experiments, we used porcine ear skin. Porcine skin is frequently used as a model for human skin [24–26]. Ears of German Land Race pigs with an age between 15 and 30 weeks and a weight of 40–65 kg were used. Pig ears were donated from the Department of Experimental Medicine, University Hospital of Tübingen. The ears were removed right after the death of the animals. Afterwards, the ears were washed with isotonic saline and postauricular skin was removed. The obtained skin sample was cleaned with cotton swabs and isotonic saline. Afterwards the surface was patted dry and packed in aluminium foil. Porcine skin was stored at

−30 °C. Before use, the skin was thawed at room temperature. Strips with adequate width were cut and attached onto a styrofoam block. A dermatom (Dermatom GA 630, Aesculap AG and Co. KG, Tuttlingen, Germany) was used to obtain skin samples with a defined thickness of 1 mm. This method is described in previous work of our group [1,2,9,10,27]. For ex vivo substantivity tests pieces with a diameter of 30 mm, and for penetration experiments discs with a diameter of 25 mm were punched out of the skin.

2.5. Ex Vivo Substantivity Test

To test the substantivity of the formulations, a method of Herrmann et al. [10] was used. Two heatable steel cylinders were fixed to a texture analyser (Type BDO-FB0.5TS, Zwick Roell GmbH and Co. KG, Ulm, Germany). Both parts were heated to 32 °C (skin surface temperature). The lower part was rigid, while the second cylinder was placed above the other and was movable. A piece of dermatomed pig ear skin was fixed to the lower cylinder and about 4 mg of formulation was applied to the skin surface. To this end, approximately 8 mg of the formulation was put on a plastic cylinder and weighed exactly. By pressing down and rotating, the formulation was transferred to the skin. Afterwards the application aid was weighed again. The mass difference gave the applied mass of formulation. Subsequently, the formulation had 10 min to dry. Another piece of skin or a piece of cloth was fixed to the upper steel cylinder. Then, the two devices were pressed together with a defined force of 10 N for 50 s. The skin surface was cleaned twice with a cotton swab, then soaked with 2 mL of phosphate-buffered saline (PBS) with pH 7.4. The swabs were collected in a 50 mL centrifuge tube and 4 mL of methanol was added to extract the API. Clothing was extracted in a mixture of methanol and PBS in equal parts. Nonivamide was quantified by HPLC. Experiments were performed in triplicate.

2.6. In Vivo Substantivity Test

A square of 9 cm^2 was marked on the upper right arm of female Caucasian volunteers. All subjects (aged 29 ± 6 years) gave their informed consent for inclusion before they participated in the study. The study was conducted in accordance with the Declaration of Helsinki, and the protocol was approved by the local Ethics Committee on Human Research (University of Belgrade, Faculty of Pharmacy, Serbia; approval number: 2298/2, issued on December 2017). Approximately 18 mg of formulation was applied and the exact mass was obtained by difference weighing. After 10 min drying time, a piece of cloth (6 × 6 cm) was fixed in the inner side of the clothing item with safety pins, such that the applied formulation was covered. Afterwards the participants had 3 h at their disposal, to return to their normal physical activities. Then the formulation was washed away twice with a cotton swab soaked with 2 mL of purified water. The two swabs were collected in a centrifuge tube and 10 mL of methanol was added to extract the API. The piece of cloth was put into a second centrifuge tube and 10 mL of methanol and 4 mL of purified water were added. Subsequently, the centrifuge tubes were shaken for 1 min and then put into an ultrasonic bath for 60 min. The amount of formulation was analysed using a UV/Vis spectrometer. All formulations contained 0.9% of avobenzone. This sun protection factor remained on the skin surface and the penetrated amount was negligible [28]. Only volunteers with a recovery within 65–125% of the applied amount of avobenzone were included. The actual determined amount of avobenzone was set as 100%.

2.7. Ex Vivo Penetration Experiments

The dermatomed pig ear skin with a thickness of 1 mm was placed on the top of the acceptor compartment of a Franz diffusion cell with 2 cm^2 penetration area (Gauer Glas, Puettlingen, Germany). The acceptor compartment was filled with a solution of 4% bovine serum albumin in phosphate-buffered saline with pH 7.4. This acceptor medium is equivalent to whole blood with regard to the permeation rate for lipophilic compounds [29]. The diffusion cells were placed in a water bath and heated to 32 °C for 30 min before the formulation was applied. The acceptor medium was stirred at 500 rpm during the incubation time. The experiments were performed under finite dose conditions. To this end, about 4 mg of formulation was applied to the skin surface in the same way as described for substantivity testing (Section 2.5). After 4 h the skin was removed from the diffusion cell. To remove the remaining formulation, skin surface was washed twice with a cotton swab soaked with 2 mL saturated magnesium sulphate solution. The actual penetration area was punched out, directly weighed and frozen in liquid nitrogen. The skin was sectioned horizontally with a cryo-microtome (HM 560 Cryo-Star; Thermo Fisher Scientific, Inc., Waltham, MA, USA) into thin sections with a thickness of 16 µm. The first incomplete cuts and the first complete cut were collected in a 2 mL tube, representing the stratum corneum. The next 14 sections were collected in a second container, representing the viable epidermis. The last fraction, the dermis, was also cut in 16 µm thin sections and put in a third vial. This method has been described in detail by Lunter and Daniels [2]. To extract the API from the skin tissue, 1 mL saturated solution of magnesium sulphate was added. This aqueous phase was covered with 200 µL acetonitrile. The organic liquid contained avobenzone as an internal standard. The tubes were shaken for 60 min at 1000 rpm (BioShake iQ, Analytik Jena AG, Jena, Germany). To achieve complete phase separation, the samples were centrifuged for 15 min at 13,400 rpm (MiniSpin, Eppendorf AG, Hamburg, Germany). Afterwards, 80 µL of the upper organic phase was transferred into a HPLC vial. Nonivamide was quantified by HPLC. This procedure was performed to concentrate nonivamide in the organic phase in order to improve quantification. Experiments were performed in triplicate.

2.8. UV/Vis Detection of Avobenzone

The concentration of avobenzone was quantified using a UV/Vis Spectrophotometer Evolution 300 in combination with Visionpro Software (Thermo Scientific, Waltham, MA, USA). The solution was filled in a quartz cuvette. The detection wavelength was 360 nm. If the signal was outside the calibration range, the stock solution was diluted with fresh solvent. The coefficient of determination was >0.999, the limit of detection was 0.009 µg/mL and the limit of quantification 0.033 µg/mL.

2.9. HPLC Analytics

The used HPLC system had the following components: Dionex P680 HPLC Pump, Dionex Autosampler ASI-100 Automated Sample Injector, Gynkotek UVD170U Detector (Dionex Corporation, Sunnyvale, CA, USA) and the column-oven SunTherm 5-100 (SunChrom Wissenschaftliche Geräte GmbH, Friedrichsdorf, Germany). For nonivamide quantification in methanol 50% (substantivity measurements), a multistep gradient with acetonitrile and phosphoric acid (pH 3.0) was performed. The amount of acetonitrile was raised from 30 to 75% within 8 min and was then held constant for 2 min. Afterwards the amount was reduced to 30% within 2 min and equilibrated for 3 min. The flow rate was set to 1.15 mL/min, the injection volume was 200 µL and the oven temperature was 40 °C. The retention time of nonivamide was approximately 5.6 min. The HPLC column Nucleosil 100-5 C8 EC 125/4 (Macherey-Nagel GmbH and Co. KG, Dueren, Germany) was used together with the HPLC-precolumn EC 4/3 Universal RP (Macherey-Nagel GmbH and Co. KG, Dueren, Germany). Avobenzone was used as an internal standard. Calibration data are given in Table 2.

Table 2. Calibration data for nonivamide in methanol 50% and acetonitrile; $n = 3$.

Solvent	Calibration Range (µg/mL)	Coefficient of Determination (R^2)	Limit of Detection (µg/mL)	Limit of Quantification (µg/mL)
Methanol 50%	0.01–0.10	0.9868	0.014	0.042
Methanol 50%	0.1–1.0	0.9953	0.029	0.103
Methanol 50%	1.0–10.0	0.9949	0.304	1.066
Acetonitrile	0.05–0.50	0.9878	0.023	0.079
Acetonitrile	0.1–1.0	0.9911	0.042	0.146
Acetonitrile	1.0–10.0	0.9994	0.109	0.390

To separate and quantify nonivamide and avobenzone in acetonitrile (penetration experiments) the HPLC column Nucleosil 100-5 C18 EC 125/4 (Macherey-Nagel GmbH and Co. KG, Dueren, Germany) was used together with the HPLC-precolumn EC 4/3 Universal RP (Macherey-Nagel GmbH and Co. KG, Dueren, Germany). A multistep gradient with methanol and phosphoric acid (pH 3.0) was performed. At the beginning, the organic amount was set to 45%, reaching 99% after 15 min, and it was then held constant for 2 min. The gradient returned within 2 min to initial conditions and was equilibrated for 5 min. The pump was set to 1.0 mL/min, the injection volume was 60 µL and the oven temperature was 30 °C. The retention time was approximately 8.6 min for nonivamide and approximately 15.1 min for avobenzone. Calibration data are given in Tables 2 and 3.

Table 3. Calibration data for avobenzone in acetonitrile; $n = 3$.

Solvent	Calibration Range (µg/mL)	Coefficient of Determination (R^2)	Limit of Detection (µg/mL)	Limit of Quantification (µg/mL)
Acetonitrile	0.05–0.50	0.9971	0.011	0.040
Acetonitrile	0.1–1.0	0.9954	0.031	0.109
Acetonitrile	1.0–10.0	0.9975	0.230	0.816

2.10. Droplet Size Measurements

Droplet size was measured by laser diffraction using Mastersizer® 2000 with Hydro 2000s (Malvern Panalytical Ltd., Malvern, UK). Therefore, 200 µL of the emulsion was added to about 10 mL of purified water and mixed manually. The mixture was put in Hydro 2000s under stirring (2000 rpm) until an obscuration between 10% and 20% was reached. After 60 s the measurement was started. One measurement cycle recorded the signal three times for 30 s. For each emulsion three aliquots were measured. For each aliquot three repetitions were performed.

2.11. Statistical Analysis

The data were obtained from repeated measurements ($n \geq 3$). The diagrams show mean ± standard deviation (SD). The data were analysed by unpaired *t*-test ($p < 0.05$) or, if multiple groups were to be compared, by one-sided one factorial analysis of variance (ANOVA) ($p < 0.05$) followed by the Student–Newman–Keuls test.

3. Results and Discussion

The aim of this work was to develop methyl cellulose-stabilised emulsions that show enhanced substantivity due to thermogelation. We thus investigated the effect of different methyl cellulose concentrations and different macrogol types on rheological properties and substantivity. The semi-solid Hydrophilic Nonivamide Cream (HNC) that is used as a therapy for chronic itch was used for comparison. To determine loss and storage modulus, oscillatory experiments were performed. The results gave information on the viscoelastic properties of the formulation. Figure 1 exemplarily shows the results of the oscillatory experiments at 5 and at 32 °C, which are equivalent to storage temperature and skin surface temperature, respectively. At 5 °C the presented emulsion has a higher loss modulus compared to its storage modulus and thus the formulation is a liquid preparation at this temperature. By increasing the temperature to 32 °C, the rheological parameters change. Storage and loss modulus reach higher values. Here, the storage modulus is higher than the loss modulus. This means that the preparation has semi-solid properties at skin surface temperature. Therefore, it can be concluded that the developed formulations show thermogelling properties. The emulsion has a dissipation factor of about 0.1 and thus, compared to HNC, it is approximately six times smaller. Therefore, the elastic properties of the emulsion are more pronounced compared to those of HNC.

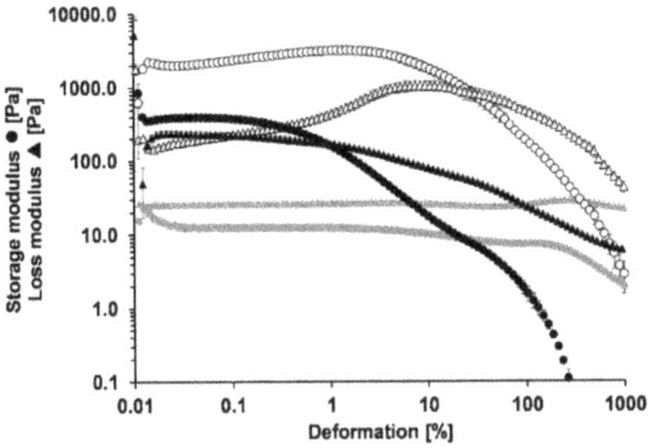

Figure 1. Oscillatory measurements of HNC at 32 °C (black icons) and the emulsion containing 4.8% methyl cellulose at 5 °C (grey icons) and 32 °C (open icons), mean ± SD, $n = 3$.

In Table 4, the rheological parameters of different emulsions are listed (for more detailed information the reader is kindly referred to supplementary material Figures S1–S5). With increasing methyl cellulose concentration, the storage and loss modulus increase, but no effect on the dissipation factor appears. The emulsions have a dissipation factor of about 0.1. Apart from different methyl cellulose concentrations, we also investigated the impact of short-chain versus long-chain macrogols. The emulsions with an amount of 0.5% or 1.0% of methyl cellulose but different types of macrogol did not differ in their rheological properties. The emulsion with 4.8% methyl cellulose and macrogol 200 had a higher storage and loss modulus than the emulsion containing macrogol 4000. The latter finding is somewhat contrary to our expectation that the long-chain macrogol that is solid at skin surface temperature might also lead to a more solid gel character. Presumably the short-chain macrogol interacts more strongly with methyl cellulose and thus exhibits a stronger impact on the rheological properties of the emulsion.

Table 4. Rheological parameters of thermogelling emulsions and HNC at 32 °C, mean ± SD, $n \geq 3$.

Formulation	Storage Modulus (Pa)	Loss Modulus (Pa)	Dissipation Factor
HNC	396.73 (±32.32)	233.37 (±16.95)	0.59 (±0.01)
4.8% Methyl cellulose, macrogol 4000	284.00 (±147.55)	25.43 (±8.96)	0.09 (±0.01)
1.0% Methyl cellulose, macrogol 4000	5.64 (±1.11)	0.61 (±0.27)	0.10 (±0.04)
0.5% Methyl cellulose, macrogol 4000	4.28 (±2.07)	0.44 (±0.23)	0.14 (±0.12)
4.8% Methyl cellulose, macrogol 200	2123.33 (±51.32)	200.00 (±6.24)	0.09 (±0.00)
1.0% Methyl cellulose, macrogol 200	3.52 (±0.62)	0.42 (±0.08)	0.12 (±0.04)
0.5% Methyl cellulose, macrogol 200	2.00 (±0.31)	0.44 (±0.23)	0.23 (±0.12)

The droplet size of the emulsions was determined directly after preparation. The results are shown in Table 5. The emulsions with high methyl cellulose concentrations showed the smallest droplet size. Upon decreasing the polymer concentration, the values for d10, d50 and d90 rose. Methyl cellulose is the emulsifying agent and a direct correlation between droplet size and methyl cellulose concentration was expected. Our results do not show any effect of the macrogol chain length on the droplet size. The emulsions with the same amount of methyl cellulose but different macrogol types were comparable with respect to their droplet size. The macroscopic and microscopic appearances of the emulsions are shown in supplementary Figure S6.

Table 5. Droplet size of the emulsions with different methyl cellulose concentrations and different macrogol types. Formulations were prepared without nonivamide, mean ± SD, $n = 3$.

Formulation	d10	d50	d90
4.8% Methyl cellulose, macrogol 4000	1.34 (±0.01)	2.37 (±0.00)	3.82 (±0.01)
1.0% Methyl cellulose, macrogol 4000	1.93 (±0.01)	4.88 (±0.01)	9.33 (±0.03)
0.5% Methyl cellulose, macrogol 4000	3.32 (±0.04)	6.70 (±0.07)	12.37 (±0.16)
4.8% Methyl cellulose, macrogol 200	1.40 (±0.00)	2.26 (±0.01)	3.45 (±0.02)
1.0% Methyl cellulose, macrogol 200	2.74 (±0.06)	5.95 (±0.08)	11.14 (±0.21)
0.5% Methyl cellulose, macrogol 200	3.09 (±0.11)	6.49 (±0.11)	11.99 (±0.21)

Furthermore, the effect of different methyl cellulose concentrations and macrogols on substantivity was investigated. The results of the ex vivo substantivity test are shown in Figure 2. It can be seen that skin-to-formulation or clothing-to-formulation contact removes about one third of HNC. Formulations with 0.5% or 1.0% methyl cellulose showed comparable results. About 70% of the applied emulsion remained at skin surface after simulated contact. The two emulsions with a methyl cellulose concentration of 4.8% showed residual amounts of 86% and 100%. This shows that neither skin-to-formulation nor clothing-to-formulation removed a substantial share of the applied emulsion.

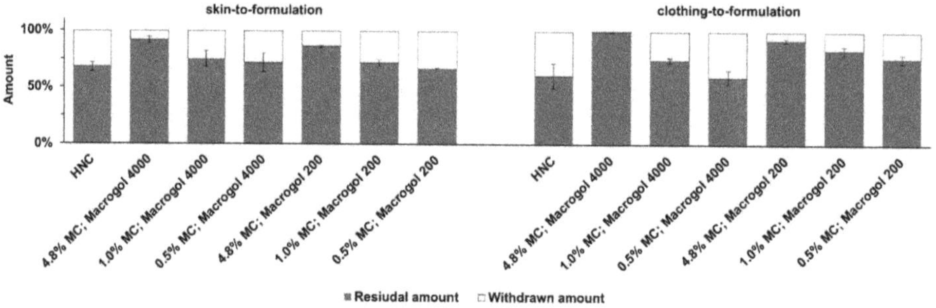

Figure 2. Ex vivo substantivity tests simulating skin-to-formulation and clothing-to-formulation contact. Results of HNC and developed emulsions, mean ± SD, $n = 3$.

The results of the ex vivo substantivity tests show that with a methyl cellulose concentration of 4.8% and macrogol 4000 or 200, high residual fractions were obtained—i.e., the withdrawn amount was not more than 14% when skin-to-formulation contact was simulated. Moreover, a residual amount up to 100% was obtained, when clothing-to-formulation was simulated. A lower methyl cellulose concentration resulted in higher withdrawn amounts. Emulsions with the same amount of methyl cellulose but different types of macrogol were comparable. The emulsions with a high methyl cellulose concentration were neither affected by simulating skin-to-formulation nor clothing-to-formulation contact. Statistical results of the ex vivo substantivity test are given in the supplementary material (Tables S1 and S2). These results can be explained by the rheological behaviour of the formulations. Emulsions that showed similar rheological behaviour also showed similar substantivity. Emulsions with high methyl cellulose concentration were characterised by their high storage modulus and a low dissipation factor and thus showed high substantivity. On the other hand, emulsions with low methyl cellulose concentration showed low storage modulus and a higher dissipation factor, resulting in lower substantivity. The substantivity of the developed emulsions is comparable to that of previously developed film-forming formulations [9,10]. This finding is remarkable, as the emulsions do not form a deductible, cohesive film.

The droplet size plays a minor role in resistance against contact with other surfaces. Formulations with 4.8%, 1.0% and 0.5% methyl cellulose showed differences in their droplet size, though we could not find a clear trend in their substantivity.

The next step was to investigate the skin penetration of nonivamide from the developed emulsions. The nonivamide site of action is located in the viable epidermis. Thus, ex vivo permeation experiments were not informative in this case as they reflect transdermal absorption. We thus focused on ex-vivo penetration experiments that enabled the measurement of the nonivamide concentration in the different strata of the skin. Penetration from the emulsion was compared to penetration from HNC, which contained nonivamide in a concentration that is clinically used (0.05%). The aim was to achieve drug levels at the site of action that were comparable to this reference. The emulsion contained 0.9% nonivamide, as this concentration had been found to give similar drug concentrations in skin to HNC 0.05% in earlier work by our group [2,3,27].

Figure 3 shows the penetrated amount of nonivamide from HNC 0.05% and an emulsion with 0.9% in the different skin layers. From HNC 0.05%, about 70 ng/cm^2 penetrated in the stratum corneum after 4 h incubation time. In both the viable epidermis and dermis we could find about 25 ng/cm^2. The new emulsion with an API concentration of 0.9% resulted in a mean of 250 ng/cm^2 nonivamide in the stratum corneum, 100 ng/cm^2 in the viable epidermis and 60 ng/cm^2 in the dermis. The penetrated amount in the stratum corneum and viable epidermis was about three to four times higher compared to that achieved using HNC 0.05%. Therefore, the drug concentration was set to 0.3% in a subsequent experiment. A reduced API concentration of 0.3% led to a reduced penetrated amount (Figure 4). Drug concentration in the viable epidermis, the site of action, was about 14 ng/cm^2 from the emulsion and 12 ng/cm^2 from HNC, and was thus comparable to HNC 0.05%. Although the emulsion contained a higher concentration of API, the penetrated amount was almost the same. This can be explained by the composition of the two formulations. HNC contained 15% of propylene glycol and 9% of ethanol, which are both known as penetration enhancers [30–32], whereas the emulsion did not contain propylene glycol. Differences in penetrated amount from HNC 0.05% between the two experiments were related to the use of skin from different donors. It can thus be concluded that the emulsion delivers an amount of the active ingredient to the skin that is suitable for therapy. The penetrated amount can be tuned by adjusting the drug concentration in the emulsion.

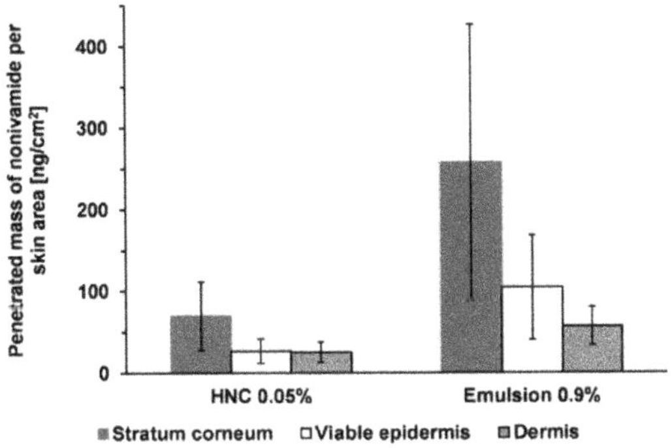

Figure 3. Penetrated amount of nonivamide after 4 h from HNC 0.05% and a developed emulsion containing 0.9% nonivamide, mean ± SD, $n \geq 3$.

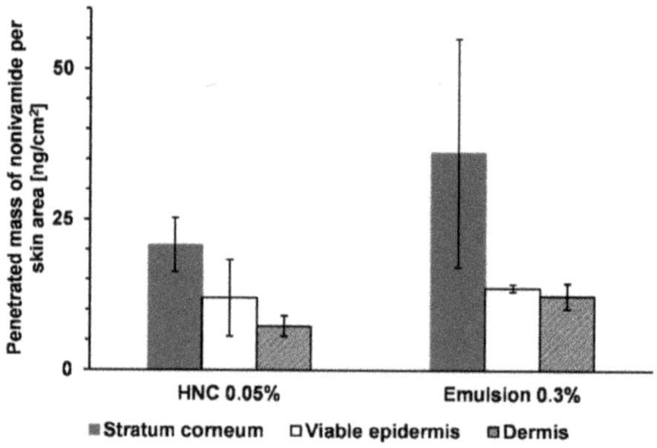

Figure 4. Penetrated amount of nonivamide after 4 h from HNC 0.05% and a developed emulsion containing 0.3% nonivamide, mean ± SD, $n = 3$.

Finally, the in vivo substantivity of the thermogelling emulsion was compared to that of HNC. The results are given in Figure 5. It can clearly be seen that from HNC, 67% of the formulation was transferred to the clothing, whereas from the emulsion only 37% was removed. This is in accordance with the ex vivo substantivity test, which had already shown that the emulsion was superior to HNC. Nevertheless, the SDs were higher and the differences between the two formulations were slightly less evident in the in vivo experiment. We believe that this was to be expected as a higher degree of variability is typical for in vivo experiments. As our study group was very homogeneous regarding age, gender and ethnicity, we believe that the variability manly reflects different physical activity among the volunteers, who were not given any restriction on to how to behave during the application interval. Therefore, the in vivo experiment better reflects real life conditions compared to the ex vivo experiment. As we could still find a significant difference between substantivity in the in vivo experiment, we are convinced that the emulsion will be superior to HNC under real-life conditions.

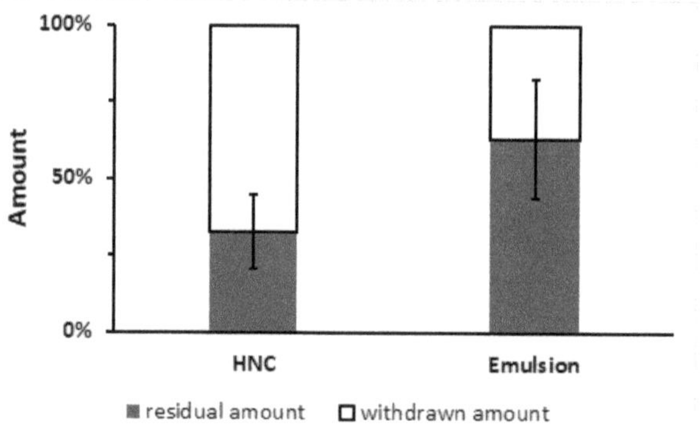

Figure 5. In vivo substantivity tests simulating clothing-to-formulation contact. Results of HNC and the developed emulsion, mean ± SD, $n = 5$ or 6.

4. Conclusions

Thermogels or formulations that form a gel in situ are promising dosage forms for different applications. Ophthalmic, injectable as well as dermal preparations are described in the literature. Lin et al. investigated thermogels containing mixtures of alginate and pluronics for ophthalmic application [33]. Zhang et al. used PLGA-PEG_PLGA-block-copolymers as injectable and biodegradable delivery systems [34]. In the context of dermal application, Hemelrijk et al. employed poloxamer to form thermogels for the enhanced delivery of 5-ALA into keratotic skin [35]. Takeuchi et al. investigated methyl cellulose-based thermogels and characterised the impact of different excipients on rheological parameters [22]. Their gels contained no oil phase and no studies concerning the dermal uptake of pharmaceutical actives from the gels were conducted. Further, the question of substantivity has not been investigated in publications dealing with methyl cellulose thermogels. Although researchers and practitioners are aware of the fact that a substantial amount of formulations is removed from the skin after application, research on the rational development of formulations with enhanced substantivity is scarce.

The presented work illustrates that the developed thermogelling emulsions are more substantive than the tested conventional semi-solid cream. With a high methyl cellulose concentration, almost the entire applied formulation stays at the application site. The results suggest that a connection between rheological characteristics and substantivity exists. High storage modulus and low dissipation factor increase the residual amount of topical formulations. Thus, it is possible to combine the advantages of the high substantivity of film-forming formulations and the beneficial characteristics of conventional semi-solid creams with regard to skin care. While in film-forming formulations the oil is immobilised in mesoporous silica particle [1], in the presented emulsions the medium-chain triglycerides are available for skin care. The penetrated amount of nonivamide is comparable to the monographed HNC 0.05%. The thermogelling emulsions may therefore provide an alternative to conventional creams in the therapy of chronic skin diseases. With enhanced substantivity, they may reduce application frequency and the contamination of patients' environment with the active ingredients. They may also be used as a formulation platform for other pharmaceutical actives. Future research will focus on the impact of further excipients on thermogelation and on the selection of optimal additives for the enhancement of in vivo substantivity. As differences were found between ex vivo and in vivo substantivity, we will further improve the ex vivo method of substantivity determination to better reflect the in vivo situation. Furthermore, the optimisation of drug delivery properties will be investigated.

Supplementary Materials: The following are available online at http://www.mdpi.com/1999-4923/11/8/361/s1, Figure S1: Oscillatory measurements methyl cellulose stabilised emulsion at 5 °C (grey icons) and 32 °C (open icons). The emulsion contains Macrogol 4000, quantities corresponds to emulsion A in Table 1, mean ± SD, $n = 3$; Figure S2: Oscillatory measurements methyl cellulose stabilised emulsion at 5 °C (grey icons) and 32 °C (open icons). The emulsion contains Macrogol 4000, quantities corresponds to emulsion B in Table 1, mean ± SD, $n = 3$; Figure S3: Oscillatory measurements methyl cellulose stabilised emulsion at 5 °C (grey icons) and 32 °C (open icons). The emulsion contains Macrogol 4000, quantities corresponds to emulsion C in Table 1, mean ± SD, $n = 3$; Figure S4: Oscillatory measurements methyl cellulose stabilised emulsion at 5 °C (grey icons) and 32 °C (open icons). The emulsion contains Macrogol 200, quantities corresponds to emulsion A in Table 1, mean ± SD, $n = 3$; Figure S5: Oscillatory measurements methyl cellulose stabilised emulsion at 5 °C (grey icons) and 32 °C (open icons). The emulsion contains Macrogol 200, quantities corresponds to emulsion B in Table 1, mean ± SD, $n = 3$; Figure S6: left: macroscopic image of a thermogelling emulsion; right: microscopic image of a thermogelling emulsion; Table S1: Statistically significance for residual amount simulating skin-to formulation contact. Emulsions are named by their methyl cellulose concentration and the molecular weight of the used macrogol. The data were analysed by one-sided one factorial analysis of variance (ANOVA) ($p < 0.05$) followed by Student-Newman-Keuls test. Lines which are not linked with the same letter are significant different; Table S2: Statistically significance for residual amount simulating clothing-to formulation contact. Emulsions are named by their methyl cellulose concentration and the molecular weight of the used macrogol. The data were analysed by one-sided one factorial analysis of variance (ANOVA) ($p < 0.05$) followed by Student-Newman-Keuls test. Lines which are not linked with the same letter are significant different.

Author Contributions: Conceptualisation, M.S. and D.L.; Data curation, M.S. and I.N.; Funding acquisition, D.J.L.; Investigation, M.S., I.N. and I.P.; Methodology, M.S., I.P. and D.J.L.; Project administration, D.J.L.; Supervision, I.P.; Writing—original draft, M.S., Writing—review and editing, D.J.L.

Funding: In this research Dominique Lunter was funded by the European Social Fund and the Ministry of Science, Research and Arts Baden-Württemberg. Furthermore, this project was partially financed by a bilateral project funded by the German Academic Exchange Service (DAAD) (grant number: 57334785) and the Serbian Ministry of Education, Science and Technological Development (grant number 451-03-01413/2016-09/10). The APC was partially funded by Deutsche Forschungsgemeinschaft and Open Access Publishing Fund of University of Tübingen.

Acknowledgments: The authors would like to thank Martin Schenk from the Department of Experimental Medicine at the University Hospital of Tübingen for providing pig ears and Shin-Etsu Chemical Co. for the generous donation of methyl cellulose. Thanks also go to Symrise AG for kindly providing avobenzone.

Conflicts of Interest: The authors declare no conflict of interest.

References

1. Heck, R.; Hermann, S.; Lunter, D.J.; Daniels, R. Film-forming formulations containing porous silica for the sustained delivery of actives to the skin. *Eur. J. Pharm. Biopharm.* **2016**, *108*, 1–8. [CrossRef]
2. Lunter, D.; Daniels, R. In vitro Skin Permeation and Penetration of Nonivamide from Novel Film-Forming Emulsions. *Skin Pharmacol. Physiol.* **2013**, *26*, 139–146. [CrossRef] [PubMed]
3. Rottke, M.; Lunter, D.J.; Daniels, R. In vitro studies on release and skin permeation of nonivamide from novel oil-in-oil-emulsions. *Eur. J. Pharm. Biopharm.* **2014**, *86*, 260–266. [CrossRef] [PubMed]
4. Lunter, D.J.; Daniels, R. New film forming emulsions containing Eudragit® NE and/or RS 30D for sustained dermal delivery of nonivamide. *Eur. J. Pharm. Biopharm.* **2012**, *82*, 291–298. [CrossRef] [PubMed]
5. Gomes, S.F.D.O.; Nunan, E.D.A.; Ferreira, L.A.M. Influence of the formulation type (o/w, w/o/w emulsions and ointment) on the topical delivery of paromomycin. *Rev. Bras. Cienc. Farm.* **2004**, *40*, 345–352. [CrossRef]
6. Zhang, Z.; Lukic, M.; Savic, S.; Lunter, D.J. Reinforcement of barrier function-skin repair formulations to deliver physiological lipids into skin. *Int. J. Cosmet. Sci.* **2018**, *40*, 494–501. [CrossRef]
7. Daniels, R.; Knie, U. Galenics of dermal products-vehicles, properties and drug release. *J. Dtsch. Dermatol. Ges.* **2007**, *5*, 367–383. [CrossRef]
8. McNamara, T.F.; Steinbach, L. Skin Substantivity as a Criterion. *J. Soc. Cosmet. Chem.* **1965**, *16*, 499–506.
9. Schmidberger, M.; Daniels, R.; Lunter, D.J. Method to determine the impact of substantivity on ex vivo skin-permeation. *Eur. J. Pharm. Biopharm.* **2018**, *131*, 1–7. [CrossRef]
10. Herrmann, S.; Daniels, R.; Lunter, D.J. Methods for the determination of the substantivity of topical formulations. *Pharm. Dev. Technol.* **2017**, *22*, 487–491. [CrossRef]
11. Dickinson, E. Hydrocolloids as emulsifiers and emulsion stabilizers. *Food Hydrocoll.* **2009**, *23*, 1473–1482. [CrossRef]
12. Gaonkar, A.G. Surface and interfacial activities and emulsion characteristics of some food hydrocolloids. *Food Hydrocoll.* **1991**, *5*, 329–337. [CrossRef]
13. Huang, X.; Kakuda, Y.; Cui, W. Hydrocolloids in emulsions: Particle size distribution and interfacial activity. *Food Hydrocoll.* **2001**, *15*, 533–542. [CrossRef]
14. Wollenweber, C.; Makievski, A.; Miller, R.; Daniels, R. Adsorption of hydroxypropyl methylcellulose at the liquid/liquid interface and the effect on emulsion stability. *Colloids Surfaces A Physicochem. Eng. Asp.* **2000**, *172*, 91–101. [CrossRef]
15. Desbrières, J.; Hirrien, M.; Ross-Murphy, S. Thermogelation of methylcellulose: Rheological considerations. *Polymer* **2000**, *41*, 2451–2461. [CrossRef]
16. Caterina, M.J.; Schumacher, M.A.; Tominaga, M.; Rosen, T.A.; Levine, J.D.; Julius, D. The capsaicin receptor: A heat-activated ion channel in the pain pathway. *Nature* **1997**, *389*, 816–824. [CrossRef] [PubMed]
17. Ständer, S.; Moormann, C.; Schumacher, M.; Buddenkotte, J.; Artuc, M.; Shpacovitch, V.; Brzoska, T.; Lippert, U.; Henz, B.M.; Luger, T.A.; et al. Expression of vanilloid receptor subtype 1 in cutaneous sensory nerve fibers, mast cells, and epithelial cells of appendage structures. *Exp. Dermatol.* **2004**, *13*, 129–139. [CrossRef]
18. Ständer, S.; Luger, T.; Metze, D. Treatment of prurigo nodularis with topical capsaicin. *J. Am. Acad. Dermatol.* **2001**, *44*, 471–478. [CrossRef]
19. Nakagawa, H.; Hiura, A. Four Possible Itching Pathways Related to the TRPV1 Channel, Histamine, PAR-2 and Serotonin. *Malays. J. Med Sci.* **2013**, *20*, 5–12.
20. Pereira, M.P.; Ständer, S. Chronic Pruritus: Current and Emerging Treatment Options. *Drugs* **2017**, *96*, 50–1007. [CrossRef]
21. Anand, P.; Bley, K. Topical capsaicin for pain management: Therapeutic potential and mechanisms of action of the new high-concentration capsaicin 8% patch. *Br. J. Anaesth.* **2011**, *107*, 490–502. [CrossRef] [PubMed]
22. Takeuchi, M.; Kageyama, S.; Suzuki, H.; Wada, T.; Notsu, Y.; Ishii, F. Rheological properties of reversible thermo-setting in situ gelling solutions with the methylcellulose?polyethylene glycol?citric acid ternary system. *Colloid Polym. Sci.* **2003**, *281*, 1178–1183. [CrossRef]

23. DAC/NRF. Hydrophile Capsaicinoid Creme 0.025%/0.05%/0.1% (NRF 11.125). In *Neues Rezepturformularium®*; ABDA, Ed.; Govi Verlag: Eschborn, Germany, 2013.
24. Jacobi, U.; Kaiser, M.; Toll, R.; Mangelsdorf, S.; Audring, H.; Otberg, N.; Sterry, W.; Lademann, J. Porcine ear skin: An in vitro model for human skin. *Skin Res. Technol.* **2007**, *13*, 19–24. [CrossRef] [PubMed]
25. Barbero, A.M.; Frasch, H.F. Pig and guinea pig skin as surrogates for human in vitro penetration studies: A quantitative review. *Toxicol. Vitr.* **2009**, *23*, 1–13. [CrossRef] [PubMed]
26. Jung, E.C.; Maibach, H.I. Animal models for percutaneous absorption. *J. Appl. Toxicol.* **2015**, *35*, 1–10. [CrossRef] [PubMed]
27. Heck, R.; Lukić, M. Ž.; Savić, S.D.; Daniels, R.; Lunter, D.J. Ex vivo skin permeation and penetration of nonivamide from and in vivo skin tolerability of film-forming formulations containing porous silica. *Eur. J. Pharm. Sci.* **2017**, *106*, 34–40. [CrossRef] [PubMed]
28. Chantelain, E.; Gabard, B.; Surber, C. Skin penetration and sun protection factor of five UV filters: effect of the vehicle. *Skin Pharmacol. Appl. Skin Physiol.* **2003**, *16*, 28–35. [CrossRef] [PubMed]
29. Delange, J. The Rate of Percutaneous Permeation of Xylene, Measured Using the "Perfused Pig Ear" Model, Is Dependent on the Effective Protein Concentration in the Perfusing Medium. *Toxicol. Appl. Pharmacol.* **1994**, *127*, 298–305. [CrossRef]
30. Williams, A.; Barry, B.; Williams, A. Urea analogues in propylene glycol as penetration enhancers in human skin. *Int. J. Pharm.* **1989**, *56*, 43–50. [CrossRef]
31. Good, W.R.; Powers, M.S.; Campbell, P.; Schenkel, L. A new transdermal delivery system for estradiol. *J. Control. Release* **1985**, *2*, 89–97. [CrossRef]
32. Williams, A.C.; Barry, B.W. Penetration enhancers. *Adv. Drug. Deliver Rev.* **2012**, *64*, 128–137. [CrossRef]
33. Lin, H.R.; Sung, K.C.; Vong, W.J. In Situ Gelling of Alginate/Pluronic Solutions for Ophthalmic Delivery of Pilocarpine. *Biomacromolecules* **2004**, *5*, 2358–2365. [CrossRef] [PubMed]
34. Zhang, L.; Shen, W.; Luan, J.; Yang, D.; Wei, G.; Yu, L.; Lu, W.; Ding, J. Sustained intravitreal delivery of dexamethasone using an injectable and biodegradable thermogel. *Acta Biomater.* **2015**, *23*, 271–281. [CrossRef] [PubMed]
35. Van Hemelrijck, C.; Müller-Goymann, C.C. Rheological characterization and permeation behavior of poloxamer 407-based systems containing 5-aminolevulinic acid for potential application in photodynamic therapy. *Int. J. Pharm.* **2012**, *437*, 120–129. [CrossRef] [PubMed]

pharmaceutics

MDPI

Article

Nanostructured Lipid Carrier Gel for the Dermal Application of Lidocaine: Comparison of Skin Penetration Testing Methods

Stella Zsikó [1], Kendra Cutcher [2], Anita Kovács [1], Mária Budai-Szűcs [1], Attila Gácsi [1], Gabriella Baki [2], Erzsébet Csányi [1] and Szilvia Berkó [1,*]

1 Institute of Pharmaceutical Technology and Regulatory Affairs, Faculty of Pharmacy, University of Szeged, 6720 Szeged, Hungary
2 Frederic and Mary Wolfe Center, College of Pharmacy and Pharmaceutical Sciences, University of Toledo, Toledo, OH 43614, USA
* Correspondence: berkosz@pharm.u-szeged.hu

Received: 6 May 2019; Accepted: 25 June 2019; Published: 2 July 2019

Abstract: The aim of this research was to investigate the stability of a lidocaine-loaded nanostructured lipid carrier dispersion at different temperatures, formulate a nanostructured lipid carrier gel, and test the penetration profile of lidocaine from the nanostructured lipid carrier gel using different skin penetration modeling methods. The formulations were characterized by laser diffraction, rheological measurements and microscopic examinations. Various in vitro methods were used to study drug release, diffusion and penetration. Two types of vertical Franz diffusion cells with three different membranes, including cellulose, Strat-M®, and heat separated human epidermis were used and compared to the Skin-parallel artificial membrane permeability assay (PAMPA) method. Results indicated that the nanostructured lipid carrier dispersion had to be gelified as soon as possible for proper stability. Both the Skin-PAMPA model and Strat-M® membranes correlated favorably with heat separated human epidermis in this research, with the Strat-M® membranes sharing the most similar drug permeability profile to an ex vivo human skin model. Our experimental findings suggest that even when the best available in vitro experiment is selected for modeling human skin penetration to study nanostructured lipid carrier gel systems, relevant in vitro/in vivo correlation should be made to calculate the drug release/permeation in vivo. Future investigations in this field are still needed to demonstrate the influence of membranes and equipment from other classes on other drug candidates.

Keywords: dermal drug delivery; diffusion cell; Franz diffusion; Skin-PAMPA; Strat-M® membrane; nanocarrier

---

1. Introduction

Topical and transdermal formulations are widely used for delivering drugs to the skin and underlying tissue, or through the skin for systemic action. The vast majority of topically applied formulations are semisolids, including creams, ointments and gels, which offer suitable residence time on the skin, and are usually well accepted by the patients. Topical formulations deliver the active pharmaceutical ingredients (APIs) into different layers of the skin, thus enabling several diseases to be prevented and/or cured. The beginning, duration and strength of the therapeutic effect depend on the efficacy of three consecutive processes: (1) The release of the API from the carrier system; (2) penetration/diffusion of the API into the stratum corneum or other skin layers; (3) exertion of a pharmacological effect at the target point. All these effects determine the safety-efficacy profile of a product [1–3]. For most skin problems or diseases, the target point is the stratum corneum, viable epidermis or dermis.

Modeling of penetration through the skin is discussed by numerous directives [4–8]. The in vitro method for skin penetration modeling is included in OECD Guideline 428 [5]. Advantages of the in vitro method are that measurements can be carried out on human skin samples among other potential membranes; multiple tests can be performed on a skin sample from the same donor; several formulations can be tested at the same time; there is no need for radio-labelling the test material; and there are no ethical issues.

Topical semisolid products are complex formulations with a complex structure. Physical properties of the composition depend on several factors, including particle size of dispersed particles, surface tension between the phases, fractional distribution of the drug between the phases, and rheological behavior of the product. These properties collectively determine the in vitro dissolution profile, together with other characteristics. The amount of API released in vitro is an important quality characteristic of a product. Modeling of penetration through the skin is a complex challenge. The device and the membrane, along with the properties of the product influence how the system can be tested most effectively. There are various types of equipment with which the diffusion and penetration of drug carrier systems can be studied. Human skin tests give the most relevant information; however, because of the high cost, it is a generally accepted approach to choose simpler methods in the early stages of formulation development. Previously, several simple, reliable, reproducible and validated methods were described for drug liberation by a vertical diffusion cell (VDC) using a synthetic membrane [9–11]. In vitro drug release testing is a widely used and reliable tool for evaluating products.

The use of Franz diffusion cells to evaluate skin permeability has developed into a major research methodology. With Franz diffusion studies, diffusion and penetration of an API through the skin and the relationships among the skin, drug and formulation can be investigated [12–19]. Franz diffusion cells are available with multiple types of automatic sampler systems. A lot of different membranes, including artificial and biological membranes can be applied on the Franz cells. Artificial membranes provide a simple and reproducible alternative way to study the basic physicochemical mechanisms of the drug diffusion, including interactions between the carrier and the membrane. They are suitable for early-stage drug development studies [13]. The Strat-M® membrane, built by two polyether sulfone layers, was specifically designed for skin penetration studies. The layers are impregnated with a mixture of synthetic lipids, and a polyolefin layer is located underneath. Moving downwards into the membrane layers, the size of the pores increases [20]. Transdermal diffusion and safety of APIs, excipients, functional cosmetic ingredients, cosmetic active substances, and finished products can be tested using the Strat-M® membrane. Advantages include that its diffusion properties are highly correlated with human diffusion studies, and it is characterized by minimal variability. It is also long-lasting and requires no special storage conditions or preparation for its use [20–24]. In addition to synthetic membranes, human skin membranes can also be used to model skin penetration. In the development of dermal preparations, it is not sufficient to perform membrane diffusion studies. It is necessary to do permeation studies through the biological membrane since the interaction of the API and carrier system with the skin can also be investigated, and it can be determined whether and to what extent the skin acts as a reservoir for the API. Usually, skin sections are obtained from plastic surgery, and a heat-separated epidermis is used as a membrane [13,25,26].

The parallel artificial membrane permeability assay (PAMPA) is a device that is adapted to simulate penetration of a product into the skin. For Skin-PAMPA, the bottom part of the PAMPA sandwich is substituted by a special donor plate, which was designed to study semi-solid products. It contains synthetic ceramides and has similar penetration properties to full-thickness skin. Synthetic lipids are easier to store, and their stability is more favorable [27–30]. The biomimetic model is able to determine in vitro human skin data based on the tests and can be a good alternative to skin permeability testing [17,28,31].

Lidocaine is a commonly used numbing agent before local interventions. Delivering lidocaine to the skin from a specific vehicle provides a numbing/pain relief effect to that area. It is possible to localize the numbing effect onto a smaller skin area without reaching the muscle. By concentrating the numbing effect to the skin, the patient is able to retain full motor function of the area to which lidocaine is applied.

Our research group previously formulated and compared different drug carrier systems for the dermal delivery of lidocaine, including a conventional hydrogel, an oleogel, a lyotropic liquid crystalline gel and nanostructured lipid carrier (NLC) gel. It was concluded that the penetration of lidocaine from the NLC gel was the most significant, and the skin hydrating and occlusive effect made it a favorable carrier system [25,32]. In addition, several articles in the literature featured lidocaine-filled NLCs or NLC gels [33–37]. Therefore, a lidocaine-loaded NLC and NLC gel was selected for the current investigations.

In this study, our aims were to investigate the stability of a lidocaine-loaded NLC dispersion at various storage temperatures, formulate an NLC gel, and evaluate the penetration profile of lidocaine from the NLC gel. Two types of vertical Franz diffusion cells with three different membranes, including a cellulose membrane, Strat-M® membrane, and heat separated human epidermis were used to study the drug release and permeation. Additionally, the NLC gels were evaluated using the Skin-PAMPA method, and the three methods were compared.

2. Materials and Methods

2.1. Materials

Lidocaine base and glycerol were obtained from Hungaropharma Ltd. (Budapest, Hungary). Miglyol® 812 N (caprylic/capric triglyceride) was a gift from Sasol GmbH (Hamburg, Germany). Cremophor® RH 60 (PEG-60 Hydrogenated Castor Oil; HLB value: 15–17) was kindly supplied by BASF SE Chemtrade GmbH (Ludwigshafen, Germany). Apifil® (PEG-8 Beeswax) was a gift from Gattefossé (St. Priest, France). Methocel™ E4M (hydroxypropyl methylcellulose) was from Colorcon (Budapest, Hungary). The water used was purified and deionized with the Milli-Q system from Millipore (Milford, MA, USA). The cellulose acetate filter (Porafil membrane filter, cellulose acetate, pore diameter: 0.45 μm) was obtained from Macherey-Nagel GmbH & Co. KG (Düren, Germany). The Strat-M® membrane (Strat-M® Membrane, Transdermal Diffusion Test Model, 25 mm) was from Merck KGaA (Darmstadt, Germany). Excised human skin was obtained from a Caucasian female patient by routine plastic surgery procedure in the Department of Dermatology and Allergology, University of Szeged. The ex vivo skin penetration test does not need ethical permission, and patient's consent according to the Act CLIV of 1997 on health, Section 210/A in Hungary. The local ethical committee (Ethical Committee of the University of Szeged, Albert Szent-Györgyi Clinical Center) was informed about the ex vivo skin penetration studies (Human Investigation Review Board license number: 83/2008). The Skin-PAMPA sandwiches (P/N: 120657), hydration solution (P/N: 120706) and stirring bars (P/N: 110066) were purchased from Pion, Inc (Woburn, MA, USA). The UV plates (UV-star micro plate, clear, flat bottom, half area) were from Greiner Bio-one (Kremsmünster, Austria).

2.2. Methods

2.2.1. Preparation of the NLC

NLCs are colloidal carriers which were introduced in the early 1990s. They are derived from o/w emulsions by replacing the liquid lipid with a solid lipid at room temperature. The lipophlic phase of NLC included Apifil, Cremophor RH 60 and Miglyol 812 N, which were melted at 60 °C under controlled stirring. Then lidocaine was added to the melted lipid phase under similar conditions. Then purified water was added to the lipid phase to form the pre-emulsion. The pre-emulsion was ultrasonicated using a Hielscher UP200S compact ultrasonic homogenizer (Hielscher Ultrasonics GmbH, Teltow, Germany) for 10 min at 70% amplitude. At the end, the sample was cooled in ice to obtain the solid lipid particles (LID-NLC) [38]. For dermal application, a gel was formed at room temperature with glycerol and Methocel E4M. In the last step, the NLC dispersion was added to the gel (LID-NLC gel). A blank-NLC and blank-NLC gel were also prepared using the same procedure, but without adding lidocaine. Table 1 summarizes the formulations. The NLC formulations were stored at different temperatures 7 °C (cold) and 25 °C (room temperature).

Table 1. Compositions of the test preparations.

LID-NLC	Blank NLC	LID-NLC Gel	Blank NLC-Gel
Apifil 11.8%	Apifil 11.8%	LID-NLC 89%	Blank NLC 89%
Cremophor RH 60.8%	Cremophor RH 60.8%	Glycerin 8%	Glycerin 8%
Miglyol 812 N 5%	Miglyol 812 N 5%	Methocel E4M 3%	Methocel E4M 3%
Purified water 69.2%	Purified water 75.2%		
Lidocaine 6%			

2.2.2. Laser Diffraction

Laser diffraction analysis was performed with a Malvern Mastersizer 2000 particle size analyzer provided with the Hydro SM wet dispersion unit (Malvern Instruments, Worcestershire, UK) to determine the particle size and stability of the NLC formulation at different temperatures (cold and room temperature). A few drops of the sample were placed inside the Hydro SM loaded with purified water, and the speed of the stirrer was set to 2000 rpm. Three values, namely d(0.1), d(0.5), and d(0.9), were evaluated, indicating that 10%, 50%, and 90% of the analyzed particles were below a certain size (diameter). The span value describing the width of the particle size distribution curve ((d(0.9) − d(0.1))/d(0.5)) was calculated as well.

2.2.3. Rheological Measurements

Rheological measurements were performed with a Physica MCR101 rheometer (Anton Paar GmbH, Graz, Austria), employing a parallel plate geometry PP25 with a measuring gap of 0.1 mm to verify the proper consistency of the LID-NLC gel system for topical application. The blank-NLC gel was studied as well. Flow curves, viscosity curves and frequency sweep tests were obtained. The shear rate was increased from 0.1 to 100 1/s (up-curve) and then decreased from 100 to 0.1 1/s (down-curve) in CR mode. The shearing time in was 300 s. The measurements were carried out at 25 °C [39].

2.2.4. Microscopic Examinations

The structure of the NLC samples was examined with a microscope (LEICA DM6 B, Leica Microsystems GmbH, Wetzlar, Germany) at room temperature. Magnifications were 100× and 200×.

2.2.5. pH Measurements

For pH measurement, 10 g of each sample (NLC dispersion and NLC gel) was placed in a beaker, and the surface pH was measured using a Testo 206 pH meter (Testo SE & Co. KGaA, Lenzkirch, Germany) with a pH2 probe. Three parallel measurements were carried out at room temperature.

2.2.6. Drug Diffusion and Penetration Studies

Three different methods were used to model and compare drug release and diffusion through the membrane and penetration into the skin from the LID-NLC gel (Table 2). The methods included two types of vertical Franz diffusion cells, namely Hanson Microette TM Topical & Transdermal Diffusion Cell System, and Logan Automated Dry heat sampling system. The third method used was the Skin-PAMPA method. On the Franz cells, the donor and acceptor phases were separated by either a synthetic cellulose acetate membrane, a Strat-M® membrane or heat-separated human epidermis (HSE). A 0.3 g portion of sample was placed in the donor chamber on the membrane. The human skin was placed in a water bath (60 ± 0.5 °C), and the epidermis was separated from the dermis. Thermostated phosphate buffer solution (PBS pH 7.4 ± 0.15), made in-house, kept at

32 ± 0.5 °C was used as the acceptor phase. Membrane diffusion and skin penetration experiments lasted 24 h (sampling times: 0.5; 1; 2; 3; 4; 5; 6; 8; 10; 12; 16; 20; and 24 h). The stirring speed was 400 rpm. The concentration of the drug was measured spectrophotometrically with a Thermo Scientific Evolution 201 spectrometer with Thermo Insight v1.4.40 software package (Thermo Fisher Scientific, Waltham, MA, USA) at a wavelength of 262 nm (analytical parameters: Slope: 0.001738 ± 0.000016; SE: 4.554×10^{-5}; SD: 0.0001205; LOD: 0.2339 μg/mL; LOQ: 0.7088 μg/mL). The Skin-PAMPA sandwiches were used after a 24-hour hydration period (Hydration Solution, Pion, Inc., Billerica, MA, USA). 70 μL of the NLC gels were applied to the well of the formulation plate as the donor phase. Phosphate buffer solution (PBS pH 7.4 ± 0.15), made in-house, was used as the acceptor phase. The top plate was filled with 250 μL of fresh acceptor solution, and a stirring bar was also used in each well. The Gut-Box™ from Pion, Inc. was used for stirring; the resultant sandwich was incubated at 32 °C for six hours. The Skin-PAMPA membrane is not designed for 24-h measurements, the membrane can provide relevant values for a shorter time. Therefore, the acceptor solution was examined after 0.5, 1, 2, 3, 4, 5 and 6 h of incubation. The quantity of the API was determined by UV spectroscopy at 262 nm using a Synergy HT UV plate reader by KC4 (BIO-TEK Instruments, Inc., Winooski, VT, USA) software. The quantity of the permeated API was expressed as μg/cm^2 units.

Table 2. The experimental design of drug diffusion and penetration studies.

Device	Hanson	Logan	Skin-PAMPA
Membrane	Cellulose acetate Strat-M® HSE	Cellulose acetate Strat-M® HSE	Skin-PAMPA membrane

2.2.7. Statistical Analysis

Two-way ANOVA analysis of variance (Bonferroni post-test), working with Prism for Windows software (GraphPad Software Inc., La Jolla, CA, USA), was used to analyze the statistical difference between the samples. Results are shown as average of six parallel experiments and standard deviation (SD). Variations were considered significant if $p < 0.05$ *, $p < 0.01$ ** and $p < 0.001$ *** versus the control.

3. Results and Discussion

3.1. Particle Size Analysis

Usually light scattering methods, such as photon correlation spectroscopy and/or laser diffraction (LD) are used for particle size determination of lipid nanoparticles. LD is a powerful method that has a wider detection spectrum (20 nm–2.000 μm), and it is considered a better option for lipid nanoparticles in the upper nanometer and micrometer size ranges.

All NLC dispersions were in the nanosize range, between 97 and 163 nm (d(0.5)). The particle size of LID-NLC stored at room temperature was the smallest (97 nm), and it was stable for three days (the values of d(0.5) and d(0.9) were below 200 nm). On the fourth day, the d(0.9) values showed a significant increase (41.749 μm). The particle size of the NLC dispersion stored in the refrigerator increased after one day. The reason for this instability was that lidocaine crystallized in the refrigerator, and the formulation was not stable under these conditions. The exact parameters are summarized in Table 3. According to the particle size analysis, the holding time of the preparation was three days at room temperature.

Table 3. Particle size of nanostructured lipid carrier (NLC) dispersions stored at different conditions.

Day	NLC Dispersion	d(0.1) μm	d(0.5) μm	d(0.9) μm	Span
1st day	Blank-NLC, room temperature	0.066	0.131	0.320	1.950
	Blank-NLC, cooled	0.066	0.130	0.302	1.821
	LID-NLC, room temperature	0.069	0.098	0.145	0.787
	LID-NLC, cooled	0.069	0.098	0.146	0.790
2nd day	Blank-NLC, room temperature	0.065	0.127	0.266	1.584
	Blank-NLC, cooled	0.065	0.127	0.266	1.587
	LID-NLC, room temperature	0.068	0.097	0.144	0.782
	LID-NLC, cooled	0.073	0.114	0.259	1.625
3rd day	Blank-NLC, room temperature	0.065	0.126	0.258	1.542
	Blank-NLC, cooled	0.065	0.126	0.262	1.564
	LID-NLC, room temperature	0.069	0.098	0.146	0.791
	LID-NLC, cooled	0.079	0.130	0.300	1.698
4th day	Blank-NLC, room temperature	0.065	0.128	0.289	1.746
	Blank-NLC, cooled	0.065	0.128	0.298	1.814
	LID-NLC, room temperature	0.090	0.163	41.749	255.201
	LID-NLC, cooled	-	-	-	-

3.2. *Microscopic Study*

Parallel to the particle size analysis, microscopic studies were performed as well on the NLC dispersions. As it can be seen in Figure 1, in cooled circumstances lidocaine crystals appeared on the second day, while at room temperature they appeared on the third day. Based on the microscopic examination, the holding time of the NLC dispersion was two days at room temperature.

The structure of the LID-NLC gel was examined with a polarized light microscope as well. The formula had a homogenous structure after two weeks, no API crystals were detected (Figure 2). It can be concluded based on these results that it is very important to gelify the NLC dispersion as soon as possible for proper stability.

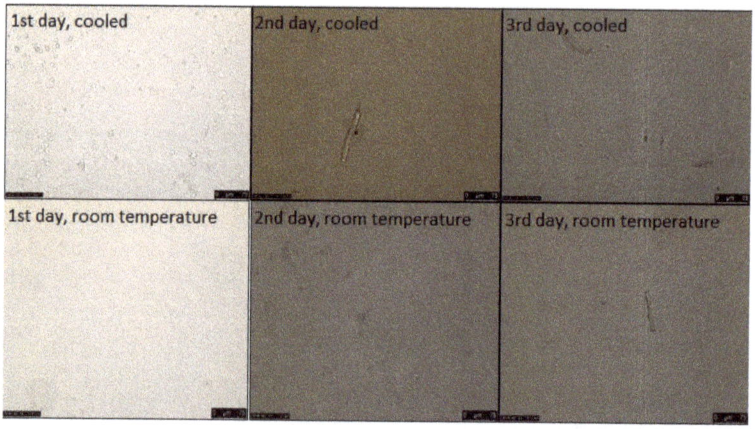

Figure 1. The NLC dispersions' stability over the course of three days at different storage conditions. (The magnification was 200×).

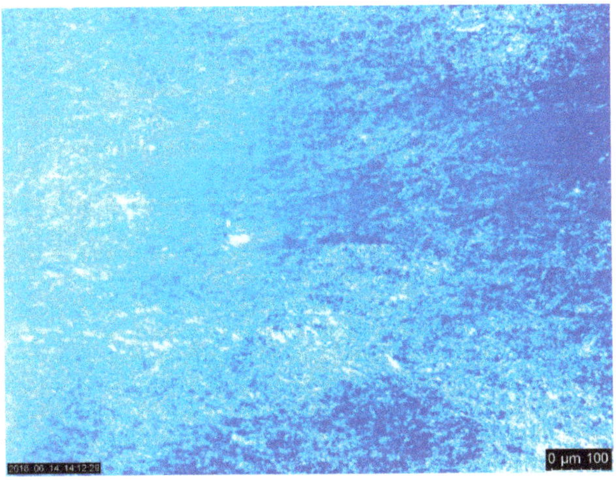

Figure 2. The solid lipid particles (LID-NLC) gel in polarized light at week two. (The magnification was 100×).

3.3. Rheological Studies

The LID-NLC gel had a shear thinning behavior (Figure 3A), which means the shear stress increased continuously with the shear rate, but the rate of the increase decreased. Slight thixotropy was observed, meaning that structure regeneration was time-dependent. The viscosity value of the LID-NLC gel at the shear rate of 100 1/s was 6.72 Pa·s at 25 °C. According to the rheological measurements, the consistency of the formulation was suitable for dermal use. The viscosity value of the blank-NLC gel at the shear rate of 100 1/s was 5.58 Pa·s at 25 °C. Based on the rheological curves, it can be stated that incorporation of the API into the formulation made the system more viscous. Viscosity values increased and consistency improved. The frequency sweep test (Figure 3B) showed a viscoelastic behavior, where the elastic characteristic dominated (G′ higher than G″); with a relatively large frequency dependence of the moduli (G′ and G″) which is a typical feature of a so-called weak gel.

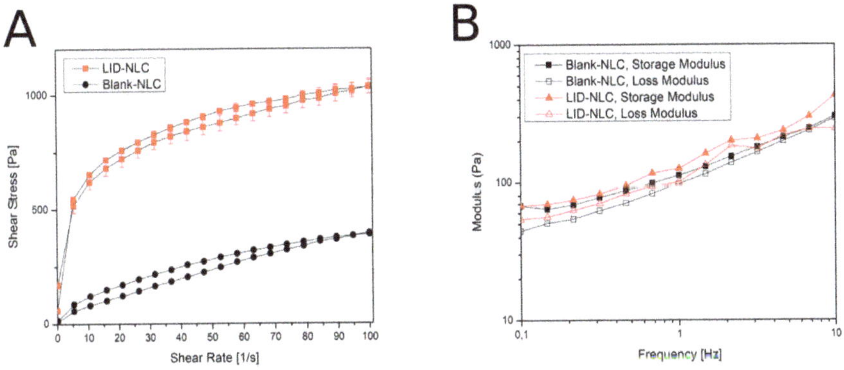

Figure 3. Rheological behavior of the NLC gel. (**A**): flow curves; (**B**): frequency sweep test.

3.4. pH Measurement

pH of the blank-NLC dispersion was 5.2 ± 0.2 and the blank-NLC gel 5.3 ± 0.3. pH of the LID-NLC dispersion was 8.0 ± 0.3 and the LID-NLC gel 7.9 ± 0.4. Due to its basic characteristics, the active ingredient increased the pH value of the preparation.

3.5. Drug Release, Diffusion and Penetration Studies

The in vitro diffusion/penetration of lidocaine from the LID-NLC gel through the two synthetic and one biological membranes and the Skin-PAMPA membrane were calculated in terms of the mean cumulative amount and percentage diffused/penetrated ± SD by 6 or 24 h (Table 4).

The cellulose acetate membrane is a non-barrier, non-skin like membrane, which was used to measure the in vitro release of lidocaine from the NLC gel. As expected, a high amount of lidocaine released through this membrane over the course of 24 h from both Franz cell types (Figure 4A). Differences between the Logan and Hanson Franz cell results were not significant, however, a lower standard deviation was observed with the Hanson method.

Table 4. The mean cumulative amount and percentage (%) diffused or penetrated at 6 and 24 h (μg/cm^2).

Time of Experiment	Cellulose		Strat-M®		HSE		Skin-PAMPA
	Hanson	Logan	Hanson	Logan	Hanson	Logan	
6 h (μg/cm^2)	3808.82 ± 448.91	3355.40 ± 320.70	304.20 ± 113.40	514.89 ± 209.69	1778.25 ± 483.81	670.85 ± 189.05	696.32 ± 20.50
6 h (%)	41.35 ± 18.8	27.73 ± 0.83	3.45 ± 1.21	7.72 ± 2.89	11.61 ± 2.95	8.785 ± 2.03	13.93 ± 0.41
24 h (μg/cm^2)	8014.05 ± 471.89	6878.13 ± 1172.21	1079.27 ± 304.36	1847.08 ± 335.19	3094.60 ± 829.73	1222.69 ± 358.70	-
24 h (%)	70.40 ± 13.72	58.66 ± 4.28	12.96 ± 3.52	27.89 ± 5.17	19.44 ± 5.05	16.00 ± 3.81	-

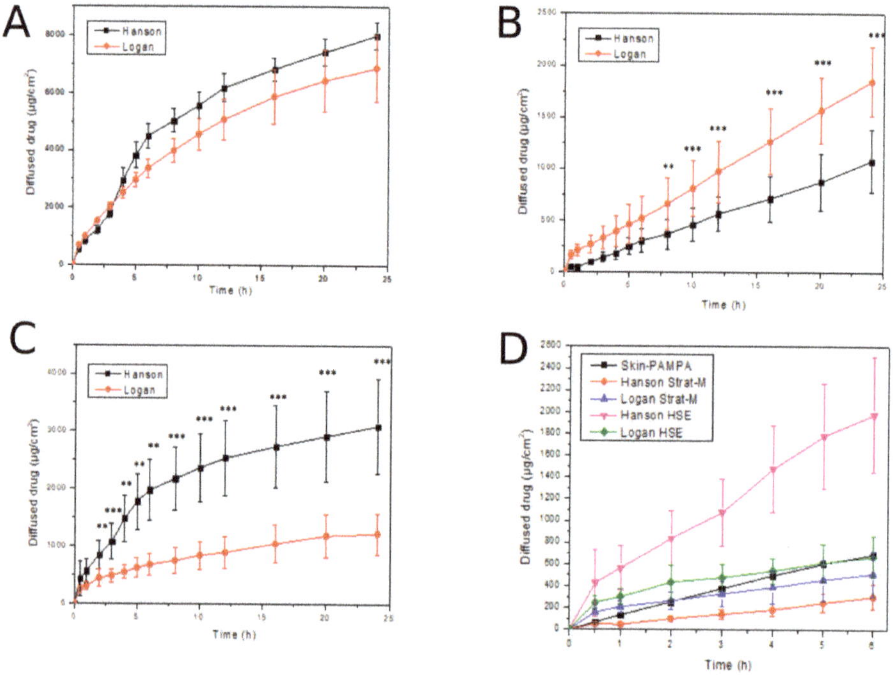

Figure 4. In vitro drug diffusion and ex vivo skin penetration studies. (**A**): In vitro release of lidocaine through cellulose acetate membrane (24 h); (**B**): In vitro penetration of lidocaine through Strat-M® membrane (24 h); (**C**): Ex vivo penetration of lidocaine through HSE (24 h); (**D**): Comparison of various penetration methods with various membranes (6 h). $p < 0.05$ *, $p < 0.01$ ** and $p < 0.001$ *** compared to each other within each one figure.

The Strat-M® membrane and HSE were skin-like and acted as barriers to API penetration. Figure 4B shows the penetration of lidocaine via the synthetic Strat-M® membrane, which Figure 4C shows the penetration via HSE. As for the Strat-M® membrane, differences between the Logan and Hanson Franz cells were significant after eight hours. Penetration via the HSE was higher than via the Strat-M® membrane, especially on Hanson device over the 24 h. In the case of HSE, differences between the Logan and Hanson Franz cells were significant from two hours. This significant difference between the two types of Franz cells can be explained by the difference in structure of the two devices. The Logan cell was open from above, therefore the measurement runs on atmospheric pressure. However, the cell of the Hanson device was closed from the top and the pressure is higher leading to significantly higher penetration. The standard deviation was similar with the two methods. Figure 4D presents the diffusion/penetration data via the three different membranes (Strat-M®, Skin-PAMPA, HSE) tested on the Franz cells and Skin-PAMPA system. A lower standard deviation was observed with the PAMPA model than with the Franz cell method. This may be caused by the diversity in the membrane structure of the two methods. However, the penetration profiles of the Skin PAMPA and in vitro and ex vivo Franz cell methods were in good balance. If comparing the results at 6 h, the values obtained with Logan cells and Skin-PAMPA method were close to each other. Our results demonstrated that a novel Strat-M® synthetic membrane and the Skin-PAMPA method have the potential to be used as an early screening tool to select the best dermal lidocaine-loaded nanoformulation.

4. Conclusions

A lidocaine-loaded NLC dispersion and a lidocaine-loaded, NLC gel were formulated to study their stability at various temperatures and evaluate their in vitro release as well as in vitro and ex vivo skin penetration. The NLC dispersions were found to be stable at room temperature, with acceptable changes in particle characteristics, for two days. Microscopic evaluations further verified the stability of the NLC dispersion at room temperature. It can be concluded that two days is a reasonable time period to create a gel from this NLC dispersion. The microscopic and rheological measurements verified that the consistency of the formulation was well suitable for dermal use, and the gel was stable for at least two weeks at room temperature.

Synthetic membranes are useful tools to examine and determine which formulation is the most promising for in vivo human skin studies. There are numerous commercial membranes available, all of which may have different drug diffusion properties. Cellulose membranes were used to study in vitro drug release, while the Skin-PAMPA membranes and Strat-M® membranes were used for modeling in vitro skin penetration. Both the Skin-PAMPA and Strat-M® membranes correlated well with HSE in this study, but the Strat-M® membranes shared the most similar drug permeability profile to an ex vivo human skin model. Our results can be used to guide formulators in selecting vehicles in early development in the pharmaceutical, personal care and cosmetic industries. Overall, researchers must carefully select the most suitable membrane to be used with Franz cells for topical quality control testing.

Modeling of penetration through the skin is a complex challenge. The drug release profiles of the LID-NLC gel obtained with the different techniques were not fully equivalent. The device and the membrane, along with the properties of the product itself, influence how the system can be tested most effectively. Based on our results, we can select the best in vitro test for modeling human skin penetration of NLC gel systems, but appropriate in vitro/in vivo correlation should be performed to calculate the drug release in vivo. Future studies in this field are still needed to explain the influence of membranes and equipment from other classes on other drug candidates.

Author Contributions: Conceptualization, S.Z. and S.B.; methodology, S.Z. and S.B.; software, M.B.-S.; validation, A.K.; formal analysis, S.Z. and K.C.; investigation, S.Z. and K.C.; writing—original draft preparation, S.Z.; writing—review and editing, G.B., E.C.; visualization, A.G.; supervision, S.B. and E.C.

Funding: This research received no external funding.

Acknowledgments: The authors would like to thank Sasol GmbH, Gattefossé and BASF SE for the gift samples. We are grateful for the financial support of the "GINOP 2.2.1-15-2016-00023" as they have made this article possible.

Conflicts of Interest: The authors declare no conflicts of interest.

References

1. Shah, V.P.; Yacobi, A.; Rădulescu, F.Ş.; Miron, D.S.; Lane, M.E. A science based approach to topical drug classification system (TCS). *Int. J. Pharm.* **2015**, *491*, 21–25. [CrossRef] [PubMed]
2. Dragicevic, N.; Maibach, H.I. *Percutaneous Penetration Enhancers Drug Penetration Into/Through the Skin*; Springer Berlin Heidelberg: Berlin/Heidelberg, Germany, 2017; ISBN 978-3-662-53268-3.
3. Ruela, A.L.M.; Perissinato, A.G.; Lino, M.E.D.S.; Mudrik, P.S.; Pereira, G.R. Evaluation of skin absorption of drugs from topical and transdermal formulations. *Br. J. Pharm. Sci.* **2016**, *52*, 527–544. [CrossRef]
4. OECD. *Guidance Notes on Dermal Absorption, Series on Testing and Assessment No. 156*; OECD: Paris, France, 2011.
5. OECD. *Test Guideline 428: Skin Absorption: In vitro Method*; OECD: Paris, France, 2004.
6. OECD. *Test Guideline 427: Skin Absorption: In vivo Method*; OECD: Paris, France, 2004.
7. OECD. *Guidance Document for the Conduct of Skin Absorption Studies*; OECD: Paris, France, 2004.
8. European Food Safety Authority (EFSA); Buist, H.; Craig, P.; Dewhurst, I.; Hougaard Bennekou, S.; Kneuer, C.; Machera, K.; Pieper, C.; Court Marques, D.; Guillot, G.; et al. Guidance on dermal absorption. *EFSA J.* **2017**, *15*, 4873. [CrossRef]
9. Shah, V.P.; Elkins, J.; Shaw, S.; Hanson, R. In Vitro Release: Comparative Evaluation of Vertical Diffusion Cell System and Automated Procedure: RESEARCH ARTICLE. *Pharm. Dev. Technol.* **2003**, *8*, 97–102. [CrossRef] [PubMed]
10. Hauck, W.W.; Shah, V.P.; Shaw, S.W.; Ueda, C.T. Reliability and Reproducibility of Vertical Diffusion Cells for Determining Release Rates from Semisolid Dosage Forms. *Pharm. Res.* **2007**, *24*, 2018–2024. [CrossRef]
11. Franz, T.J. Percutaneous Absorption. On the Relevance of in Vitro Data. *J. Invest. Dermatol.* **1975**, *64*, 190–195. [CrossRef]
12. Bakonyi, M.; Gácsi, A.; Berkó, S.; Kovács, A.; Csányi, E. Stratum corneum lipid liposomes for investigating skin penetration enhancer effects. *RSC Adv.* **2018**, *8*, 27464–27469. [CrossRef]
13. Flaten, G.E.; Palac, Z.; Engesland, A.; Filipović-Grčić, J.; Vanić, Ž.; Škalko-Basnet, N. In vitro skin models as a tool in optimization of drug formulation. *Eur. J. Pharm. Sci.* **2015**, *75*, 10–24. [CrossRef]
14. Intarakumhaeng, R.; Alsheddi, L.; Wanasathop, A.; Shi, Z.; Li, S.K. Skin Permeation of Urea Under Finite Dose Condition. *J. Pharm. Sci.* **2019**, *108*, 987–995. [CrossRef]
15. Trombino, S.; Russo, R.; Mellace, S.; Varano, G.P.; Laganà, A.S.; Marcucci, F.; Cassano, R. Solid lipid nanoparticles made of trehalose monooleate for cyclosporin-A topic release. *J. Drug Deliv. Sci. Technol.* **2019**, *49*, 563–569. [CrossRef]
16. Soriano-Ruiz, J.L.; Suñer-Carbó, J.; Calpena-Campmany, A.C.; Bozal-de Febrer, N.; Halbaut-Bellowa, L.; Boix-Montañés, A.; Souto, E.B.; Clares-Naveros, B. Clotrimazole multiple W/O/W emulsion as anticandidal agent: Characterization and evaluation on skin and mucosae. *Coll. Surf. B Biointerfaces* **2019**, *175*, 166–174. [CrossRef] [PubMed]
17. Zhang, Y.; Lane, M.E.; Hadgraft, J.; Heinrich, M.; Chen, T.; Lian, G.; Sinko, B. A comparison of the in vitro permeation of niacinamide in mammalian skin and in the Parallel Artificial Membrane Permeation Assay (PAMPA) model. *Int. J. Pharm.* **2019**, *556*, 142–149. [CrossRef] [PubMed]
18. Montenegro, L.; Castelli, F.; Sarpietro, M. Differential Scanning Calorimetry Analyses of Idebenone-Loaded Solid Lipid Nanoparticles Interactions with a Model of Bio-Membrane: A Comparison with In Vitro Skin Permeation Data. *Pharmaceuticals* **2018**, *11*, 138. [CrossRef] [PubMed]
19. Dahlizar, S.; Futaki, M.; Okada, A.; Yatomi, C.; Todo, H.; Sugibayashi, K. Combined Use of N-Palmitoyl-Glycine-Histidine Gel and Several Penetration Enhancers on the Skin Permeation and Concentration of Metronidazole. *Pharmaceutics* **2018**, *10*, 163. [CrossRef] [PubMed]
20. Haq, A.; Goodyear, B.; Ameen, D.; Joshi, V.; Michniak-Kohn, B. Strat-M® synthetic membrane: Permeability comparison to human cadaver skin. *Int. J. Pharm.* **2018**, *547*, 432–437. [CrossRef] [PubMed]
21. Balázs, B. Investigation of the Skin Barrier Function and Transdermal Drug Delivery Techniques. Ph.D. Thesis, Unviersity of Szeged, Szeged, Hungary, 2016.
22. Simon, A.; Amaro, M.I.; Healy, A.M.; Cabral, L.M.; de Sousa, V.P. Comparative evaluation of rivastigmine permeation from a transdermal system in the Franz cell using synthetic membranes and pig ear skin with in vivo-in vitro correlation. *Int. J. Pharm.* **2016**, *512*, 234–241. [CrossRef] [PubMed]

23. Uchida, T.; Kadhum, W.R.; Kanai, S.; Todo, H.; Oshizaka, T.; Sugibayashi, K. Prediction of skin permeation by chemical compounds using the artificial membrane, Strat-M^{TM}. *Eur. J. Pharm. Sci.* **2015**, *67*, 113–118. [CrossRef] [PubMed]
24. Kim, K.-T.; Kim, M.-H.; Park, J.-H.; Lee, J.-Y.; Cho, H.-J.; Yoon, I.-S.; Kim, D.-D. Microemulsion-based hydrogels for enhancing epidermal/dermal deposition of topically administered 20(S)-protopanaxadiol: In vitro and in vivo evaluation studies. *J. Ginseng Res.* **2018**, *42*, 512–523. [CrossRef] [PubMed]
25. Bakonyi, M.; Berkó, S.; Kovács, A.; Budai-Szűcs, M.; Kis, N.; Erős, G.; Csóka, I.; Csányi, E. Application of quality by design principles in the development and evaluation of semisolid drug carrier systems for the transdermal delivery of lidocaine. *J. Drug Deliv. Sci. Technol.* **2018**, *44*, 136–145. [CrossRef]
26. Sütő, B.; Berkó, S.; Kozma, G.; Kukovecz, Á.; Budai-Szűcs, M.; Erős, G.; Kemény, L.; Sztojkov-Ivanov, A.; Gaspar, R.; Csányi, E. Development of ibuprofen-loaded nanostructured lipid carrier-based gels: Characterization and investigation of in vitro and in vivo penetration through the skin. *Int. J. Nanomed.* **2016**, *11*, 1201–1212.
27. Sinkó, B.; Garrigues, T.M.; Balogh, G.T.; Nagy, Z.K.; Tsinman, O.; Avdeef, A.; Takács-Novák, K. Skin–PAMPA: A new method for fast prediction of skin penetration. *Eur. J. Pharm. Sci.* **2012**, *45*, 698–707. [CrossRef] [PubMed]
28. Köllmer, M.; Mossahebi, P.; Sacharow, E.; Gorissen, S.; Gräfe, N.; Evers, D.-H.; Herbig, M.E. Investigation of the Compatibility of the Skin PAMPA Model with Topical Formulation and Acceptor Media Additives Using Different Assay Setups. *AAPS PharmSciTech* **2019**, *20*, 89. [CrossRef] [PubMed]
29. Vizserálek, G.; Berkó, S.; Tóth, G.; Balogh, R.; Budai-Szűcs, M.; Csányi, E.; Sinkó, B.; Takács-Novák, K. Permeability test for transdermal and local therapeutic patches using Skin PAMPA method. *Eur. J. Pharm. Sci.* **2015**, *76*, 165–172. [CrossRef] [PubMed]
30. Sinkó, B.; Vizserálek, G.; Takács-Novák, K. Skin PAMPA: Application in practice. *ADMET DMPK* **2015**, *2*, 191–198. [CrossRef]
31. Luo, L.; Patel, A.; Sinko, B.; Bell, M.; Wibawa, J.; Hadgraft, J.; Lane, M.E. A comparative study of the in vitro permeation of ibuprofen in mammalian skin, the PAMPA model and silicone membrane. *Int. J. Pharm.* **2016**, *505*, 14–19. [CrossRef] [PubMed]
32. Bakonyi, M.; Gácsi, A.; Kovács, A.; Szűcs, M.-B.; Berkó, S.; Csányi, E. Following-up skin penetration of lidocaine from different vehicles by Raman spectroscopic mapping. *J. Pharm. Biomed. Anal.* **2018**, *154*, 1–6. [CrossRef] [PubMed]
33. Puglia, C.; Sarpietro, M.G.; Bonina, F.; Castelli, F.; Zammataro, M.; Chiechio, S. Development, Characterization, and In Vitro and In Vivo Evaluation of Benzocaine- and Lidocaine-Loaded Nanostructrured Lipid Carriers. *J. Pharma. Sci.* **2011**, *100*, 1892–1899. [CrossRef]
34. Ribeiro, L.N.M.; Breitkreitz, M.C.; Guilherme, V.A.; da Silva, G.H.R.; Couto, V.M.; Castro, S.R.; de Paula, B.O.; Machado, D.; de Paula, E. Natural lipids-based NLC containing lidocaine: From pre-formulation to in vivo studies. *Eur. J. Pharm. Sci.* **2017**, *106*, 102–112. [CrossRef]
35. Muller, R.H.; Radtke, M.; Wissing, S.A. Solid lipid nanoparticles (SLN) and nanostructured lipid carriers (NLC) in cosmetic and dermatological preparations. *Adv. Drug Deliv. Rev.* **2002**, *54*, 131–155. [CrossRef]
36. Rincón, M.; Calpena, A.; Fabrega, M.-J.; Garduño-Ramírez, M.; Espina, M.; Rodríguez-Lagunas, M.; García, M.; Abrego, G. Development of Pranoprofen Loaded Nanostructured Lipid Carriers to Improve Its Release and Therapeutic Efficacy in Skin Inflammatory Disorders. *Nanomaterials* **2018**, *8*, 1022. [CrossRef]
37. You, P.; Yuan, R.; Chen, C. Design and evaluation of lidocaine- and prilocaine-coloaded nanoparticulate drug delivery systems for topical anesthetic analgesic therapy: A comparison between solid lipid nanoparticles and nanostructured lipid carriers. *Drug Design Dev. Ther.* **2017**, *11*, 2743–2752. [CrossRef] [PubMed]
38. Li, Q.; Cai, T.; Huang, Y.; Xia, X.; Cole, S.; Cai, Y. A Review of the Structure, Preparation, and Application of NLCs, PNPs, and PLNs. *Nanomaterials* **2017**, *7*, 122. [CrossRef] [PubMed]
39. *Draft Guideline on Quality and Equivalence of Topical Products*; EMA/CHMP/QWP/708282/2018; European Medicines Agency: Amsterdam, The Netherlands, 2018.

MDPI
St. Alban-Anlage 66
4052 Basel
Switzerland
Tel. +41 61 683 77 34
Fax +41 61 302 89 18
www.mdpi.com

Pharmaceutics Editorial Office
E-mail: pharmaceutics@mdpi.com
www.mdpi.com/journal/pharmaceutics

www.ingramcontent.com/pod-product-compliance
Lightning Source LLC
LaVergne TN
LVHW070653100526
838202LV00013B/952